AN INTERDISCIPLINARY APPROACH TO PSORIASIS

Edited by **Anca Chiriac**

An Interdisciplinary Approach to Psoriasis
http://dx.doi.org/10.5772/65196
Edited by Anca Chiriac

Contributors

Francisco Capani, Rodolfo Köllilker-Frers, Matilde Otero-Losada, Vanesa Cosentino, Eduardo Kersberg, Sevgi Akarsu, Ceylan Avci, Meliha Merve Hiz, Sevilay Oguz Kılıc, Ceren Canbey Göret, Başak Büyük, Tuba Demirci, Cüneyt Akı, Sibel Oymak, Carolina Negrei, Daniel Boda, Luis Santamaria-Babí, Ester Ruiz-Romeu, Mario E. Cancino-Diaz, Sandra Rodríguez-Martínez, Juan C. Cancino-Diaz, Sonia M Pérez-Tapia, Isaí Martínez-Torres, Maria Crisan, Sorin Marian Dudea, Radu Badea, Horatiu Colosi, Stefan Strilciuc, Diana Crisan, Mayumi Komine, Mamitaro Ohtsuki, Jitlada Meephansan, Urairack Subpayasarn, Vita Dolžan, Sara Redenšek, Cristian Podoleanu

Published by InTech
Janeza Trdine 9, 51000 Rijeka, Croatia

Publishing Process Manager Mirena Calmic
Technical Editor SPi Global
Cover InTech Design team

First published June, 2017
Printed in Croatia
Legal deposit, Croatia: National and University Library in Zagreb

Additional hard copies can be obtained from orders@intechopen.com

An Interdisciplinary Approach to Psoriasis, Edited by Anca Chiriac
p. cm.
Print ISBN 978-953-51-3251-6
Online ISBN 978-953-51-3252-3

For EU product safety concerns:
IN TECH d.o.o., Prolaz Marije Krucifikse Kozulić 3, 51000 Rijeka, Croatia,
info@intechopen.com or visit our website at intechopen.com.

Meet the editor

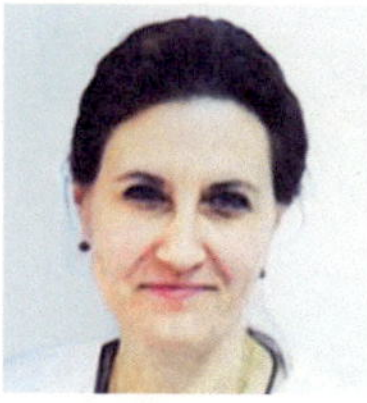

Dr. Anca Chiriac, MD, PhD, is a clinical dermatologist whose research interests are focused on psoriasis, clinical aspects, and pathogenic mechanisms. Dr. Anca Chiriac received her MD degree from Grigore T. Popa University of Medicine and Pharmacy in 1991 and PhD degree in 2005 in Medicine from Carol Davila University of Medicine and Pharmacy, Bucharest, Romania. She completed her postdoctoral studies at Necker-Enfants Malades Hospital, Paris, France; Ed. Herriot Hospital Lyon, France; and A. Sygros Hospital University of Athens, European Center for Allergy and Research Foundation Berlin, Germany. From 2013, she is a professor of Dermatology at Apollonia University, Iasi, and an associate researcher at P. Poni Institute of Macromolecular Chemistry, Romanian Academy. She has published over 150 articles and book chapters and has been involved in many international research projects.

Contents

Preface

It is a great pleasure and honor to present this book.

Psoriasis is a chronic systemic disease that occurs worldwide, affecting people of all ages and gender and all ethnic origins, with a negative impact on patient's quality of life.

The etiology of psoriasis remains unclear, although substantial efforts have been focused on all aspects of psoriasis during the last decades.

A genetic predisposition is well documented, as well as external and internal triggers.

The role of the immune system in psoriasis is the main topic of research nowadays.

New and noninvasive methods of diagnosing and severity evaluation have been applied in daily clinical practice.

Epidemiology of psoriasis, its incidence, and prevalence on the global level could be a key factor in clinical research.

Retrospective controlled studies have been done in order to elucidate the association of psoriasis with different comorbidities.

National and international guidelines regarding the diagnosis of psoriasis and treatment are of utmost importance and should have an interdisciplinary approach.

All these concepts are presented within the pages of this book, aiming to raise questions and to give answers to some issues related to psoriasis.

I am grateful to the authors for their remarkable contributions to this book. The chapters have been written by clinicians and experts from different fields of activity, from renowned institutions with the aim of providing new insights into psoriasis.

I am indebted to the team from InTech for all the support in making this publication possible. In particular I would like to thank Ms. Mirena Calmic for her assistance in the preparation of the book.

Professor Anca Chiriac
Apollonia University
Nicolina Medical Center
P. Poni Institute of Macromolecular Chemistry, Romanian Academy
Iasi, Romania

Section 1

Etiopathogenesis

Chapter 1

Psoriasis and Genetics

Hız Meliha Merve, Kılıç Sevilay, Oymak Sibel,
Büyük Başak, Canbey Göret Ceren,
Tuba Demirci and Akı Cüneyt

Additional information is available at the end of the chapter

http://dx.doi.org/10.5772/intechopen.68344

Abstract

Psoriasis is an erythematous, scaly chronic inflammatory dermatosis and occurs due to altered epidermal differentiation and hyperproliferation due to faulty signals that speed up the growth cycle of skin cells. Psoriasis reduces quality of life, and psoriatic patients generally have higher risk for metabolic disease. Psoriasis is associated with many burdening comorbidities, which often share similar pathogenic features and follow a progressive pattern. Genetic variation in human genome causes specific kind of disease, and nowadays, research is focused on metabolic pathways that trigger psoriasis and related comorbidities. In addition, genetic variations are also important for psoriasis treatment regime and response. The purpose of this section is to shown to genetic epidemiology, pharmacogenetics, immune genetics of psoriasis and related comorbidities.

Keywords: psoriasis, genetics, variations, SNP

1. Introduction

Psoriasis was first thought to originate from a biochemical imbalance due to excessive proliferation of keratinocytes; yet recent researches focused on the investigation of the genetic basis of this immunological condition.

Psoriasis, a chronic inflammatory disease, is thought to be closely related to metabolic and cardiovascular diseases; however, mortality rate of the disease is rare. Genetic and epidemiologic studies have also pointed out that cardiovascular and metabolic diseases are more prevalent in the community than psoriasis cases in psoriasis cases. Thus, determination of genetic variation on genome that triggers both psoriasis and related comorbidities is crucial.

In addition, personal genomic variations are important for diagnosis and treatment of the psoriasis and related comorbidities effectively.

2. Epidemiology of psoriasis

Psoriasis can affect people of all ages, ethnic origins and genders around the world. There are very literatures showing the incidence of the disease, since there is no compulsory retention of psoriasis case recordings and reliable source constraints. On the other hand, prevalence varies among different countries in Europe [1]. Although psoriasis may affect 2% of the world population, the incidence of disease varies 0.09–11.4% between different countries and races [1–4]. The reasons for the variability of prevalence are that the epidemiological methods and limitations of the studies differ [2]. Psoriasis is not evident among Latin American indigenous, people of Samoa and New Zealand, and in contrast, the prevalence is increasing up to 12% in Kasachy [5]. The prevalence of psoriasis in Asian countries or Asians common countries is 0.4% in China, 0.3–1% in Japan, and 0.8% in India, while the prevalence of West African and American black population was reported as 0.3–0.7% and 0.7%, respectively [6].

The results have shown that there is a very weak correlation between geographical latitude and psoriasis [2, 7]. In contrast, psoriasis is more commonly seen in places where the upper latitudes of that are colder and Caucasians are more frequent[5, 8–10]. For example, in twin studies carried out in Australia, it has a higher prevalence of psoriasis in southern region of cold than the northern region where is warmer [8, 9]. When investigating the regional distribution of psoriasis cases in Norway, the incidence of disease has been found to increase inversely proportional to the temperature rise in the country [10].

According to the global disease burden study conducted in 2010 [11], it has been reported that the disability-adjusted life year increases with age, especially the highest burden of disease shown between the ages of 50–69 [2, 11]. Psoriasis is associated with many burdening comorbidities, which often share similar pathogenic features and follow a progressive pattern, and thus, direct and indirect cost of psoriasis has significant effects on both patients and health care systems.

3. Psoriasis as a genetic disease

Genetic factors play a role in psoriasis development; yet, the exact mechanism that triggers psoriasis is still unknown. Twin studies, familial aggregation studies, linkage studies, and population-based association studies are all important to understand the effect of the genes in heritability of the disease. Nowadays, genome-wide association studies and linkage studies are also frequently used to identify disease mechanism and risk-related genes. Association studies on genome-wide and a meta-analysis aim to reveal the potential risk genes and loci of genome that emerged comorbidities as a result of these diseases such as s psoriasis.

Psoriasis is a complex disease that not simply explained by Mendelian inheritance rules. Lomholt's study that performed (1954) in an island has determined that 91% of psoriatic patients have a previous family history [12]. Earlier studies speculated psoriasis as autosomal dominant disease, but the truth is so different [13]. This speculation relies on the fact that human lymphocyte antigen gene located in a single locus thus its effects as dominant. That is why psoriasis is accepted as a dominant disease [13]. Although dominant inheritance firstly goes to foreground in studies to investigate the pattern of inheritance of psoriasis, it has been focused on the disease transition by heterogeneous or polygenic in broader studies.

The twin studies rely on the fact, if the disease occurs in monozygotic twins because of phenotypical differences between monozygotic twins. This means that environmental factors affect the disease because they have identical genetic background. In contrast, dizygotic twins have genetic background like brothers or sisters, and thus, phenotypical differences occur as a result of genetic or environmental factors or both.

The concordance of psoriasis has greater rates in monozygotic twins than dizygotic twins'; thus, genetic factors are important for disease development. In contrast, the rate is never reaching to 100% in monozygotic twins so environmental influences for disease development. Duffy et al. [8] have reported concordance for psoriasis higher in monozygotic twins (35%) when compared to dizygotic twins (12%) in Australian population. The data from National Twin Registry System of Denmark had been shown that the concordance of psoriasis in dizygotic twins was 15–30%; yet, the rates rises up to 65–72% in monozygotic twins [14]. The Danish Twin Registry System records have shown that monozygotic twins increased risk of psoriasis than in dizygotic twins [15]. A twin study has been shown that psoriasis risk has been rise up to 3 times in monozygotic twins when compared to fraternal twins [16]. Although twin studies have shown strongest genetic background of psoriasis, heritability rate of psoriasis never reaches to 100% among monozygotic twins. This missing heritability means environmental factors [15, 16] and epigenetic alterations [17] have effects on psoriasis development.

Psoriasis was diagnosed 6% in first-degree relatives of patients with psoriasis [18, 19] generations, settlement in geographical regions and ethnic group studies related to population showed that psoriasis is a complex genetic-based, multifactorial disease [6]. All these data showed why psoriasis was accepted as a heritable disease but not 100% as a genetic disease. Psoriasis was first associated with the major histocompatibility complex (MHC) region in the short arm of the 6th chromosome in 1972 [20–22]. MHC is an intense region of the genome and contains HLA-I and HLA-class human leukocyte antigens. In fact, the 80–200 kb long region in the HLA-C gene region has been accepted as the Psoriasis susceptibility gene region (PSOR1) [23]. HLA-Cw6 in PSOR1 region was associated with psoriasis in many ethnic groups and geographical regions [24–27]. However, the risk zones related to subclinical forms of the disease vary in patients with psoriasis. For example, HLA-Cw6 positivity is associated with early onset and familial transition of psoriasis [28]. HLA-CW6 gene region affects the response of ustekinumab using in the treatment of psoriasis [29]. Other gene regions (PSORS2 (17q25), PSORS3 (4q34), PSORS4 (1q), PSORS5 (3q21, PSORS6 (19p13), PSORS7 (1p) PSORS8 (16q12-13), PSORS11 (5q31.1-q33.1), PSORS12 (20q13), and PSORS13 (6q21)) related to psoriasis distribute to different chromosomes [13, 30–37].

4. Immunogenetics of psoriasis

Psoriasis is an immune-mediated disease and, for that reason, immune-mediated mechanism has been extensively studied. Genetic studies focus on identification reasons that trigger uncontrolled proliferation of keratinocytes and recruitment of T cells into the skin. In healthy individuals, T cells are originated from embryonal pluripotent cells by cytokine induction. Immature thymocytes are transferred to thymus for proliferation through clonal expansion. T cells are specified to helper T cells or cytoxic T cells by adding specific surface antigens ($CD4^+$ or $CD8^+$) and differentiating to give response for antigenic signals. In psoriatic skin samples, Th1 cell differentiation is up-regulated and that cause impaired Th1/Th2 balanced [38, 39]. Evidence indicates that Th1-delivered cytokines IL-1, IL-2, IL-6, IL-8, tumor necrosis factor-α (TNF- α), transforming growth factor (TGF) and Granulocyte-macrophage colony-stimulating factor are upregulated, while Th2-delivered cytokines IL-4, IL-5, and IL-10 are downregulated [40–44]. The cytokines IL-12 is critical for both T-cell activation and differentiation also contributes to DC/T cell interactions [45]. TNIP1, NFKBIA, IL12B and LCE3D–LCE3E are known susceptibility loci for psoriasis [46], and the variation of IL-12 is associated with psoriasis in different populations [47–49]. Meta analyses have shown that IL-12B variation (rs3212227, rs6887695) has been associated both psoriasis and psoriatic arthritis [50]. IL-12 and IL-23 are heterodynamic cytokines; both of them share same p40 subunit. IL-12 consists of p35 and p40 subunit and IL-23 consist of p19 and p40 subunits. The metabolic model for psoriasis suggests that dermal dendritic cells are secreted IL-23 by that way trigger Th17 cell line activation. IL-23 is crucial for naive T cell differentiation to Th17. Activated Th17 cells are secreted IL-17A, IL-17F, IL-22 and IL-26 and that proinflammatory cytokines effects epidermal and dermal cells gene expression and keratinocyte maturation. For that reason, IL12/IL 23 pathway seems important for psoriasis treatment and different studies are performed in that metabolic pathway [51–54].

5. Immunohistochemical parameters

The demonstration of specific markers by immunohistochemical methods in histopathological tissue specimens diagnosed as psoriasis is important in terms of supporting and confirming the diagnosis. We have evaluated most of the cytokines referred to in the pathophysiology in immunogenetic section which can be used for immunohistochemical methods. In psoriatic tissue, sample Th1-mediated cytokines IL-1, IL-2, IL-6, IL-8, tumor necrosis factor-α (TNF-α), transforming growth factor (TGF) and granulocyte-macrophage colony-stimulating factor increase and Th2-mediated cytokines IL-4, IL-5, and IL-10 decrease [40–44].

IL-17 plays an important role in psoriasis, and recently, both IL-17 inhibitors and IL-17receptor type A blockers are new monoclonal antibodies which are approved by US FDA [55]. Lee and colleagues have immunohistochemically evaluated IL-17A expressions in different types of psoriasis, and the results have shown that samples from palmoplantar and pustular type psoriasis samples were stained with IL-17A strongly, while plaque type samples were stained with IL-17A intermittently [56].

Macrophage migration inhibitory factor (MIF) is directly related to the severity of clinical symptoms, and serum MIF levels are usually high in patients with psoriasis [57]. In contrast, immunohistochemical staining by anti-MIF antibody in psoriatic lesions showed that MIF levels are very low [58]. Toll-like receptors (TLRs) are a group of molecules that play a crucial role in innate immunity and also regulate antimicrobial defense. TLR2 is immunohistochemically staining uniformly in all the layers of the normal deep epidermis that does not lose its nuclei, yet TLR2 staining differs in psoriatic skin samples [59, 60]. Panzer and colleagues have shown that TLR2 staining is lower in granular and upper spinous, whereas it was strongly observed in the lower spinous and basal strata [59]. TLR4 is normally found in all the nuclear layers, while it is more pronounced in the upper layers of the basal layer. In psoriatic skin lesions, TLR4 was stained weak in the basal layer, yet TLR4 was stained strongly in the upper spinous and granular layers [59]. IL-8 is produced in psoriatic lesions and immunohistochemical demonstration supports disease diagnosis [61]. In a study, evaluating the relationship between geographic tongue (GT) and psoriasis has been shown that anti-CD4, CD8, CD20, CD68, S100, and Ki-67 antibodies results were similar in tissue samples from both diseases, and according to that result, geographic tongue is speculates as an oral psoriasis lesion [62].

6. Pharmacokinetics of psoriasis in genetic aspect

Psoriasis is a chronic, non-curative disease, and thus, effective psoriasis treatment is important for long-term cure and inhibition of disease manifestation. Psoriasis can be treated by topical, photo(chemo)therapy, classic systemic drug(methotrexate, cyclosporine, acitretin) and biologic agents (infliximab, adalimumab, etanercept). The psoriasis treatment is affected by psoriasis type, severity, presence of comorbidities, previous response to other treatments and patients.

Ustekinumab is an anti-p40 monoclonal antibody which is effective for psoriasis treatment via its inhibitor effect of interleukin-12/23 pathway. By that way, ustekinumab inhibits T helper (Th)1 and Th17 pathway and inhibits immune cell activation. In addition, HLA-Cw+ patients have better clinical response to ustekinumab than HLACw- ones [29]. Talamonti et al. state that HLACw+ patients response to ustekinumab is 9.8 times more efficient than mutant genotype. In contrast, TNFAIP3 polymorphism and LCE3B/3C gene deletions have no effect on ustekinumab response [29].

TNF-inhibitors infliximab and adalimumab and the fusion protein, etanercept are used widely for psoriasis treatment. Nishikawa and colleagues [63] have shown that JAG2, ADRA2A and TLR10 polymorphisms are associated with TNFα response. Prieto-Pérez and colleagues [64] have shown that PGLYR4, ZNF816A, CTNNA2, IL12B, MAP3K1, and HLA-C genes are associated with anti-TNF response at 3 months, while FCGR2A, HTR2A, and CDKAL1 are related anti-TNF response at 6 months. TNF gene polymorphism is also associated with psoriasis and psoriatic arthritis due to its effects on TNF production. Murdaca and colleagues have demonstrated TNF-α polymorphism on +489 position of the gene effects efficiency of etanercept treatment on psoriatic arthritis patients (PsA) [65]. In fact, the idea simply relies on the fact that gene polymorphism affects the biological properties of encoded proteins. TNF blockers are widely used for regulation of inflammatory cascade and by that way treatment of the immune-related disease. If polymorphic product of the gene is your pharmaceutical target and has different molecular structure, then wild type its means pharmacodynamics of the drug varies due to personal variation.

Both IL-17 antagonists and IL-17 receptor blockers are accepted as effective and safe for psoriasis treatment [66]. Brodalumab is a human monoclonal antibody that binds to interleukin-17 receptor and waits for US-FDA approval for psoriasis treatment [55, 67]. IL-17 expression is upregulated in psoriatic skin samples. Both secukinumab and ixekizumab are the cytokine antagonists used for psoriasis treatment [68]. Nowadays, recent studies are focused on the relationship between IL-17 family cytokines (IL-17A, IL-17B, IL-17C, IL-17D, IL-17E, and IL-17F) and IL-17 receptor polymorphisms with psoriasis susceptibility and treatment response [69–71].

7. The link between psoriasis and comorbidities in view of genetics

Nowadays, psoriasis is accepted as a systemic disease because of higher rates of obesity, depression, psychiatric disorders, diabetes, hyperlipidemia, cardiovascular diseases, arthritis, uveitis, ulcerative colitis, Crohn's disease, and metabolic syndrome among psoriatic patients. Even if, the mortality rate of the psoriasis is low, psoriatic patients over 65 have at least two comorbidities [72]. Thus, interdisciplinary approach should be an integral part of the routine, and also the dermatologist should be careful with psoriasis and related disorders. Although the systemic inflammation process during psoriasis development is still unclear, the chronic inflammatory process may trigger development of many burden comorbidities in psoriatic patients. Many epidemiological studies revealed relationship between psoriasis and diabetes [72, 73]. Aside, the studies have shown that cardiovascular risk increases among patient with psoriasis and psoriatic arthritis [74]. In that point, dermatologist should be careful about systemic drug usage for psoriasis treatment because medications can sometime trigger maintenance factor in the pathogenesis of psoriasis [75–78].

In that section, we would like to evaluate the common mechanism between psoriasis and psoriatic comorbidities in molecular and genetic basis. For example, psoriatic patients are more prone to develop Crohn's disease more than general population [79]. The molecular basis of Crohn's disease is activation of CD4+ T cells by intestinal epithelial cells (IECs) and lamina propria immune cells and that activate both Th1 and Th17cells and cause elevated level of TNFα and Th17-related cytokine. Th1 and Th17 differentiation is common both in psoriasis and Crohn's disease; for that reason, TNF inhibitors are effective for treatment of Crohn's disease as psoriasis [80].

7.1. Psoriatic arthritis

Joint involvements in patients with psoriasis were put forward for the first time by Alibert in 1818 [81, 82]. Psoriatic arthritis is a negative spondyloarthropathy [71–83]. Important radiological findings of the psoriatic arthritis are peripheral joint involvement, destructive and proliferative changes, spinal involvement, interphalangeal joint ledge, fibroosteitis and acroostelolysis [84, 85]. Strong genetic relationship is remarkable between positive family history [81, 86] and human leukocyte antigen (HLA) class II alleles for psoriatic arthritis [87–89].

Psoriatic arthritis (PsA) is diagnosed in 25–34% of psoriatic patients [90]. Psoriasis without joint involvement (PsO) and psoriatic arthritis (PsA) occur as a result of autoimmune responses that are triggered by genetic and environmental factors. The pathogenesis of psoriasis only (PsO) and psoriatic arthritis (PsA) may be explained impaired cytokine levels [91].

To clarify immungenetics mechanism of psoriatic arthritis has been focused on human leukocyte antigen (HLA). HLA gene region is located on the short arm of chromosome 6. This region is highly polymorphic depending on mutation and recombination [92]. Psoriatic arthritis associates with various HLA risk haplotype such as HLA-B7 B57 B13, B16, B17, DR7, B38, B39, CW6, and B27 [89, 93, 94]. While CW6 HLA-alleles were associated with early onset of the disease [95], HLA-B38 and HLA-B39 were associated with polyarthritis [87], and HLA-B27 was associated with dorsal involvement. Positivity of human leukocyte antigen "HLA-B27" in psoriatic arthritis patients makes a higher risk of arthritis compared to other HLA alleles [90, 96]. In Turkish population, we have found that HLA-B27 positivity increased the risk of psoriasis and psoriatic arthritis 5 to 10 times more, respectively [97]. There are various molecular-based hypotheses such as molecular mimicry, defective immunity, heavy chain folding incorrectly, and deterioration of HLA-B27 allele for relationship between HLA-B27 and psoriatic arthritis (PsA) [97].

7.2. Obesity

Storing energy in the form of triacylglycerols is considered to be the primary task of adipocytes; but adipocytes have physically some additional functions such as preservation of internal organs, regulating temperature, storage of lipid-soluble vitamins, steroid metabolism, immunity, and being assigned in inflammatory processes [98, 99]. Adipose tissue runs like as an endocrine tissue as the sympathetic system regulators with hormone and cytokine production during the regulation of energy metabolism [100]. Adipose tissue plays also an important role in homeostasis besides production, secretion such as TNF-alpha, IL-8, monocyte chemoattractant protein 1, cytokines and chemokines and storing energy in the form of fatty acids, together with the adipokines, leptin, adiponectin, resistin, such as pro-inflammatory and anti–inflammatory factors [98, 101].

The risk of diseases such as a high rate of insulin resistance, type 2 diabetes, dyslipidemia, gout, hypertension, and cardiovascular involvement is higher in obese individuals [102–107, 110]. Adipokine tissue secretes cytokines thus increasing volume or amount of adipokine tissue cause increasing the amount of circulating cytokines. Then, elevated amount of cytokines causes arteriosclerosis and insulin resistance and to induce hypertension and type 2 diabetes [108].

In a study that investigated the risk of obesity in patients with psoriasis, same sex siblings and 88 psoriasis outpatients were compared by calculating the BMI. The result of this study has obtained a significant relationship between the severity of psoriasis and BMI [109]. Duarte et al. have found that it was a statistically significant relationship between obesity and psoriasis severity on patients with psoriasis by using different parameters, such as BMI and waist/hip ratio [110]. It was shown to be positive commensurate with psoriasis risk of weight gain and high BMI in another study performed in the United States with 809 psoriasis patients followed for 12 years [111]. Obesity was determined to be more than psoriasis only (PSO) patients [112–114], and it was determined that obesity increases the risk of psoriatic arthritis in individuals under 18 years of age [115].

7.3. The impaired glucose tolerance and diabetes

Glucose intolerance, diabetes, and obesity are more frequent in patients with psoriasis [74, 75, 116–119]. The study conducted by Onsun et al. has found that diabetes was significantly more frequent in patients with psoriasis when compared to the incidence of psoriasis in patients with diabetes [120]. Azfar and his colleagues have found that patients with severe psoriasis involvement have more risk of with diabetes; in contrast, they concluded that psoriasis was an independent risk factor for type 2 diabetes [121]. Armesto and colleagues have found that occurrence of risk of type 2 diabetes was found to have higher, late-onset, nonfamilial transmission, but in patients with joint involvement [122]. Finley et al. have shown that expression of IL-17 and IL-20 is elevated in diabetic wounds, and they emphasized the psoriasis and diabetes link via cytokines [123]. Granata et al. have demonstrated that IL-23/IL-17, and IL-18 are main cytokines that has central role for obesity, type 1 diabetes, and psoriasis [124]. Eirís et al. have demonstrated that IL12B rs6887695 and rs3212227 increase the type 2 diabetes risk approximately 3 and 6 times, respectively [125]. In addition, IL23 receptor polymorphism was also found significantly associated with diabetes in psoriatic patients [125]. Presta et al. have found that polymorphism in the 3'untranslated region of IL-18 gene increases the insulin sensitivity risk [126]. In addition to literature, we have evaluated the diabetes risk among psoriasis patients; yet, we could not find any significant relation between TNF-α-238 G/A and TNF-α-308 G/A polymorphisms with diabetes [127].

7.4. Cardiovascular diseases

The epidemiological studies have shown that cardiovascular morbidity and mortality increased in patients with psoriasis in Refs. [77, 78, 128, 129]. Inflammation located in pathogenesis of psoriasis is known to cause metabolic and cardiovascular disease. The molecular relationship between psoriasis and cardiovascular disease may be explained by T cell activation and enhance of Th1 cytokine production (TNF-α, IL-1β, IL-10, and IFN). The TNF-α and IL-1 trigger oxidative stress causes migration of leukocytes into atherosclerotic plaques [101], so TNF inhibitors have beneficial effects on prevention of cardiovascular events both in psoriasis and psoriatic arthritis [130]. Our study group has evaluated hypertension risk and psoriasis. eNOS Glu298Asp single-nucleotide polymorphism has found to be increased in hypertensive psoriatic patients when compared with healthy volunteers [131]. In contrast, we could not find relationship between TNF-α-298 and TNF-α-308 polymorphisms with hypertension and cardiovascular disease [127].

7.5. Metabolic syndrome

Metabolic syndrome is associated with conditions such as physical inactivity and improper diet, occurring nutrition changes, and daily lifestyle. It is characterized as a disease of civilization by high mortality and morbidity [132].

It is a fact that metabolic syndrome and its components are often seen in patients with psoriasis. Also, polymorphism may be triggering both psoriasis and metabolic syndrome together. Abdel Hay and Rashed have shown that leptin gene 2548G/A polymorphism increases risk of both psoriasis and metabolic syndrome [133].

7.6. Psychological trauma and addiction

Psoriasis is a chronic skin disease that negatively affects the quality of life in many ways. Patients with psoriasis reduce quality of life with comorbidities like arthritis. Psoriasis can lead not only to physical health problems, but also to mental and social health problems. Psoriatic lesions that occur especially in hands, face, and on the scalp cause shame, embarrassment, and social inhibition in social life and by that way increase the risk of depression, anxiety, lack of self-confidence, smoking and alcohol addiction, and trend of suicidal thoughts in patients with psoriasis [134].

Kurd et al. have shown that depression, anxiety, and suicidality risk increases 1.39, 1.31, and 1.44 times more in psoriatic patients than healthy people, respectively [135]. Psoriatic patients are more prone to psychiatric comorbidities and suicidal ideation than other dermatological diseases [136]. Deveci and et al. have found significantly higher depression rate and suicide attempts in cases with psoriasis when compared to patients with other dermatological problems [137].

Use of alcohol and tobacco makes difficult the therapeutic harmony and also increases the toxicity of the drug besides reducing the effectiveness of systemic anti-psoriatic drug. Excessive alcohol intake can induce production of proinflammatory cytokine in various cell types and increase the cell lymphocyte proliferation and activation [138]. Serotonin may be triggered psoriasis as a growth factor that promotes keratinocyte proliferation [139]. The serotonin transporter gene promoter region and serotonin2A receptor gene have been found associated with psoriasis in Thai population [140, 141].

8. Conclusions

What would cause the metabolic alteration among psoriatic patients? Does systemic drug usage in long term causes comorbidities in patients with psoriasis? or Is it the domino effect of impaired metabolism? It has not reached a consensus about it.

Advances in understanding the immune-mediated pathological mechanisms of psoriasis will be highlighted with the relationship between psoriasis and psoriasis-related comorbidities. Much psoriatic comorbidity may be triggered by the cytokines and chemokines, which were secreted by T-cells, keratinocytes, and antigens presenting cells after keratinocyte hyper proliferation. Hence, molecular approaches are important to identify the link immunogenic mechanism with psoriasis-related comorbidities in view of molecular pathways.

Determinations of genomic risk profile of the psoriatic patients allow diagnosing of psoriasis and its related comorbidities at an early stage; hence, the life quality can be increased by treating them earlier. In addition, evidence-based information helps physicians to make clear decision and help to minimize medical errors as well as unnecessary drug usage. As a sum, this information allows to increase treatment cost and work loss. In addition, pharmacogenomics of drugs among psoriatic patients is tightly related to personal variations on genome, and thus, complex genetic heterogeneity affects the treatment power.

Author details

Hız Meliha Merve[1]*, Kılıç Sevilay[2], Oymak Sibel[3], Büyük Başak[4], Canbey Göret Ceren[5], Tuba Demirci[6] and Akı Cüneyt[7]

*Address all correspondence to: mervemeliha@comu.edu.tr

1 Faculty of Medicine, Department of Medical Biology, Çanakkale Onsekiz Mart University, Çanakkale, Turkey

2 Faculty of Medicine, Department of Dermatology, Çanakkale Onsekiz Mart University, Çanakkale, Turkey

3 Faculty of Medicine, Department of Public Health, Çanakkale Onsekiz Mart University, Çanakkale, Turkey

4 Faculty of Medicine, Department of Histology and Embriology, Çanakkale Onsekiz Mart University, Çanakkale, Turkey

5 Faculty of Medicine, Department of Pathology, Çanakkale Onsekiz Mart University, Çanakkale, Turkey

6 Faculty of Medicine, Department of Histology and Embryology, Atatürk University, Turkey

7 Faculty of Science and Arts, Department of Biology, Çanakkale Onsekiz Mart University, Çanakkale, Turkey

References

[1] Fernandez-Obregon A. Psoriasis - A systemic disease. In: Dr. O' Daly J, editor. Psoriasis. InTech; 2012. pp. 159-216. DOI: 10.5772/25894

[2] WHO Library Cataloguing-in-Publication Data Global Report on Psoriasis. 1. Psoriasis—Epidemiology. World Health Organization. **ISBN 978** 92 4 156518 9

[3] Gibbs S. Skin disease and socioeconomic conditions in rural Africa: Tanzania. International Journalof Dermatology. 1996;**35**(9):633-639

[4] Danielsen K, Olsen AO, Wilsgaard T, Furberg AS. Is the prevalence of psoriasis increasing? A 30–year follow-up of a population–based cohort. British Journal of Dermatology. 2013;**168**:1303-1310

[5] Farber EM, Nall ML. Epidemiology: Natural history and genetics. In: Roenigk HH, Maibach HI, editors. Psoriasis. (3rd ed.). New York: Marcel; pp. 107-158

[6] Campalani E, Barker JNWN. The clinical genetics of psoriasis. Current Genomics. 2005;**6**(1):51-60

[7] Jacobson CC, Kumar S, Kimball AB. Latitude and psoriasis prevalence. Journal of the American Academy of Dermatology. 2011;**65**(4):870-873

[8] Duffy DL, Spelman LS, Martin NG. Psoriasis in Australian twins. Journal of the American Academy of Dermatology. 1993;**29**(3):428-434

[9] Neimann AL, Porter SB, Gelfand JM. The Epidemiology of Psoriasis. Expert Review of Dermatology. 2006;**1**(1):63-75

[10] Braathen DL, Botten G, Bjerkedal T. Prevalence of Psoriasis in Norway. ActaDermato-Venereologica. 1989;**142**:5-8

[11] Institute for Health Metrics and Evaluation (IHME). Global Burden of Disease Study 2010: Results by Cause 1990-2010. Seattle: IHME; 2012

[12] Lomholt G. Psoriasis on the Faroe Islands; a preliminary report. ActaDermato-Venereologica. 1954;**34**(1-2):92

[13] Tomfohrde J, Silverman A, Barnes R, Fernandez-Vina MA, Young M, Lory D, Morris L, Wuepper KD, Stastny P, Menter A, et al. Gene for familial psoriasis susceptibility mapped to the distal end of human chromosome 17q. Science. 1994;**264**(5162):1141-1145

[14] Wuepper KD, Coulter SN, Haberman A. Psoriasis vulgaris: A genetic approach. Journal of Investigative Dermatology. 1990;**95**(5):2S-4S

[15] Lønnberg AS, Skov L, Skytthe A, Kyvik KO, Pedersen OB, Thomsen SF. Heritability of psoriasis in a large twin sample. British Journal of Dermatology. 2013;**169**(2):412-416

[16] AlShobaili HA, Shahzad M, Al-Marshood A, Khalil A, SettinA, Barrimah I. Genetic background of psoriasis. International Journal of Health Sciences. 2010;**4**(1):23-29

[17] Gervin K, Vigeland MD, Mattingsdal M, Hammerø M, Nygård H, Olsen AO, Brandt I, Harris JR, Undlien DE, Lyle R. DNA methylation and gene expression changes in monozygotic twins discordant for psoriasis: Identification of epigenetically dysregulated genes. PLOS Genetics, 2012;**8**(1):e1002454

[18] Li Y, Liao W, Chang M, Schrodi SJ, Bui N, Catanese JJ, Poon A, Matsunami N, Callis-Duffin KP, Leppert MF, Bowcock AM, Kwok PY, Krueger GG, Begovich AB. Further genetic evidence for three psoriasis-risk genes: ADAM33, CDKAL1, and PTPN22. Journal of Investigative Dermatology. 2009;**129**(3):629-634

[19] Bowcock AM, Cookson WO. The genetics of psoriasis, psoriatic arthritis and atopic dermatitis. Human Molecular Genetics. 2004;**13**(1):R43-R55

[20] Trembath RC, Clough RL, Rosbotham JL, Jones AB, Camp RD, Frodsham A, Browne J, Barber R, Terwilliger J, Lathrop GM, Barker JN. Identification of a major susceptibility locus on chromosome 6p and evidence for further disease loci. Human Molecular Genetics. 1997;**6**(5):813-820

[21] White SH, Newcomer VD, Mickey MR, Terasaki PI. Disturbance of HL-Aantigen frequency in psoriasis. The New England Journal of Medicine. 1972;**287**(15):740-743

[22] Russell TJ, Schultes LM, Kuban DJ. Histocompatibility (HL-A) antigens associated with psoriasis. The New England Journal of Medicine. 1972;**287**(15):738-740

[23] Zhu KJ, Lv YM, Yin XY, Wang ZX, Sun LD, He SM, Cheng H, Hu DY, Zhang Z, Li Y, Zuo XB, Zhou YW, Yang S, Fan X, Zhang XJ, Zhang FY. Psoriasis regression analysis of MHC loci identifies shared genetic variants with vitiligo. PLoS One. 2011;**6**(11):e23089. DOI: 10.1371/journal.pone.0023089

[24] Fan X, Yang S, Huang W, Wang ZM, Sun LD, Liang YH, Gao M, Ren YQ, Zhang KY, Du WH, Shen YJ, Liu JJ, Zhang XJ. Fine mapping of the psoriasis susceptibility locus PSORS1 supports HLA-C as the susceptibility gene in the Han Chin. 2008;**4**(3):e1000038. DOI: 10.1371/journal.pgen.1000038

[25] Romphruk AV, Oka A, Romphruk A, Tomizawa M, Choonhakarn C, Naruse TK, Puapairoj C, Tamiya G, Leelayuwat C, Inoko H. Corneodesmosingene: No evidence for Psors 1 gene in North-Eastern Thai psoriasis patients. Tissue Antigens. 2003;**62**(3): 217-224

[26] Mallon E, Bunce M, Wojnarowska F, Welsh K. HLA-CW*0602 is a susceptibility factor in type I psoriasis, and evidence ala-73 is increased in male type I psoriatics. Journal of Investigative Dermatology. 1997;**109**(2):183-186

[27] Ikäheimo I Tiilikainen A, Karvonen J, Silvennoinen-Kassinen S. HLA risk haplotype Cw6,DR7,DQA1*0201 and HLA-Cw6 with reference to the clinical picture of psoriasis vulgaris. Archives of Dermatological Research. 1996;**288**(7):363-365

[28] Christophers E. Henseler T. Psoriasis type I and type II are subtypes of nonpustular psoriasis. Seminars in dermatology. 1992;**11**(4):261-266

[29] Talamonti M, Botti E, Galluzzo M, Teoli M, Spallone G, Bavetta M, Chimenti S, Costanzo A. Pharmacogenetics of psoriasis: HLA-Cw6 but not LCE3B/3C deletion nor TNFAIP3 polymorphism predisposes to clinical response to interleukin 12/23 blocker ustekinumab. British Journal of Dermatology. 2013;**169**(2):458-463. DOI: 10.1111/bjd.12331

[30] Huffmeier U., Uebe S., Ekici AB, Bowes J, Giardina E, Korendowych E, Juneblad K, Apel M, McManus R, Ho P, Bruce IN, Ryan AW, Behrens F, Lascorz J, Böhm B, Traupe H, Lohmann J, Gieger C, Wichmann HE, Herold C, Steffens M, Klaresko L, Wienker TF, Fitzgerald O, Alenius GM, McHugh NJ, Novelli G, Burkhardt H, Barton A, Reis A. Common variants at TRAF3IP2 are associated with susceptibility to psoriatic arthritis and psoriasis. Nature Genetics. 2010;**2**(11):996-999

[31] Capon F, Bijlmakers MJ, Wolf N, Quaranta M, Huffmeier U, Allen M, Timms K, Abkevich V, Gutin A, Smith R, Warren RB, Young HS, Worthington J, Burden AD, Griffiths CE, Hayday A, Nestle FO, Reis A, Lanchbury J, Barker JN, Trembath RC. Identification of ZNF313/RNF114 as a novel psoriasis susceptibility gene. Human Molecular Genetics. 2008;**17**(13):1938-1945

[32] Asumalahti K, Laitinen T, Lahermo P, Suomela S, Itkonen-Vatjus R, Jansen C, Karvonen J, Karvonen SL, Reunala T, Snellman E, Uurasmaa T, Saarialho-Kere U, Kere J. Psoriasis susceptibility locus on 18p revealed by genome scan in Finnish families not associated with PSORS1. Journal of Investigative Dermatology. 2003;**121**(4):735-740

[33] Zhang XJ, He PP, Wang ZX, Zhang J, Li YB, Wang HY, Wei SC, Chen SY, Xu SJ, Jin L, Yang S, Huang W. Evidence for a major psoriasis susceptibility locus at 6p21(PSORS1) and a novel candidate region at 4q31 by genome-wide scan in Chinese hans. Journal of Investigative Dermatology. 2002;**119**(6):1361-1366

[34] Veal CD, Clough RL, Barber RC, Mason S, Tillman D, Ferry B, Jones AB, Ameen M, Balendran N, Powis SH, Burden AD, Barker JN, Trembath RC. Identification of a novel psoriasis susceptibility locus at 1p and evidence of epistasis between PSORS1 and candidate loci. Journal of Medical Genetics. 2001;**38**(1):7-13

[35] Lee YA, Rüschendorf F, Windemuth C, Schmitt-Egenolf M, Stadelmann A, Nürnberg G, Ständer M, Wienker TF, Reis A, Traupe H. Genomewide scan in German families reveals evidence for a novel psoriasis-susceptibility locus on chromosome 19p13. The American Journal of Human Genetics. 2000;**67**(4):1020-1024

[36] Capon F, Novelli G, Semprini S, Clementi M, Nudo M, Vultaggio P, Mazzanti C, Gobello T, Botta A, Fabrizi G, Dallapiccola B. Searching for psoriasis susceptibility genes in Italy: genome scan and evidence for a new locus on chromosome 1. Journal of Investigative Dermatology. 1999;**112**(1):32-35

[37] Enlund F, Samuelsson L, Enerbäck C, Inerot A, Wahlström J, Yhr M, Torinsson A, Riley J, Swanbeck G, Martinsson T. Psoriasis susceptibility locus in chromosome region 3q21 identified in patients from Southwest Sweden. European Journal of HumanGenetics. 1999;**7**(7):783-790

[38] Jadali Z, Eslami MB, Mansouri P, Safari R, Bayatian P, Mirshafiey A,SalehiNodeh AR. Th1/Th2 cytokines in psoriasis. Iranian Journalof Public Health. 2007;**36**(2):87-91

[39] Craven NM, Jackson CW, Kirby B, Perrey C, Pravica V, Hutchinson IV, Griffiths CE. Cytokine gene polymorphisms in psoriasis. British Journal of Dermatology. 2001;**144**(4):849-853

[40] Grossman RM, Krueger J, Yourish D, Granelli-Piperno A, Murphy DP, May LT, Kupper TS, Sehgal PB, Gottlieb AB. Interleukin 6 is expressed in high levels in psoriatic skin and stimulates proliferation of cultured human keratinocytes. Proceedings of the National Academy of Sciences. 1989;**86**:6367-6371

[41] Groves RW, Allen MH, Ross EL, Barker JN, MacDonald DM. Tumournecrosis factor alpha is pro-inflammatory in normal human skin and modulates cutaneous adhesion molecule expression. British Journalof Dermatology. 1995;**132**(3):345-352

[42] Gomi T, Shiohara T, Munakata T, Imanishi K, Nagashima M. Interleukin 1a, Tumor Necrosis Factor a, and Interferon gamma in psoriasis. Archives of Dermatology. 1991;**127**(6):827-830

[43] Uyemura K, Yamamura M, Fivenson DF, Modlin RL, Nickoloff BJ. The cytokine network in lesional and lesion-free psoriatic skin is characterized by a T-Helper type 1 cell-mediated response. Journal of Investigative Dermatology. 1993;**101**(5):701-705

[44] Konstantinova NV, Duong DM, Remenyik E, Hazarika P, Chuang A, Duvic M. Interleukin-8 is induced in skin equivalents and is highest in those derived from psoriatic fibroblasts. Journal of Investigative Dermatology. 1996;**107**(4):615-621

[45] Lew W, Bowcock AM, Krueger JG. Psoriasis vulgaris: cutaneous lymphoid tissue supports T-cell activation and "Type 1" inflammatory gene expression. Trends in Immunology. 2004;**25**(6):295-305

[46] Zuo X, Sun L, Yin X, Gao J, Sheng Y, Xu J, Zhang J, He C, Qiu Y, Wen G, Tian H7, Zheng X, Liu S, Wang W, Li W, Cheng Y, Liu L, Chang Y, Wang Z, Li Z, Li L, Wu J, Fang L, Shen C, Zhou F, Liang B, Chen G, Li H, Cui Y, Xu A, Yang. Whole-exome SNP array identifies 15 new susceptibility loci for psoriasis. Nature Communications. 2015;**6**:6793. DOI: 10.1038/ncomms7793

[47] Haase O, Mosaad H, Eldarouti MA, Elramly AZ, Samir N, Abdelhady MM, Samir M, El-Gharib I, Salah S, El-Shennawy FA, Mosaad Y, Elwan N, Salem H, Abdelgaber S, Recke A, Möller S, Zillikens D, Ibrahim S. TNFAIP3 and IL12B gene polymorphisms associated with psoriasis vulgaris in an Egyptian cohort. Journal of the European Academy of Dermatology and Venereology.2015;**29**(7):1297-1301

[48] Oka A, Mabuchi T, Ikeda S, Terui T, Haida Y, Ozawa A, Yatsu K, Kulski JK, Inoko H. IL12B and IL23R gene SNPs in Japanese psoriasis. Immunogenetics. 2013;**65**(11):823-828

[49] Lee YH, Song GG. Associations between interleukin-23R and interleukin-12B polymorphisms and psoriasis susceptibility: A meta-analysis. Immunological Investigations. 2013;**42**(8):726-736

[50] Zhu KJ, Zhu CY, Shi G, Fan YM. Author informationMeta-analysis of IL12B polymorphisms (rs3212227, rs6887695) With Psoriasis and Psoriatic Arthritis. Rheumatology International. 2013;**33**(7):1785-1790. DOI: 10.1007/s00296-012-2637-4

[51] Luu M, Cordoro KM. The Evolving Role of Biologics in The Treatment of Pediatric Psoriasis. Skin Therapy Letter. 2013;**18**(2):1-4

[52] Leonardi CL, Kimball AB, Papp KA, Yeilding N, Guzzo C, Wang Y, Li S, Dooley LT, Gordon KB. Efficacy and Safety of Ustekinumab, a Human Interleukin-12/23 Monoclonal Antibody, in Patients With Psoriasis: 76-Week Results From a Randomise Double-Blind, Placebo-Controlled Trial (PHOENIX 1). Lancet. 2008;**371**(9625):1665-1674

[53] Kurzeja M, Rudnicka L, Olszewska M. New interleukin-23 pathway inhibitors in dermatology: Ustekinumab, Briakinumab, and Secukinumab. American Journal of Clinical Dermatology. 2011;**12**(2):113-125

[54] Quatresooz P, Hermanns-Lê T, Piérard GE, Humbert P, Delvenne P, Piérard-Franchimont C. Ustekinumab in psoriasis immunopathology with emphasis on the Th17-IL23 axis: A primer. Journal of Biomedicine and Biotechnology. 2012;**2012**:147413. DOI: 10.1155/2012/147413

[55] Tong Y, Peranteau AJ, Nawas Z, Tyring SK. A review of brodalumab, an IL-17 receptor antagonist, for moderate-to-severe plaque psoriasis. Skin Therapy Letter. 2017;**22**(1):1-6

[56] Lee E, Zarei M, LaSenna C, Villada G, Romanelli P. Psoriasis targeted therapy: Characterization of interleukin 17A expression in subtypes of psoriasis. Journal of Drugs in Dermatology. 2015;**14**(10):1133-1136

[57] Pazyar N, Feily A, Yaghoobi R. Macrophage migration inhibitory factor as an incriminating agent in dermatological disorders. Indian Journal of Dermatology. 2013;**58**(2):157. DOI:10.4103/0019-5154.108068

[58] Shimizu T, Nishihira J, Mizue Y, Nakamura H, Abe R, Watanabe H, Ishibashi T, Shimizu H. Histochemical analysis of macrophage migration inhibitory factor in psoriasis vulgaris. Histochemistry and Cell Biology. 2002;**118**(3):251-257

[59] Rudiger Panzer, Conrad Blobel, Regina Folster-Holst, EhrhardtProksch. TLR2 and TLR4 expression in atopic dermatitis, contact dermatitis and psoriasis. Experimental Dermatology. 2014;**23**(5):364-366. DOI: 10.1111/exd.12383

[60] Salama DM, Abdel Halim DM, Fawzy N, Rashed L. Toll-like receptor 2 (TLR2) gene expression in psoriasis vulgaris and its correlation with vitamin D3 serum level before and after NB-UVB. The Medical journal of Cairo University. 2013;**81**(2):95-101

[61] Ishimoto T, Kataoka S, Shiga T, Sano S. Increase of psoriasis-associated IL-8 in the intralesional blood despite undetectable in the peripheral blood. Journal of Dermatological Science. 2016;**84**(1):e103-e1. DOI: 10.1016/j.jdermsci.2016.08.312

[62] Picciani BLS, Carneiro S, Cantisano MH, Avelleira JCR, Azulay DR, Pinto JMN, Dias EP. Geographic tongue or oral psoriasis?. Oral Surgery, Oral Medicine, Oral Pathology and Oral Radiology. 2012;**114**(4):e108-e108

[63] Nishikawa R, Nagai H, Bito T, Ikeda T, Horikawa T, Adachi A, Matsubara T, Nishigori C. Genetic prediction of the effectiveness of biologics for psoriasis treatment. The Journal of Dermatology. 2016;**43**(11):1273-1277. DOI: 10.1111/1346-8138.13412., 2016.

[64] Prieto-Pérez R, Solano-López G, Cabaleiro T, Román M, Ochoa D, Talegón M, Baniandrés O, López-Estebaranz JL, de la Cueva P, Daudén E, Abad-Santos F. New polymorphisms associated with response to anti-TNF drugs in patients with moderate-to-severe plaque psoriasis. The Pharmacogenomics Journal. 2016; DOI: 10.1038/tpj.2016.64, 2016

[65] Murdaca G, Gulli R, Spanò F, Lantieri F, Burlando M, Parodi A, Mandich P, Puppo F. TNF-α gene polymorphisms: association with disease susceptibility and response to anti-TNF-α treatment in psoriatic arthritis. Psoriasis and Genetics. 2014;**134**(10):2503-2509. DOI: 10.1038/jid.2014.123

[66] Wu D, Hou SY, Zhao S, Hou LX, Jiao T, Xu NN, Zhang N. Efficacy and safety of interleukin-17 antagonists in patients with plaque psoriasis: A meta-analysis from phase 3 randomized controlled trials. Journal of the European Academy of Dermatology and Venereology. 2017. DOI: 10.1111/jdv.14125. [Epub ahead of print]

[67] FDA accepts AstraZeneca's brodalumab BLA for plaque psoriasis, PDUFA date November 16Valeant Announces FDA Acceptance of BLA Submission for Brodalumab in Moderate-to-Severe Plaque Psoriasis. 2016

[68] Burkett PR, Kuchroo VK. IL-17 blockade in psoriasis. Cell. 2016;**167**(7):1669. DOI: 10.1016/j.cell.2016.11.044

[69] Białecka M, Ostasz R, Kurzawski M, Klimowicz A, Fabiańczyk H, Bojko P, Dziedziejko V, Safranow K, Machoy-Mokrzyńska A, Drozdzik M. IL17A and IL17F gene polymorphism association with psoriasis risk and response to treatment in a polish population. Dermatology. 2016;**232**(5):592-596. DOI: 10.1159/000448090

[70] Kim SY, Hur MS, Choi BG1, Kim MJ, Lee YW, Choe YB, Ahn KJ. A preliminary study of new single polymorphisms in the T helper type 17 pathway for psoriasis in the Korean population. Clinical & Experimental Immunology. 2017;**187**(2):251-258. DOI: 10.1111/cei.12888

[71] Prieto-Pérez R, Solano-López G, Cabaleiro T, Román M, Ochoa D, Talegón M, Baniandrés O, LópezEstebaranz JL, de la Cueva P, Daudén E, Abad-Santos F. The polymorphism rs763780 in the IL-17F gene is associated with response to biological drugs in patients with psoriasis. Pharmacogenomics. 2015;**16**(15):1723-1731. DOI: 10.2217/pgs.15.107

[72] Gullive WP. Importance of Screening for Comorbidities in Psoriasis Patients. Expert Review of Dermatology. 2008;**3**(2):133-135

[73] Brauchli YB, Jick SS, Meier CR. Psoriasis and the RISK of incident diabetes mellitus: A population-based study. British Journal of Dermatology. 2008;**159**:1331-1337

[74] Cohen AD, Dreiher J, Shapiro Y, Vidavsky L, Vardy DA, Davidovici B, Meyerovitch J. Psoriasis and diabetes: A population-based cross-sectional study. Journal of the European Academy of Dermatology and Venereology. 2008;**22**(5):585-589. DOI: 10.1111/j.1468-3083.2008.02636.x

[75] Horreau C, Pouplard C, Brenaut E, Barnetche T, Misery L, Cribier B, Jullien D, Aractingi S, Aubin F, Joly P, Le Maître M, Ortonne JP, Paul C, Richard MA. Cardiovascular morbidity and mortality in psoriasis and psoriatic arthritis: A systematic literature review. Journal of the European Academy of Dermatology and Venereology. 2013;**3**:12-29. DOI: 10.1111/jdv.12163

[76] Abuabara K, Lee H, Kimball AB. The effect of systemic psoriasis therapies on the incidence of myocardial infarction: A cohort study. British Journal of Dermatology. 2011;**165**:1066-1073

[77] Gelfand JM, Mehta NM, Langan SM. Psoriasis and cardiovascular risk:Strenght in numbers. JAMA. 2011;**131**(5):1007-1010

[78] Friedewald VE, Cather JC, Gelfand JM, Gordon KB, Gibbons GH, Grundy SM, Jarratt MT, Krueger JG, Ridker PM, Stone N, Roberts WC. AJC editor's consensus: Psoriasis and coronary artery disease. American Journalof Cardiology. 2008;**102**(12):1631-1643. DOI:10.1016/j.amjcard.2008.10.004

[79] Najarian DJ, Gottlieb AB. Connections between psoriasis and Crohn's disease. Journal of the American Academy of Dermatology. 2003;**48**(6):805-821. quiz 822-4

[80] Skroza N, IlariaProietti, Riccardo Pampena, Giorgio La Viola, Nicoletta Bernardini, Francesca Nicolucci, ErsiliaTolino, Sara Zuber, Valentina Soccodato, and Concetta Potenza. Correlations between Psoriasis and Inflammatory Bowel Diseases. BioMed Research International. vol. 2013;**2013**:8. Article ID 983902. DOI:10.1155/2013/983902

[81] Moll JMH, Wright V. Psoriatic arthritis. Seminars in Arthritis and Rheumatism. 1973;**3**:55-78

[82] Erdem RH. PsoriatikArtrtitinKlinikÖzellikleri. Romatizma. 2000;**15**(1):31-38

[83] Gezer Albayrak I, Levendoğlu F, Özerbil ÖM. PsöriasisHastalarındaPsöriatik ArtritGörülmeSıklığıvePsöriatikArtritinKlinikÖzellikleri. Genel Tip Dergisi. 2016;**26**(2): 58-61

[84] Canpolati F, Akpinar H, Eskioğlu F. Mean Platelet Volume in Psoriasis and Psoriatic Arthritis. Clinical Rheumatology. 2010;**29**(3):325-328

[85] McHugh NJ, Laurent MR, Treadwell BLJ, Treadwell BL, Tweed JM, Dagger J. Other seronegative spondyloarthropathies. Medicine. 2009;**38**(4):190-193

[86] Pedersen OB, Svendsen AJ, Ejstrup L, Skytthe A, Junker P. On the Heritability of Psoriatic Arthritis. Disease Concordance Among Monozygotic And Dizygotic Twins. 2008;**67**(10):1417-1421

[87] Olivieri I, Padula A, D'Angelo S, Cutro MS. Psoriatic Arthritis Sine Psoriasis. The Journal of Rheumatology Supplement. 2009;**83**:28-29. DOI: 10.3899/jrheum.090218

[88] Bonfiglioli R, Conde RA, Sampaio-Barros PD, Louzada-Junior P, Donadi EA, Bertolo MB. Frequency of HLA-B27 alleles in Brazilian patients with psoriatic arthritis. Clinical Rheumatology. 2008;**27**(6):709-712

[89] Gladman DD, Farewell VT, Kopciuk KA, Cook RJ. HLA Markers and progression in psoriatic arthritis. The Journal of Rheumatology. 1998;**25**(4):730-733

[90] Gladman DD, Antoni C, Mease P, Clegg DO, Nash P. Psoriatic arthritis: Epidemiology, clinical features, course and outcome. Annals of the Rheumatic Diseases. 2005;64(2):ii14-7

[91] Brockbank J. Gladman DD. Psoriatic arthritis. Expert Opinion on Investigational Drugs. 2000;9(7):1511-1522

[92] de Bakker PI, Mc Vean G, Sabeti PC, Miretti MM, Green T, Marchini J, Ke X, Monsuur AJ, Whittaker P, Delgado M, Morrison J, Richardson A, Walsh EC, Gao X, Galver L, Hart J, Hafler DA, Pericak--Vance M, Todd JA, Daly MJ. A high-resolution HLA and SNP haplotype map for disease association studies in the extended human MHC. Nature Genetics. 2006;38(10):1166-1172

[93] Eastmond CJ. Psoriatic arthritis. Genetics and HLA Antigens. Baillière's Clinical Rheumatology. 1994;8(2):263-276

[94] Gladman DD, Anhorn KA, Schachter RK, Mervart H. HLA antigens in psoriatic arthritis. The Journal of Rheumatology. 1986;13(3):586-592

[95] Ho PY, Barton A, Worthington J, Plant D, Griffiths CE, Young HS, Bradburn P, Thomson W, Silman AJ, Bruce IN. Investigating the role of the HLA-Cw*06 and HLA-DRB1 genes in susceptibility to psoriatic arthritis: Comparison with psoriasis and undifferentiated inflammatory arthritis. Annals of the Rheumatic Diseases. 2008;67(5):677-682

[96] Veale DJ, Ritchlin C. ve FitzGerald O. Immunopathology of psoriasis and psoriatic arthritis. Annals of the Rheumatic Diseases. 2005;64(2):26-29

[97] Öğretmen Z, Hız MM, Sılan F, Koşar S, Özdemir Ö. Is the HLA B27 genotype a riscfaktor for psoriatic arthritis and psoriasis vulgaris? Türkderm 2014;48:131-134

[98] Fantuzzi G. Adipose tissue, adipokines, and inflammation. The Journal of Allergy and Clinical Immunology. 2005;115(5):911-919

[99] Kershaw EE, Flier JS. Adipose Tissue as an endocrine organ. The Journal of Clinical Endocrinology & Metabolism. 2004;**89**(6):2548-2556

[100] Frühbeck G, Gómez-Ambrosi J, Muruzábal FJ, Burrell MA. The adipocyte: A model for integration of endocrine and metabolic signaling in energy metabolism regulation. American Journal of Physiology Endocrinology Metabolism. **280**:E827-E847

[101] Russolillo A, Iervolino S, Peluso R, Lupoli R, Di Minno A, Pappone N, Di Minno MN. Obesity and psoriatic arthritis: From pathogenesis to clinical outcome and management. Rheumatology (Oxford). 2012;52(1):62-67

[102] Pessinaba S, Yayehd K, Pio M, Baragou R, Afassinou Y, Tchérou T, Damorou F. Obesity in cardiology consultation in lome: Prevalence and risk factors associated with cardiovascular disease study in 1200 patients. The Pan African Medical Journal. 2012;12:99

[103] Blüher M. The Distinction of Metabolically 'Healthy' From 'Unhealthy' Obese Individuals. Current Opinion in Lipidology. 2010;**21**(1):38-43

[104] Spiotta RT, Luma GB. Evaluating obesity and cardiovascular risk factors in children and adolescents. American Family Physician. 2008;78(9):1052-1058

[105] Nguyen S, McCulloch C, Brakeman P, Portale A, Hsu CY. Being overweight modifies the association between cardiovascular risk factors and microalbuminuria in adolescents. Pediatrics. 2008;121(1):37-45

[106] Poirier P. Targeting abdominal obesity in cardiology: Can we be effective? Canadian Journal of Cardiology. 2008;24:13D-17D

[107] Wyatt SB, Winters KP, Dubbert PM. Overweight and obesity: Prevalence, consequences, and causes of a growing public health problem. The American Journal of the Medical Sciences. 2006;331(4):166-174

[108] Steinberger J, Daniels SR. Obesity, insulin resistance, diabetes, and cardiovascular risk in children. Circulation. 2003;107:1448-1453

[109] Hansson GK, Hermansson A. The immune system in atherosclerosis. Nature Immunology. 2011;12:204-212

[110] Murray ML, Bergstresser PR, Adams-Huet B, Cohen JB. Relationship of psoriasis severity to obesity using same-gender siblings as controls for obesity. Clinical and Experimental Dermatology. 2009;34(2):140-144

[111] Duarte GV, Oliveira Mde F, Cardoso TM, Follador I, Silva TS, Cavalheiro CM, Nonato W, Carvalho EM. Association between obesity measured by different parameters and severity of psoriasis. International Journal of Dermatology. 2012;52(2):177-181

[112] Kumar S, Han J, Li T, Qureshi AA. Obesity, waist circumference, weight change and the risk of psoriasis in US women. Journal of the European Academy of Dermatology and Venereology. 2012;10:1293-1298. DOI: 10.1111/jdv.12001

[113] Love TJ, Zhu Y, Zhang Y, Wall-Burns L, Ogdie A, Gelfand JM, Choi HK. Obesity and the risk of psoriatic arthritis: A population-based study. Annals of the Rheumatic Diseases. 2012;71(8):1273-1277

[114] Husted JA, Thavaneswaran A, Chandran Eder L, Rosen CF, Cook RJ, Gladman DD. Cardiovascular and other comorbidities in patients with psoriatic arthritis: Acomparison with patients with psoriasis. Arthritis Care & Research(Hoboken). 2011;63(12):17

[115] Soltani-Arabshahi R, Wong B, Feng BJ, Goldgar DE, Duffin KC, Krueger GG. Obesity in early adulthood as a risk factor for psoriatic arthritis. Archives of Dermatology. 2010;146(7):721-726. DOI: 10.1001/archdermatol.2010.141

[116] Yang YW, Keller JJ, Lin HC. Medical comorbidity associated with psoriasis in adults: A population based study. British Journal of Dermatology. 2011;165(5):1037-1043

[117] Davidovici BB, Sattar N, Prinz J, Puig L, Emery P, Barker JN, van de Kerkhof P, Ståhle M, Nestle FO, Girolomoni G, Krueger JG. Psoriasis and systemic inflammatory diseases: Potential mechanistic links between skin disease and co-morbid conditions. Journal of Investigative Dermatology. 2010;**130**(7):1785-1796. DOI: 10.1038/jid.2010.103

[118] Qureshi AA, Choi HK, Setty AR, Curhan GC. Psoriasis and the risk of diabetes and hypertension: A prospective study of US female nurses. Archives of Dermatology. 2009;145(4):379-382

[119] Gibson SH, Perry HO. Diabetes and psoriasis. AMA Archives of Dermatology. 1956;74(5):487-488

[120] Onsun N, Su Ö, Eriş Z, Davutoğlu M, Cebeci F, Senocak M. PsoriasisteDiyabet, Diyabette Psoriasis Sıklığı. Türkderm. 2010;44(1):12-14

[121] Azfar RS, Seminara NM, Shin DB, Troxel AB, Margolis DJ, Gelfand JM. Increased risk of diabetes mellitus and likelihood of receiving diabetes mellitus treatment in patients with psoriasis. Archives of Dermatology. 2012;148(9):995-1000

[122] Armesto S, Santos-Juanes J, Galache-Osuna C, Martinez-Camblor P, Coto E, Coto-Segura P. Psoriasis and type 2 diabetes risk among psoriatic patients in a spanish population. Australasian Journal of Dermatology. 2012;53(2):128-130

[123] Finley PJ, DeClue CE, Sell SA, DeBartolo JM, Shornick LP. Diabetic wounds exhibit decreased Ym1 and arginase expression with increased expression of IL-17 and IL-20. Advances in Wound Care(New Rochelle). 2016;5(11):486-494

[124] Granata M, Skarmoutsou E, Trovato C, Rossi GA, Mazzarino MC, D'Amico F. Obesity, type 1 diabetes, and psoriasis: An autoimmune triple flip. Pathobiology. 2016;17. [Epub ahead of print]

[125] Eirís N, González-Lara L, Santos-Juanes J, Queiro R, Coto E, Coto-Segura P. Genetic variation at IL12B, IL23R and IL23A is associated with psoriasis severity, psoriatic arthritis and type 2 diabetes mellitus. Journal of Dermatological Science. 2014;75(3):167-172. DOI: 10.1016/j.jdermsci.2014.05.010. Epub 2014 Jun 11

[126] Presta I, Andreozzi F, Succurro E, Marini MA, Laratta E, Lauro R, Hribal ML, Perticone F, Sesti G. IL-18 gene polymorphism and metabolic syndrome. Nutrition, Metabolism & Cardiovascular Diseases. 2009;19(2):e5-e6. DOI: 10.1016/j.numecd.2008.10.002. Epub 2009 Jan 26

[127] Işik S, Hız MM, Kılıç S, Öğretmen Z, Silan F. Is there any increased risk of hypertension, diabetes and cardiac diseases in psoriatic patients with TNF-α G238A and G308A polymorphism? Advances in Dermatology and Allergology/PostępyDermatologiiAlergologii. 2016;33(6):440-444. DOI:10.5114/pdia.2016.58384

[128] Prodanovich S, Kirsner RS, Kravetz JD, Ma F, Martinez L, Federman DG. Asociation of psoriasis with coronaryartery, cerebrovascular and peripheral vascular diseases and mortality. 2009;**145**(6):700-703

[129] Driessen RJ, Boezeman JB, Van de Kerkhof PC, De Jong EM. Cardiovascular risk factors in high-need psoriasis patientsand its implications for biological therapies. Journal of Dermatological Treatment. 2009;20(1):42-47

[130] Yang ZS, Lin NN, Li L, Li Y. The effect of TNF inhibitors on cardiovascular events in psoriasis and psoriatic arthritis: An Updated Meta-Analysis. Clinical Reviews in Allergy & Immunology. 2016;51(2):240-247

[131] Ogretmen Z, Hiz MM, Silan F, Uludag A, Ozdemirc O. Association of endothelial nitric oxide synthase Glu298Asp gene polymorphism in psoriasis cases with hypertension. Annals of Saudi Medicine. 2014;34(4):340-345. DOI: 10.5144/0256-4947.2014.340

[132] Bricker LA, Greydanus DE. The Metabolic Syndrome: a Gathering Challenge in a Time of Abundance. Adolescent Medicine: State of the Art Reviews. 2008;19:475-497

[133] Abdel Hay RM, Rashed LA. Association between the leptin gene 2548G/A polymorphism, the plasma leptin and the metabolic syndrome with psoriasis. Experimental Dermatology. 2011;20(9):715-719

[134] Cohen BE, Martires KJ, Ho RS. Psoriasis and the risk of depression in the US population: National Health and Nutrition Examination Survey 2009-2012. JAMA Dermatology. 2016;152(1):73-79

[135] Kurd SK, Troxel AB, Crits-Christoph P, Gelfand JM. The risk of depression, anxiety and suicidality in patients with psoriasis: A population-based cohort study. Archives of Dermatology. 2010;146(8):891-895. DOI:10.1001/archdermatol.2010.186

[136] Pompili M, Innamorati M, Trovarelli S, Narcisi A, Bellini S, Orsini D, Forte A, Erbuto D, Botti E, Lamis DA, Girardi P, Costanzo A. Suicide risk and psychiatric comorbidity in patients with psoriasis. Journal of International Medical Research. 2016;44(1):61-66

[137] Deveci A, Ermertcan AT, Deniz F, Madak BG, Öztürkcan S. PsoriasisliHastalardaAlkol KullanımıveİntiharOlasılığıTürkiye'dePsikiyatri. 2007;9(2):103-107

[138] Farkas A, Keměny L. Psoriasis and alcohol: Is cutaneous ethanol one of the missing links? British Journal of Dermatology. 2010;162(4):711-716

[139] Younes SF, Bakry OA. Immunohistochemicalevaluation of role of serotonin in pathogenesis of psoriasis. Journal of Clinical and Diagnostic Research. 2016;10(10):EC05-EC09

[140] Tencomnao T, Wongpiyabovorn J. An investigation of the relationship between serotonin transporter gene promoter polymorphism and psoriasis susceptibility in a Thai population. Genetics and Molecular Research. 2010;9(4):2275-2282

[141] Ronpirin C, Tencomnao T, Wongpiyabovorn J. Association between the -1438A/G polymorphism of the serotonin 2A receptor gene and late-onset psoriasis in a Thai population. Genetics and Molecular Research. 2010;9(1):208-214

Chapter 2

A Review of Possible Triggering or Therapeutic Effects of Antimicrobial Vaccines on Psoriasis

Sevgi Akarsu and Ceylan Avcı

Additional information is available at the end of the chapter

http://dx.doi.org/10.5772/67691

Abstract

Psoriasis is a chronic, immune-mediated disease resulting from interactions of genetic background with environmental triggering factors, such as trauma, infections and drugs. Dendritic cells, activated T-cells toward a Th1 and Th17 response and inflammatory cytokines [tumor necrosis factor (TNF)-alpha, IL-6, -12, -17, -22 and -23] are the key factors in psoriasis pathogenesis. Patients diagnosed with psoriasis are at increased risk of infection due to the nature of disease and immunosuppressive therapies. Vaccination is recommended to prevent infections in patients with psoriasis. Additionally, vaccines such as *Mycobacterium vaccae,* live attenuated varicella zoster virus and Leishmania amastigotes have been reported to induce improvement in psoriasis patients. It has been suggested that vaccines, targeting molecules in the immunopathogenesis of psoriasis, may be a new treatment option for psoriasis patients without any serious side effects. However, induction or worsening of the psoriasis and psoriatic arthritis followed by some vaccines (e.g., influenza, rubella, tetanus, BCG) has also been reported in the literature. In this review, we focus on the vaccines in psoriasis in terms of their both triggering and therapeutic effects.

Keywords: psoriasis, antimicrobial vaccination, recommended vaccines, triggering vaccines, therapeutic vaccines

1. Introduction

Psoriasis is a chronic, immune-mediated disease with a prevalence of 2–3% in adult population. Psoriatic arthritis affects approximately 11% of psoriasis patients, and cardiovascular disease is increased [1]. Psoriasis disease is caused by the interactions of genetic background with various environmental triggering factors. HLA-Cw6 allele in PSORS1, the most associated gene with psoriasis, encodes a major histocompatibility complex I allele that is the major factor for antigen presentation of intracellular peptides to the immune system [2].

Several environmental factors, such as trauma (Koebner effect), infections, obesity, smoking and some medications, play a role in the onset of psoriasis. Guttate psoriasis is related to streptococcal throat infections as two-thirds of patients have a history of throat infection nearly 2 weeks before the eruption [3, 4]. A homology between streptococcal M protein and human keratin 17, which is upregulated in the skin of psoriasis, has been reported. In the basis of this finding, T-cells cross-reacting with human keratin and streptococci have been detected in HLA-CW6-positive psoriasis patients, raising the possibility that psoriasis is an autoimmune disease [5].

In the initial phase of the disease, certain dendritic cell (DC) populations such as plasmacytoid DCs (pDC) and dermal myeloid DCs are activated and produce the key psoriasis effector cytokines IL-12 and IL-23. Self-DNA or self-RNA from damaged keratinocytes and the antimicrobial peptide LL37 stimulate pDCs, through Toll-like receptor (TLR) 9 or TLR7/8 and IFN-alpha production is triggered. The stimulation of pDCs is followed by differentiation and activation of myeloid DCs, which express cytokines IL-12, tumor necrosis factor (TNF)-alpha, TGF-beta and IL-6. These cytokines induce T-cells to polarize into Th1 and Th17 subtypes, with suppressing of regulatory T-cells [1, 2, 6, 7]. CD4+ T-cells secreting IL-17 are classified as a different T-helper population called Th17 cells, which are critical in psoriasis pathogenesis. Th17 cells produce IL-17A and IL-17F, and Th1 cells produce TNF-alpha, IFN-gamma, IL-12, IL-22 and IL-23 that promote the pathological changes in psoriasis skin lesions [2, 8].

For psoriasis patients with localized disease, topical treatments including corticosteroids, vitamin D derivatives, tazarotene, anthralin, tar, calcineurin inhibitors, keratolytic agents and urea are the first-line therapy [9]. Phototherapy is a mainstay option particularly for patients resistant to topical treatments with widespread disease [10]. In cases with moderate-to-severe psoriasis resistant to any of these treatments, conventional systemic therapy is done with methotrexate (MTX), cyclosporine, fumaric acid esters and acitretin. In patients who have failed to respond to conventional systemic therapies and phototherapy or the person is intolerant to, or has a contraindication to these treatments, biologic immunotherapy is used. There are several agents such as TNF-alpha inhibitors (etanercept, infliximab and adalimumab) and ustekinumab that are available in the treatment of psoriasis [11].

Vaccination is a proven way of reducing the incidence of serious or life-threatening infectious disease in general population and in patients with immune-mediated inflammatory disease. Vaccines are recommended for psoriasis patients due to their susceptibility to infections [12]. The data emphasize that especially some types of vaccines may trigger an exacerbation of psoriatic skin lesions or induce improvement in psoriasis [1, 13].

In this review, we aim to summarize the vaccines in psoriasis in terms of their both triggering and therapeutic effects.

http://dx.doi.org/10.5772/67691

2. Vaccines recommended for psoriasis patients

Patients diagnosed with psoriasis are at risk of infections owing to the nature of disease and immunosuppressive therapies [12, 14]. Therefore, the medical board of the National Psoriasis Foundation recommends vaccinations in compliance with recommendations of the Advisory Committee for Immunization Practices to prevent infections [12]. Types of vaccines can be categorized as live and inactivated vaccines (**Table 1**) [12, 14].

Live vaccines, which contain attenuated natural pathogens, are contraindicated in immunocompromised patients and should be given 2 or 4 weeks before the immunosuppressive therapy. Additionally, immunosuppressive medications should be stopped generally 3 months before the immunization with live vaccines [12, 14]. However, a few reports suggest that some live vaccines such as yellow fever vaccine in patients receiving MTX may be safe [15]. More research is needed for safety of live vaccines in immunocompromised patients [12, 15]. Inactivated vaccines are safe for patients on immunomodulatory therapy due to their noninfectious content but vaccine response may be suboptimal [12, 14, 16]. It has been reported that the antibody response ratio following seven-valent conjugate pneumococcal vaccination was significantly higher in controls when compared to patients treated with MTX or MTX combined with TNF inhibitors. On the other hand, in the same study, patients treated with TNF inhibitors as monotherapy had numerically lower but not significantly different antibody levels, compared to controls [17]. In a study, ustekinumab did not impair the immune response to pneumococcal and tetanus toxoid vaccines in psoriasis patients [18]. In another study, efalizumab caused a nearly threefold decrease in the antibody response to tetanus toxoid vaccine while not changing the immune response to pneumococcal polysaccharide vaccine [19]. Immune responses to pneumococcal polysaccharide vaccine in patients with chronic plaque psoriasis treated with alefacept were similar to those seen in healthy subjects [20].

Inactivated or inert vaccines	Live vaccines
Salk poliomyelitis vaccine	Vaccinia/smallpox
Most influenza vaccines (injectable)	Rotavirus
Hepatitis A	Measles-mumps-rubella
Hepatitis B	Yellow fever
Human papillomavirus	Oral poliomyelitis
Diphtheria-tetanus-pertussis	Varicella zoster vaccine
Haemophilus influenza type b conjugate vaccine	Herpes zoster
Pneumococcal	Intranazal influenza virus
Meningococcal	BCG
Rabies	Oral typhoid
Parenteral typhoid	
Anthrax	
Japanese encephalitis	

Table 1. Types of vaccines.

In a study assessing the seasonal 2012 influenza vaccination among patients with psoriatic arthritis and psoriasis, usage of TNF-alpha blockers or disease-modifying antirheumatic drugs did not affect the response rate [21]. Annual immunization with inactivated influenza vaccine is recommended for psoriasis patients on immunosuppressive treatment due to high mortality rates of seasonal influenza [12, 22]. In a French study on 1308 psoriasis patients, Sbidian et al. reported that 19% of patients received the 2009 monovalent H1N1 vaccine. Only 33% of the patients treated with biologics were vaccinated [23]. The vaccination rate of influenza vaccine in 2010/2011 was found 28% among 1299 patients with psoriasis or psoriatic arthritis in Germany. Thirty-eight percent of the patients were on biological therapy at the time of vaccination [22]. Despite the recommendations, the vaccination coverage was low in psoriasis patients in both studies [22, 23].

Zoster vaccine, a live attenuated vaccine, is recommended for use in immunocompetent individuals 60 years of age or older to reduce the risk and severity of herpes zoster (HZ) [12]. Increased incidence of HZ has been reported in psoriasis patients receiving combination treatment with biologic medications and MTX while biologic or systemic agents as monotherapy did not increase the risk of HZ [24]. Zhang et al. reported that zoster vaccination was not related to increased risk of HZ in patients with immune-mediated disease including psoriasis under biological therapy [25, 26]. However, it was emphasized that infliximab increases the risk of HZ in most of the cohort studies while the risk of HZ in patients receiving etanercept, adalimumab or ustekinumab therapy is not clear [27]. Yun et al. indicated that the use of biologic agents and systemic steroids in patients with autoimmune and inflammatory diseases increased the risk of HZ [28]. Consequently, HZ vaccination should be considered for patients who are going to receive biological agents especially infliximab and combination treatment with MTX therapy. Additionally, the vaccine should be administered before initiation of the immunosuppressive therapy [24, 27].

As a conclusion, it has been reported that immunization status, including *Haemophilus influenza*, hepatitis A and B, human papillomavirus, influenza, *Neisseria meningitides* and *Streptococcus pneumoniae* should be assessed in all patients with moderate-to-severe psoriasis [12]. Recommendations for vaccination of patients diagnosed with psoriasis are given in **Table 2** [12, 14].

Type of vaccine	Before therapy	On therapy
Inactivated vaccines		
Influenza	Vaccinate with inactivated or live attenuated vaccine	Annual inactivated influenza
Human papillomavirus	Recommended for male and female < age 26 years	Same
Hepatitis A	For selected individuals at high risk (diabetes, liver disease, injecting drug users, homosexual men, employees or residents in institutional settings)	Same, test for serology after vaccination
Hepatitis B	For individuals at high risk and without evidence of disease and immunity	Use high-dose vaccine, test for serology after vaccination
Pneumococcal	Immunization with 23-valent pneumococcal polysaccharide vaccine	Immunization with 13-valent pneumococcal conjugate vaccine followed by 23-valent pneumococcal polysaccharide vaccine if not given prior

http://dx.doi.org/10.5772/67691

Type of vaccine	Before therapy	On therapy
Haemophilus influenza type b	Unvaccinated individuals can be vaccinated	Same
Diphtheria-tetanus-pertussis	Booster is recommended every 10 years and for high-risk wounds, offer before therapy	Same
Meningococcal	For selected individuals at high risk (asplenia, complement deficiency, group living situation)	Same
Poliomyelitis	For selected individuals at high risk (healthcare workers or laboratory personnel)	Same
Live vaccines		
Varicella zoster	Test for serology before initiation of therapy, if negative, offer vaccination	Contraindicated
Herpes zoster	1 dose for adults ≥50 years	Contraindicated
Measles-mumps-rubella	Assessment of immunization by history and serology before initiation of therapy, if negative, offer vaccination	Contraindicated

Table 2. Recommendations for vaccination of patients diagnosed with psoriasis before or on systemic immunosuppressants.

3. Triggering effect of vaccines on psoriasis

As mentioned above, basis on a genetic predisposition, various environmental factors may cause development of psoriasis in patients who are in latent period. Physical or chemical factors, infections and various types of medications are the most important among these, and they may affect the course of psoriasis by many different mechanisms [13]. Triggering vaccines on psoriasis and psoriatic arthritis are summarized below.

3.1. Koebner effect

Various types of skin trauma with subsequent development of new psoriasis lesions about 10 days later are known as 'Koebner-phenomenon' [29]. In a study evaluating the relation between 'Koebner-phenomenon' and intradermal antigens, 30 psoriasis patients and 20 control subjects were firstly determined for Koebner status and then were tested with intradermal injections of purified protein derivative, Candida, mumps; mixed respiratory vaccine and saline control solutions. Two psoriasis patients were Koebner positive and developed psoriasis at all five injection sites. Besides, in five Koebner negative patients, local psoriasis lesions were observed in at least one injection site of different antigens. These findings were interpreted that some psoriatic patients may have individually specific sensitivity to different antigens to trigger the cellular immune response in psoriasis [30].

Additionally, in a recent placebo-controlled study, evaluating the 'nontypeable Haemophilus influenza protein vaccine', a psoriasis case was reported to be associated with injection of saline placebo at 114 days post-dose 3 in the placebo group indicating the Koebner effect [31].

3.2. BCG vaccination

BCG is a live attenuated strain of *Mycobacterium bovis*, which has been used as local immunotherapy for bladder cancer since 1976 [32]. In 1955, a psoriasis case was described following BCG vaccination under the name of 'psoriasis vaccinalis' [33]. A male with psoriatic arthropathy after BCG immunotherapy for bladder carcinoma and a psoriasis case after BCG vaccination are the other early reports associated with BCG vaccination [34, 35]. Koca et al. also defined a 7-year-old boy with guttate psoriasis-like lesions developed 1 week after the BCG vaccination [35]. Takayama et al. presented a 6-month-old girl with psoriatic skin lesions initially appeared on the vaccination site 1 month after the BCG vaccination. In that case, expression of activated phospho-Stat-3 was found in the epidermal keratinocytes of the lesional skin. Mycobacterial heat shock proteins have been reported to stimulate IL-6, which promotes the development of Th17 cells. Thus, the authors speculated that BCG vaccination might mediate the generation of IL-22-producing Th17 cells and lead to activation of epidermal Stat-3 and psoriatic skin lesions [36]. In addition, an 80-year-old man with bladder carcinoma was reported with erythrodermic pustular psoriasis triggered by intravesical BCG immunotherapy. The similar mechanism with Th1 and Th17 cells generation after BCG vaccination was thought to play an important role in the pathogenesis of psoriasis [32].

3.3. Tetanus-diphtheria (Td) vaccination

A case of 50-year-old psoriasis patient in remission was described as guttate psoriasis 1 week after the Td vaccination [37]. Td vaccine has shown to induce IL-6 production, which stimulates Th17 cells, having a key role in psoriasis pathogenesis [37, 38]. It was suggested that this mechanism was the triggering cause in this case [37]. In a case-control study evaluating the potential risk factors for the onset of psoriatic arthritis, exposure to rubella (OR = 12.4, 95% CI = 1.2–122.14) and tetanus (OR = 1.9, 95% CI = 1.0–3.7) vaccines was reported at a higher frequency in psoriatic arthritis group as compared to the psoriasis group without arthritis [39].

3.4. Influenza vaccination

Shin et al. described a 26-year-old woman with multiple erythematous scaly macules scattered on the extremities and trunk compatible with guttate psoriasis following injection of an inactivated split-virus influenza A/H1N1 vaccine without adjuvant [40]. Güneş et al. reported 43 patients suffering from psoriasis in that 36 of them had exacerbation of pre-existing psoriasis while disease first appeared in the remaining seven patients after influenza vaccination in the 2009–2010 season. Thirty-seven of these patients had mixed plaque type and guttate psoriasis, three of them suffered from palmoplantar psoriasis, and another three of them had scalp psoriasis. Although there is the lack of control group and follow-up evaluations in that study, they suggested that their observations may support the association between influenza vaccination and the development of psoriasis due to the short-time onset of psoriasis after vaccination and the lack of other possible triggers [13].

There is also a cross-sectional study investigating a total of 1125 cases for the onset or flare of psoriasis occurring within 3 months following the 2009 monovalent H1N1/seasonal vaccination through a national survey in France. The overall influenza vaccine coverage was found 19% in this population. Ten patients were reported with a psoriasis of new onset ($n = 7$) or with a worsening of previously diagnosed psoriasis ($n = 3$) within a median time period of 8 days after vaccination. Due to the uncertainties about the actual number of psoriatic patients undergoing vaccination, underestimation of the incidence due to underreporting and underdiagnosis and the lack of control group, the data could not provide a definitive conclusion about an association between vaccination and the psoriasis. However, the authors claimed that even if it is not a very strong risk, influenza vaccination is associated with psoriasis flare [41].

In another study, the effects of seasonal influenza vaccination in psoriatic arthritis patients under anti-TNF-alpha therapy were evaluated. 1 month after the vaccination (T1), patients ($n = 25$) had statistically significant increase in tender joint count (TJC) ($p = 0.009$) and erythrocyte sedimentation rate (ESR) ($p = 0.046$) as compared to baseline. Statistically significant difference was observed only in TJC (p = 0.01) 3 months after the vaccination (T3). Additionally, vaccinated patients showed a significant increase in TJC ($p = 0.004$), ESR ($p = 0.007$), Health Assessment Questionnaire ($p = 0.023$), patient global assessment ($p = 0.013$) and physician global assessment ($p = 0.026$) when compared to nonvaccinated patients ($n = 25$) at T1. At T3, similar findings were observed for only ESR ($p = 0.006$) and physician global assessment ($p = 0.013$) when data were analyzed between two groups. In conclusion, the authors suggested that influenza vaccine may have a short lasting triggering effect on psoriatic arthritis patients [42].

3.5. Adenovirus vaccination

In a retrospective study, which evaluated the possible side effects related to adenovirus types 4 and 7 in military recruits, psoriasis (21 versus 7 cases) was found more frequently (RR = 2.44, 95% CI = 1.13–5.31) in the vaccinated group ($n = 100,000$) when compared to unvaccinated group ($n = 100,000$) [43].

4. Therapeutic effects of vaccines on psoriasis

Both conventional systemic treatments and biologic agents are related to serious side effects. The biologic immunotherapy agents act by inhibiting over-expressed T-cell activity by reducing T-cell numbers, T-cell trafficking or immune deviation and blocking the activities of proinflammatory cytokines, which may lead to severe infections, myelodegenerative and autoimmune disorders [29]. Additionally, over the past few years, various John Cunningham virus (JCV) associated brain syndromes have been reported as a result of increased usage of the immunomodulatory medications [44]. The progression in the enlightenment of the immunopathogenesis of psoriasis may provide new therapeutic options that do not have immunosuppressive side effects. Vaccination is a progressing therapy option for psoriasis and the other chronic inflammatory disorders such as multiple sclerosis, rheumatoid arthritis and atherosclerosis, which are termed as noncommunicable diseases [1, 45, 46]. It has clearly demonstrated that vaccines have the ability to activate effectors such as dendritic cells and T lymphocytes, which are also involved in psoriasis pathogenesis [41]. Noncommunicable disease vaccines target cells, proteins or other molecules that are related to these disorders and modulate the immune system, similar to traditional vaccines [45].

Approximately two-thirds of guttate psoriasis patients and a quarter of chronic psoriasis patients have an association with streptococcal throat infections. Fry et al. claimed that vaccination against Streptococcus pyogenes as well as the other possible microorganisms that trigger psoriasis may be a new way to prevent psoriasis [3, 4]. It has also been suggested that psoriasis may benefit from development of a T-cell receptor peptide vaccine [47].

As we mentioned before, IL-17 has been shown to play an important role as a proinflammatory cytokine in psoriasis. IL-17 is demonstrated as a 'target antigen' for the treatment of autoimmune disorders and psoriasis in preclinical experiments in animal models and in clinical trials [48]. Dallenbach et al. showed that immunization with Qβ-IL-17, a virus-like particle-based vaccine, generated IL-17-specific IgG in mice. In order to evaluate the role of hypermutation and affinity maturation, they mutated the hypermutated antibody back to germline sequence, producing a set of two antibodies with VH regions differing in three aminoacids, but recognizing the same epitope. They showed that both the hypermutated and the germline antibody significantly neutralized IL-17 and blocked its biological activity *in vivo*. They also demonstrated that both antibodies were able to reduce imiquimod-induced psoriatic skin inflammation, indicating that vaccination against IL-17 may be a new therapeutic option for psoriasis [49].

Over-expression of ß-defensin 2, known as a skin antimicrobial peptide, has been reported to be associated with psoriasis [50]. In a recent study, serum ß-defensin 2 levels have been found to correlate with IL-17A levels and psoriasis area severity index (PASI) scores in psoriatic patients [51]. Additionally, García-Valtanen et al. demonstrated that ß-defensin 2 improves the DNA vaccine efficacy due to its adjuvant-like effects besides its antiviral and immunomodulatory properties in a study of zebrafish. They claimed that this psoriasis-related peptide might be used as an adjuvant in DNA vaccination to improve the efficacy of viral vaccines [50].

The TNF-alpha-induced protein 3 (TNFAIP3) is an anti-inflammatory factor that inhibits NF-κB activation in T-cells. In a few studies, it was reported that expression of TNFAIP3 mRNA was significantly higher in patients with mild psoriasis than in the patients with severe psoriasis, suggesting that TNFAIP3 gene may be a 'target' molecule for psoriasis therapy [52, 53]. There are also reported studies, which are mentioned below, about the usage of vaccines on psoriasis.

4.1. Mycobacterium vaccae

Mycobacterium vaccae, a nonpathogenic organism usually applied as a heat-killed suspension, has been used as an adjunct immunotherapy for tuberculosis and leprosy [54]. The immunotherapy trials began after discovery of the therapeutic effect of *M. vaccae* injection in psoriasis skin lesions of leprosy patients with concomitant psoriasis [55].

A placebo-controlled study in patients with chronic plaque psoriasis evaluated the potential beneficial effects of *M. vaccae* immunotherapy. The study group of 31 patients received a dose of *M. vaccae*, and placebo group of 24 patients were given a dose of tetanus toxoid. The mean PASI values at both 3 and 6 months for the *M. vaccae* group were significantly lower than their entry values ($p < 0.001$ and $p < 0.005$), while the tetanus toxoid group did not reach this significance at any time. The failure of the patients to return for follow-up visits and the selection of tetanus toxoid as a placebo were the problems of the study. In spite of these limitations, the authors claimed that the study showed a significant improvement ($p < 0.005$) in the PASI after a single injection of *M. vaccae* [56]. A subsequent study of 24 patients, PASI scores of whom showed significant reduction ($p < 0.001$) at 12 and 24 weeks in comparison with the initial PASI score after two intradermal inoculations of *M. vaccae*, confirmed these findings [56].

A study performed on 36 patients with psoriatic arthritis randomized the patients to receive two intradermal injections of 50 μg delipidated, deglycolipidated *M. vaccae* (PVAC) or placebo and followed up them for 24 weeks. The psoriatic arthritis response criteria at either 12 or 24 weeks were achieved by 50% (9/18) in both placebo and PVAC group. There was only a significant change in the visual analogue scale over time between the two groups. The mean score had decreased by 19.2 mm in the PVAC group and increased by 4.8 mm in the placebo group ($p = 0.006$). Consequently, the authors claimed that PVAC was not an effective immunotherapy for psoriatic arthritis [57]. Likewise, a placebo-controlled study did not show a clearly efficacy of PVAC in the treatment of psoriasis patients, because 75% PASI was similar among the studied groups at week 12 [55].

Mycobacterium w is a nonpathogenic, rapidly growing, cultivable strain of atypical mycobacteria and has been used as an adjuvant immunotherapy for leprosy, tuberculosis and human immunodeficiency virus, like *M. vaccae* [58]. The efficacy of Mycobacterium w in psoriasis was also evaluated by some trials [58, 59]. In a study of 36 psoriasis patients, 24 of them were in the study group and received two doses of 0.1 ml of heat-killed Mycobacterium w at 3 weekly intervals. The remaining 12 patients in the control group were given of normal saline at the same weeks. The study showed marked improvement (>50% reduction in PASI score) in the four of 24 cases (16.6%) and moderate improvement (25–50% reduction) in 15 cases (62.5%) at the end of the 4 months. No improvement was seen in the 4 of 24 patients, and the disease got worse in 1 patient. There were no significant side effects, although five patients had new lesions at the site of injection [59]. On the other hand, in another study that included 45 psoriasis patients who received a total of four doses of Mycobacterium w, the percentage reduction of PASI score was only 33% at the end of 12 weeks. Additionally, at the beginning of the study, PASI scores showed increase in nine patients, four of whom were severe and received an alternative therapy [58]. The results were in contrast to findings of the prior study by Rath et al. [58, 59].

The mechanism of mycobacterium immunotherapy leads to improvement in psoriasis is not known exactly. Lehrer et al. suggested that the decreasing effect of TNF-alpha might cause clinical improvement in psoriasis patients treated with *M. vaccae* immunotherapy [56]. According to Dalbeth et al., increased IL-10 levels after the PVAC injection may lead to improvement in psoriasis due to inhibition of T-cell function and reduction of IFN-gamma and TNF-alpha production [57].

4.2. Leishmania amastigotes

In a trial about a vaccine for cutaneous leishmaniasis, O'Daly et al. observed 100% clinical remission of a psoriatic lesion in one patient after third vaccination. After this discovery, they performed an open-label, single-center study to evaluate the leishmaniasis vaccine (AS100®) in 2770 psoriasis patients. When baseline PASI values were compared with the post-treatment values, PASI 100 was achieved in 23%, PASI 75 in 45%, PASI 50 in 13%, PASI 10 in 9% and <PASI 10 was determined in 3% of patients. The most common adverse effects were pain and nodule formation, which were injection side related. The other systemic adverse effects were considered as mild and moderate in severity. Similar results were observed in a second, double-blind, placebo-controlled study, performed by the same group [60]. In a subsequent study, O'Daly et al. evaluated further purified vaccines, resulting in seven chromatography fractions per four Leishmania species. They suggested that three fractions from *L. brasiliensis* and four fractions from *L. chagasi* demonstrated the maximal therapeutic effect on psoriasis [61]. O'Daly et al. also revealed that regarding to PASI values, certain lymphocyte subtypes decreased in peripheral blood cells suggesting migration from the blood to the skin while others increased suggesting activation by unknown antigens. After injection seven doses of AS100 vaccine, lymphocyte subtypes CD3+CD8−, CD8+CD3−, HLA+CD8−, CD8+HLA+ and CD4+CD8− increased as PASI values decreased and clinical improvement was seen, while CD8+CD3+, CD8+HLA−, CD19 and CD8+CD4+ decreased in peripheral blood cells. These results suggested that treatment with Leishmania antigens leads lymphocytes to traffic between blood and skin and activates T-cells in skin plaques, contrary to current treatments killing T-cells in psoriasis patients [62]. Another open-label, single-center study conducted by O'Daly et al. showed clinical remission in patients with psoriatic arthritis after the average number of 9.9 ± 4.8 doses of AS100 treatment [63].

4.3. Live attenuated varicella vaccine

A placebo-controlled study was conducted by El-Darouti et al. to evaluate the adjuvant effect of live attenuated varicella vaccine (Varilrix®) in patients with resistant severe psoriasis after their observation of improvement in one patient with severe psoriasis following a chickenpox infection. Study group received four doses of Varilrix® once every 3 weeks before low-dose cyclosporine (2.5 mg/kg/day) while control group received four doses of subcutaneous saline as placebo. Study group demonstrated significantly higher improvement in their PASI values. According to El-Darouti et al., the hypotheses explaining the mechanism of live attenuated varicella vaccine on psoriasis are given as below [64]:

- The stimulating effect of varicella zoster virus on the humoral response by Th-2 cells and subsequent downregulation of the Th-1 response,
- The inhibitory effect of IFN-alpha on Th-17 cells by peripheral blood cells exposed to varicella zoster virus antigen,
- The upregulation of regulatory T-cells that have inhibitory effects on psoriasis after receiving varicella vaccine.

Subsequently, El-Darouti et al. reported that live attenuated varicella vaccine is effective in psoriasis when used with low-dose cyclosporine by acting possibly on the Th17/ regulatory T-cells balance [65].

http://dx.doi.org/10.5772/67691

5. Conclusion

Vaccination is an effective tool for reducing the incidence of serious or life-threatening infectious disease [45]. Patients diagnosed with psoriasis are at risk of infections due to the nature of disease and immunosuppressive therapies [12, 14]. For this reason, the medical board of the National Psoriasis Foundation recommends vaccination for patients diagnosed with psoriasis in compliance with recommendations of the Advisory Committee for Immunization Practices [12]. Besides, vaccines such as *M. vaccae*, live attenuated varicella zoster virus and Leishmania amastigotes have been reported to be effective in the treatment of psoriasis. Vaccines, regulating the inflammatory response in psoriasis, may be a new therapeutic option for psoriasis patients without any serious side effects. On the other hand, the data emphasize that especially some types of vaccines may trigger an exacerbation of psoriatic skin lesions. The very low incidence of psoriasis following vaccination reveals the safe profile but some authors recommend the follow-up of such individuals [13]. Further large-sized and controlled clinical research studies need to be carried out to confirm the relationships between psoriasis and the vaccination.

Author details

Sevgi Akarsu[1]* and Ceylan Avcı[2]

*Address all correspondence to: sevgi.akarsu@deu.edu.tr

1 Department of Dermatology, Faculty of Medicine, Dokuz Eylul University, Izmir, Turkey

2 Department of Dermatology, Bilecik State Hospital, Bilecik, Turkey

References

[1] Kaffenberger BH, Lee GL, Tyler K, Chan DV, Jarjour W, Ariza ME, et al. Current and potential immune therapies and vaccines in the management of psoriasis. Human Vaccines & Immunotherapeutics. 2014;**10**(4):876–86. doi:10.4161/hv.27532

[2] Alexander H, Nestle FO. Pathogenesis and immunotherapy in cutaneous psoriasis: what can rheumatologists learn? Current Opinion in Rheumatology. 2017;**29**(1):71–8. doi:10.1097/BOR.0000000000000358

[3] Fry L, Baker BS, Powles AV. Psoriasis—a possible candidate for vaccination. Clinical & Developmental Immunology. 2006;**13**(2–4):361–7. doi:10.1080/17402520600800861

[4] Fry L, Baker BS, Powles AV. Psoriasis—a possible for vaccination. Autoimmunity Reviews. 2007;**6**(5):286–9. doi:10.1016/j.autrev.2006.09.007

[5] Valdimarsson H, Thorleifsdottir RH, Sigurdardottir SL, Gudjonsson JE, Johnston A. Psoriasis—as an autoimmune disease caused by molecular mimicry. Trends in Immunology. 2009;**30**(10):494–501. doi:10.1016/j.it.2009.07.008

[6] Eberle FC, Brück J, Holstein J, Hirahara K, Ghoreschi K. Recent advances in understanding psoriasis. F1000Research. 2016;**5**:1–9. doi:10.12688/f1000research.7927.1

[7] Haniffa M, Gunawan M, Jardine L. Human skin dendritic cells in health and disease. Journal of Dermatological Science. 2017;**77**(2):85–92. doi:10.1016/j.jdermsci.2014.08.012

[8] Strzępa A, Szczepanik M. IL-17-expressing cells as a potential therapeutic target for treatment of immunological disorders. Pharmacological Reports: PR. 2011;**63**(1):30–44.

[9] Samarasekera EJ, Sawyer L, Wonderling D, Tucker R, Smith CH. Topical therapies for the treatment of plaque psoriasis: systematic review and network meta-analyses. British Journal of Dermatology. 2013;**168**(5):954–67. doi:10.1111/bjd.12276

[10] Wong T, Hsu L, Liao W. Phototherapy in psoriasis: a review of mechanisms of action. Journal of Cutaneous Medicine Surgery. 2013;**17**(1):6–12.

[11] Nast A, Gisondi P, Ormerod AD, Saiag P, Smith C, Spuls PI, et al. European S3-Guidelines on the systemic treatment of psoriasis vulgaris--Update 2015 – Short version – EDF in cooperation with EADV and IPC. Journal of European Academy of Dermatology and Venereology. 2015;**29**(12):2277–94. doi:10.1111/jdv.13354

[12] Wine-Lee L, Keller SC, Wilck MB, Gluckman SJ, Van Voorhees AS. From the Medical Board of the National Psoriasis Foundation: Vaccination in adult patients on systemic therapy for psoriasis. Journal of American Academy of Dermatology. 2013;**69**(6):1003–13. doi:10.1016/j.jaad.2013.06.046

[13] Gunes AT, Fetil E, Akarsu S, Ozbagcivan O, Babayeva L. Possible triggering effect of influenza vaccination on psoriasis. Journal of Immunology Research. 2015;**2015**(2015):ID 258430. doi:10.1155/2015/258430

[14] Rahier JF, Moutschen M, Van Gompel A, Van Ranst M, Louis E, Segaert S, et al. Vaccinations in patients with immune-mediated inflammatory diseases. Rheumatology (Oxford, England). 2010;**49**(10):1815–27. doi:10.1093/rheumatology/keq183

[15] Stuhec M. Yellow fever vaccine used in a psoriatic arthritis patient treated with methotrexate: a case report. Acta Dermatovenerologica Alpina Pannonica, et Adriatica. 2014;**23**(3):63–4. doi:10.15570/actaapa.2014.15

[16] Lebwohl M, Bagel J, Gelfand JM, Gladman D, Gordon KB, Hsu S, et al. From the Medical Board of the National Psoriasis Foundation: monitoring and vaccinations in patients treated with biologics for psoriasis. Journal of the American Academy of Dermatology. 2008;**58**(1):94–105. doi:10.1016/j.jaad.2007.08.030

[17] Kapetanovic MC, Roseman C, Jönsson G, Truedsson L, Saxne T, Geborek P, et al. Antibody response is reduced following vaccination with 7-valent conjugate pneumococcal vaccine in adult methotrexate-treated patients with established arthritis, but not those treated with tumor necrosis factor inhibitors. Arthritis and Rheumatism. 2011;**63**(12):3723–32. doi:10.1002/art.30580

[18] Brodmerkel C, Wadman E, Langley RG, Papp KA, Bourcier M, Poulin Y, et al. Immune response to pneumococcus and tetanus toxoid in patients with moderate-to-severe psoriasis following long-term ustekinumab use. Journal of Drugs in Dermatology. 2013;**12**(10):1122–9.

[19] Marmon S, Strober BE. Balancing immunity and immunosuppression: vaccinating patients receiving treatment with efalizumab. The Journal of Investigative Dermatology. 2008;**128**(11):2567–9. doi:10.1038/jid.2008.291

[20] Lynde C, Krell J, Korman N, Mathes B; Vaccine Study Investigators. Immune response to pneumococcal polysaccharide vaccine in adults with chronic plaque psoriasis treated with alefacept. Journal of American Academy of Dermatology. 2011;**65**(4):799–806. doi:10.1016/j.jaad.2010.04.040

[21] Polachek A, Korobko U, Mader-Balakirski N, Arad U, Levartovsky D, Kaufman I, et al. Immunogenecity and safety of vaccination against seasonal 2012 influenza virus among patients with psoriatic arthritis and psoriasis. Clinical and Experimental Rheumatology. 2015;**33**(2):181–6.

[22] Radtke MA, Rustenbach SJ, Reusch M, Strömer K, Augustin M. Influenza vaccination rate among patients with moderate to severe psoriasis. Journal of the German Society of Dermatology. 2013;**11**(9):837–44. doi:10.1111/ddg.12010

[23] Sbidian E, Tubach F, Pasquet B, Paul C, Jullien D, Sid-Mohand D, et al. Factors associated with 2009 monovalent H1N1 vaccine coverage: a cross sectional study of 1,308 patients with psoriasis in France. Vaccine. 2012;**30**(39):5701–7. doi:10.1016/j.vaccine.2012.07.014

[24] Shalom G, Zisman D, Bitterman H, Harman-Boehm I, Greenberg-Dotan S, Dreiher J, et al. Systemic therapy for psoriasis and the risk of herpes zoster: A 500,000 Person-year Study. JAMA. 2015;**151**(5):533–8. doi:10.1001/jamadermatol.2014.4956

[25] Zhang J, Delzell E, Xie F, Baddley JW, Spettell C, McMahan RM, et al. The use, safety, and effectiveness of herpes zoster vaccination in individuals with inflammatory and autoimmune diseases: a longitudinal observational study. Arthritis Research & Therapy. 2011;**13**(5):R174. doi:10.1186/ar3497

[26] Zhang J, Xie F, Delzell E, Chen L, Winthrop KL, Lewis JD, et al. Association between vaccination for herpes zoster and risk of herpes zoster infection among older patients with selected immune-mediated diseases. JAMA. 2012;**308**(1):43–9. doi:10.1001/jama.2012.7304

[27] Adelzadeh L, Jourabchi N, Wu JJ. The risk of herpes zoster during biological therapy for psoriasis and other inflammatory conditions. Journal of the European Academy of Dermatology and Venereology. 2014;**28**(7):846–52. doi:10.1111/jdv.12307

[28] Yun H, Yang S, Chen L, Xie F, Winthrop K, Baddley JW et al. Risk of herpes zoster in autoimmune and inflammatory diseases: implications for vaccination. Arthritis & Rheumatolgy. 2016;**68**(9):2328–37. doi:10.1002/art.39670

[29] Burgdorf WHC, Plewig G, Wolf HH, Landthaler M, editors. Braun-Falco's Dermatology. 4th ed. Heidenberg: Springer; 2009. 506–526 p.

[30] Dogan B, Harmanyeri Y. Intradermal antigen tests and the Koebner phenomenon in psoriasis. International Journal of Dermatology. 1997;**36**(4):263–5.

[31] Leroux-Roels G, Van Damme P, Haazen W, Shakib S, Caubet M, Aris E, et al. Phase I, randomized, observer-blind, placebo-controlled studies to evaluate the safety, reactogenicity and immunogenicity of an investigational non-typeable Haemophilus influenzae (NTHi) protein vaccine in adults. Vaccine. 2016;**34**(27):3156–63. doi:10.1016/j.vaccine.2016.04.051

[32] Wee JS, Natkunarajah J, Moosa Y, Marsden RA. Erythrodermic pustular psoriasis triggered by intravesical bacillus Calmette-Guérin immunotherapy. Clinical and Experimental Dermatology. 2012;**37**(4):455–7. doi:10.1111/j.1365-2230.2011.04183.x

[33] Raaschou-Nielsen W. Psoriasis vaccinalis; report of two cases, one following B.C.G. vaccination and one following vaccination against influenza. Acta Dermato-Venereologica. 1955;**35**(1):37–42.

[34] Queiro R, Ballina J, Weruaga A, Fernández JA, Riestra JL, Torre JC, et al. Psoriatic arthropathy after BCG immunotherapy for bladder carcinoma. British Journal of Rheumatology. 1995;**34**(11):1097.

[35] Koca R, Altinyazar HC, Numanoğlu G, Unalacak M. Guttate psoriasis-like lesions following BCG vaccination. Journal of Tropical Pediatrics. 2004;**50**(3):178–9.

[36] Takayama K, Satoh T, Hayashi M, Yokozeki H. Psoriatic skin lesions induced by BCG vaccination. Acta Derm-Venereologica. 2008;**88**(6):621–2. doi:10.2340/00015555-0496

[37] Macias VC, Cunha D. Psoriasis triggered by tetanus-diphtheria vaccination. Cutaneous and Ocular Toxicology. 2013;**32**(2):164–5. doi:10.3109/15569527.2012.727936

[38] Bettelli E, Carrier Y, Gao W, Korn T, Strom TB, Oukka M et al. Reciprocal developmental pathways for the generation of pathogenic effector TH17 and regulatory T cells. Nature. 2006;**441**(7090):235–8. doi:10.1038/nature04753

[39] Pattison E, Harrison BJ, Griffiths CE, Silman AJ, Bruce IN. Environmental risk factors for the development of psoriatic arthritis: results from a case-control study. Annals of Rheumatic Diseases. 2008;**67**(5):672–6. doi:10.1136/ard.2007.073932

[40] Shin MS, Kim SJ, Kim SH, Kwak YG, Park HJ. New onset Guttate psoriasis following pandemic H1N1 influenza vaccination. Annals of Dermatology. 2013;**25**(4):489–92. doi:10.5021/ad.2013.25.4.489

[41] Sbidian E, Eftekahri P, Viguier M, Laroche L, Chosidow O, Gosselin P, et al. National survey of psoriasis flares after 2009 monovalent H1N1/seasonal vaccines. Dermatology (Basel, Switzerland). 2014;**229**(2):130–5. doi:10.1159/000362808

[42] Caso F, Ramonda R, Del Puente A, Darda MA, Cantarini L, Peluso R, et al. Influenza vaccine with adjuvant on disease activity in psoriatic arthritis patients under anti-TNF-α therapy. Clinical and Experimental Rheumatology. 2016;**34**(3):507–12.

[43] Choudhry A, Mathena J, Albano JD, Yacovone M, Collins L. Safety evaluation of adenovirus type 4 and type 7 vaccine live, oral in military recruits. Vaccine. 2016;**34**(38):4558–64. doi:10.1016/j.vaccine.2016.07.033

[44] Miskin DP, Koralnik IJ. Novel syndromes associated with JC virus infection of neurons and meningeal cells: no longer a gray area. Current Opinion in Neurology. 2015;**28**(3):288–94. doi:10.1097/WCO.0000000000000201

[45] Darrow JJ, Kesselheim AS. A new wave of vaccines for non-communicable diseases: what are the regulatory challenges? Food Drug Law Journal. 2015;**70**(2):243–58.

[46] García-González V, Delgado-Coello B, Pérez-Torres A, Mas-Oliva J. Reality of a vaccine in the prevention and treatment of atherosclerosis. Archives of Medical Research. 2015;**46**(5):427–37. doi:10.1016/j.arcmed.2015.06.004

[47] Medi BM, Singh J. Prospects for vaccines for allergic and other immunologic skin disorders. American Journal of Clinical Dermatology. 2006;**7**(3):145–53.

[48] Foerster J, Bachman M. Beyond passive immunization: toward a nanoparticle-based IL-17 vaccine as first in class of future immune treatments. Nanomedicine (London, England). 2015;**10**(8):1361–9. doi:10.2217/nnm.14.215

[49] Dallenbach K, Maurer P, Röhn T, Zabel F, Kopf M, Bachmann MF. Protective effect of a germline, IL-17-neutralizing antibody in murine models of autoimmune inflammatory disease. European Journal of Immunology. 2015;**45**(4):1238–47. doi:10.1002/eji.201445017

[50] García-Valtanen P, Martinez-Lopez A, Ortega-Villaizan M, Perez L, Coll JM, Estepa A. In addition to its antiviral and immunomodulatory properties, the zebrafish ß-defensin 2 (zfBD2) is a potent viral DNA vaccine molecular adjuvant. Antiviral Research. 2014;**101**:136–47. doi:10.1016/j.antiviral.2013.11.009

[51] Kolbinger F, Loesche C, Valentin MA, Jiang X, Cheng Y, Jarvis P, et al. ß-Defensin 2 is a responsive biomarker of IL-17A-driven skin pathology in patients with psoriasis. The Journal of Allergy and Clinical Immunology. Forthcoming. doi:10.1016/j.jaci.2016.06.038

[52] Jiang X, Tian H, Fan Y, Chen J, Song Y, Wang S, et al. Expression of tumor necrosis factor alpha-induced protein 3 mRNA in peripheral blood mononuclear cells negatively correlates with disease severity in psoriasis vulgaris. Clinical and Vaccine Immunology. 2012;**19**(12):1938–42. doi:10.1128/CVI.00500-12

[53] Zhang X, Xia P, Zhang L, Zhang Z. Upregulation of tumor necrosis factor alpha-induced protein 3 mRNA in mildpsoriasis vulgaris. Clinical and Vaccine Immunology. 2013;**20**(8):1341. doi:10.1128/CVI.00267-13

[54] Balagon MV, Tan PL, Prestidge R, Cellona RV, Abalos RM, Tan EV, et al. Improvement in psoriasis after intradermal administration of delipidated, deglycolipidated *Mycobacterium vaccae* (PVAC): results of an open-label trial. Clinical and Experimental Dermatology. 2001;**26**(3):233–41. doi:10.1046/j.1365–2230.2001.00804.x

[55] Netto EM, Takahashi D, de Fátima Paim de Oliveira M, Barbosa P, Ferraz N, Paixão A, et al. Phase II randomized, placebo-controlled trial of M. vaccae-derived protein (PVAC) for the treatment of psoriasis. Vaccine. 2006;**24**(23):5056–63. doi:10.1016/j.vaccine.2006.03.047

[56] Lehrer A, Bressanelli A, Wachsmann V, Bottasso O, Bay ML, Singh M, et al. Immunotherapy with *Mycobacterium vaccae* in the treatment of psoriasis. FEMS Immunology and Medical Microbiology. 1998;**21**(1):71–7. doi:10.1111/j.1574-695X.1998.tb01151.x

[57] Dalbeth N, Yeoman S, Dockerty JL, Highton J, Robinson E, Tan PL, et al. A randomised placebo controlled trial of delipidated, deglycolipidated *Mycobacterium vaccae* as immunotherapy for psoriatic arthritis. Annals of Rheumatic Diseases. 2004;**63**(6):718–22. doi:10.1136/ard.2003.007104

[58] Kumar B, Sandhu K, Kaur I. Role of Mycobacterium w vaccine in the management of psoriasis. The British Journal of Dermatolgy. 2005;**152**(2):380–2. doi:10.1111/j.1365-2133.2005.06343.x

[59] Rath N, Kar HK. Efficacy of intradermal heat-killed Mycobacterium w in psoriasis: a pilot study. International Journal of Dermatology. 2003;**42**(9):756–7.

[60] O'Daly JA, Lezama R, Rodriguez PJ, Silva E, Indriago NR, Peña G, et al. Antigens from Leishmania amastigotes induced clinical remission of psoriasis. Archieves of Dermatological Research. 2009;**301**(1):1–13. doi:10.1007/s00403-008-0883-9

[61] O'Daly JA, Lezama R, Gleason J. Isolation of Leishmania amastigote protein fractions which induced lymphocyte stimulation and remission of psoriasis. Archieves of Dermatological Research. 2009;**301**(6):411–27. doi:10.1007/s00403-009-0940-z

[62] O'Daly JA, Rodriguez B, Ovalles T, Pelaez C. Lymphocyte subsets in peripheral blood of patients with psoriasis before and after treatment with leishmania antigens. Archieves of Dermatological Research. 2010;**302**(2):95–104. doi:10.1007/s00403-009-0992-0

[63] O'Daly JA, Gleason J, Lezama R, Rodriguez PJ, Silva E, Indriago NR. Antigens from Leishmania amastigotes inducing clinical remission of psoriatic arthritis. Archieves of Dermatological Research. 2011;**303**(6):399–415. doi:10.1007/s00403-011-1133-0

[64] El-Darouti MA, Hegazy RA, Abdel Hay RM, Abdel Halim DM. Live attenuated varicella vaccine: a new effective adjuvant weapon in the battlefield against severe resistant psoriasis, a pilot randomized controlled trial. Journal of the American Academy of Dermatology. 2012;**66**(3):511–3. doi:10.1016/j.jaad.2011.07.032

[65] El-Darouti MA, Hegazy RA, Abdel Hay RM, Rashed LA. Study of T helper (17) and T regulatory cells in psoriatic patients receiving live attenuated varicella vaccine therapy in a randomized controlled trial. European Journal of Dermatology. 2014;**24**(4):464–9. doi:10.1684/ejd.2014.2377

Chapter 3

Pathogenic Role of Cytokines and Effect of Their Inhibition in Psoriasis

Jitlada Meephansan, Urairack Subpayasarn,
Mayumi Komine and Mamitaro Ohtsuki

Additional information is available at the end of the chapter

http://dx.doi.org/10.5772/intechopen.68421

Abstract

The pathogenesis of psoriasis is complex, and cytokines play an important role in mediating cell-cell interactions that result in abnormal structures and functions of many cell types in psoriasis, such as abnormal proliferation and differentiation of keratinocytes, abnormal proliferation of blood vessels, stimulation of immune cells, and driving abnormal immune reactions. In this chapter, we summarize the roles and functions of inflammatory cytokines that play a crucial role in psoriasis such as tumor necrosis factor (TNF)-α, interleukin (IL)-12/IL-23, and IL-17, as well as their inhibitors that are used to treat psoriasis.

Keywords: psoriasis, inflammation, cytokine, biologic drugs, pathogenesis

1. Introduction

Psoriasis is a common chronic inflammatory disease characterized by abnormal proliferation of keratinocytes, increased dermal vascularity, and multiple inflammatory cell infiltration. It is an immune-mediated skin disease influenced by genetic and epigenetic variations, which can be triggered by environmental factors. Psoriasis affects approximately 2% of people worldwide [1, 2].

Psoriasis typically presents as indurated scaly erythematous plaques and is easily diagnosed; however, variable clinical manifestations may be presented. As a result, psoriasis remains a clinical diagnosis defined by morphologic findings and appearances. The major clinical manifestations include characteristic cutaneous lesions, including whitish scaly erythematous plaques and/or pustular or guttate lesions. There are several clinical forms of psoriasis, including plaque psoriasis, psoriasis guttate, psoriasis arthropathica, pustular psoriasis, psoriasis erythroderma, and inverse psoriasis. The most common type of psoriasis is psoriasis vulgaris, which accounts for 85–90% of all cases [1, 3].

Histologically, psoriasis is characterized by hyperproliferation and abnormal differentiation of keratinocytes; dilated, hyperplastic blood vessels; and inflammatory infiltration of lymphocytes mainly into the dermis. The skin patches are typically erythematous and scaly, which, in addition to the physical appearance, may result in psychological stress and poor quality of life. Like other systemic inflammatory diseases, psoriasis affects far more organs than the skin and often presents with chronic inflammatory responses in joints, nails, and other organs.

Immunological dysfunction in psoriasis involves cross talk between immune cells and non-immune cells with cytokines. Several important types of immune cells in psoriasis have been found to play a role in pathogenesis, including Th1, Th17, and regulatory T cells. Corresponding cytokines that may be involved include interferon (IFN)-γ, tumor necrosis factor (TNF)-α, interleukin (IL)-23, and IL-17. More recently, IL-9-secreting Th9 cells have been identified, and the inflammatory responses of keratinocytes, $\gamma\delta$T cells, T regulatory cells, and other cell types in psoriasis have been explored. Emerging evidence indicates that new genetic variations and epigenetic modifications are associated with psoriatic disease [4, 5].

2. Immunological changes in psoriasis

Psoriasis is characterized by keratinocyte hyperproliferation and the abnormal infiltration of effector T cells, dendritic cells, neutrophils, and macrophages [6]. The effect of multiple cell types involved in psoriasis is mediated by a complex network of cytokines and their interactions.

3. Role of inflammatory cytokines in psoriasis

3.1. Interferons (IFN)

Type I interferons (IFNs), IFN-α and IFN-β, can suppress viral replication and stimulate immune reactions in response to viral infections; thus, they are potential mediators of antiviral host defense. Activated plasmacytoid dendritic cells (pDCs) preferentially produce type I IFNs following interactions between intracellular TLR7 and TLR9 with viral RNA and DNA [7, 8]. Type I IFN-α and IFN-β are not expressed in the normal skin but are produced in virally infected skin where pDCs are present, as well as in skin wounds where mechanical injury stimulates infiltration of pDCs and in lesional psoriatic skin where pDC-derived type I IFNs are sustained [9]. This stimulates myeloid DC phenotypic maturation and activation, enabling T-cell priming. Several studies have demonstrated that these cytokines are most relevant in the early phase of psoriasis, as demonstrated by the IFN-α signature in primary psoriatic plaques. Albanesi et al. [10] found that pDC infiltration in psoriatic skin correlates with the expression of markers typical of early stage of disease, whereas it is notably absent in chronic lesions. In this regard, blocking of type I IFN signaling may prevent the upregulation of T cells and development of non-lesional to lesional skin [9]. For downstream inflammatory pathways, type I IFNs modulate the production of IFN-γ and IL-17 and are involved in the differentiation and activation of T cells, particularly Th1 and Th17 cells [11] (**Figure 1**).

Th1 cells are a potential source of IFN-γ, a type II interferon. Previously, the Th1 pathway was proposed to be the predominant pathogenic path for psoriasis [12]. Th1 cells, producing IFN-γ, are increased in the psoriatic lesional skin and peripheral blood and can be decreased by effective therapy. However, the potential role of IFN-γ became less important after the identification of a new key cytokine, Th17-producing IL-17 [13]. Selective blockage of IL-23-induced IL-17 leads to full recovery of psoriasis based on clinical, histological, and molecular markers [14].

IFN-γ acts on psoriatic keratinocytes and endothelial cells, leading to the activation and production of antimicrobial peptides (e.g., LL-37 cathelicidin and β-defensins). IFN-γ induces the cross phosphorylation of Janus kinase 1 (JAK1) and JAK3, resulting in the downstream activation of STAT3. Subsequent activation of STAT transcription factors is important for cell growth and is efficient for regulating many genes expressed in psoriatic lesions [15]. IFN-γ promotes the release of cytokines (IL-23, IL-1) and chemokines (CXCL10, CXCL11), as well as the expression of adhesion molecules from DCs, T cells, keratinocytes, and endothelial cells [16], thus promoting the recruitment of inflammatory cells to lesional plaques. Studies suggest that IFN-γ can be used as a biomarker for determining psoriasis severity and therapy evaluation because of the positive correlation between serum IFN-γ levels and PASI scores [17].

However, direct blockage of IFN-γ with a neutralizing antibody in patients with psoriasis was shown to have little or no therapeutic effect, indicating that IFN-γ does not directly participate the psoriasis phenotype [18]. It has been suggested that the IL-12/IFN-γ axis acts to suppress IL-17-modulated tissue injury [19, 20]. Consequently, continued expression of the IL-12/IFN-γ axis in disease while Th17 circuits are inhibited through IL-23 or IL-17 blockage may lead to better suppression and improvement of psoriasis [5].

3.2. TNF-α

TNF-α is involved in many inflammatory cutaneous diseases, including psoriasis. Several different cells can produce TNF-α in the context of skin inflammation, including keratinocytes, macrophages, T cells (Th1, Th17, and Th22 cells), and psoriatic DCs (particularly TIP-DCs) [5, 21, 22]. Several studies showed that circulating levels of TNF-α (in addition to IFN-γ and IL-12) are elevated in psoriasis patients and correlate with severity of disease [23, 24], although different studies have shown varying results [25].

The key effects of TNF-α are regulating the antigen-presenting ability of DCs and stimulation of T-cell infiltration. It has a variety of effects because there are two types of TNF receptors (TNFR), TNFR1 and TNFR2. TNFR1 is expressed on nearly all cell types, whereas TNFR2 is present predominantly on endothelial cells and hematopoietic cells. TNF-α acts in part

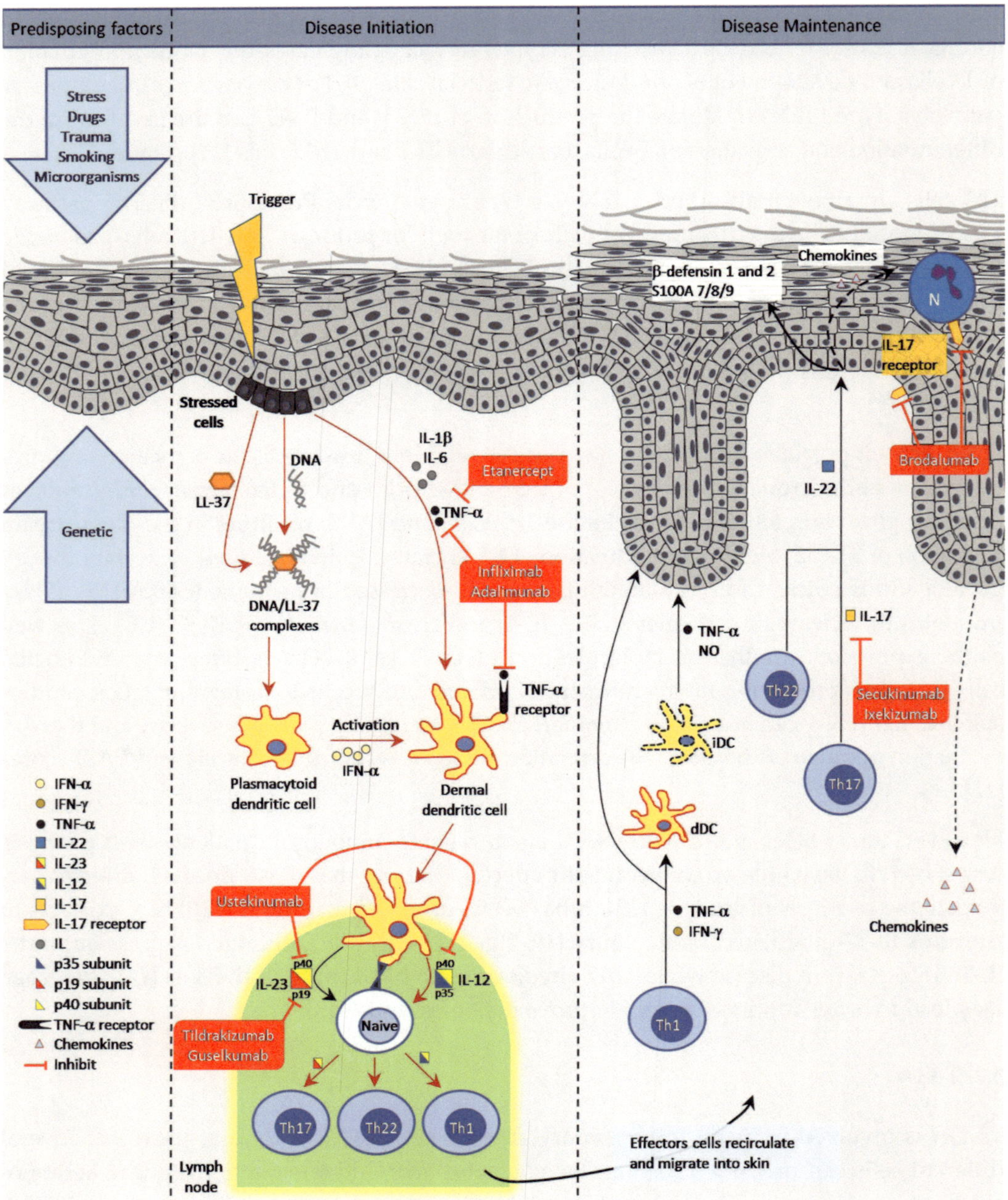

Figure 1. The scheme of cytokine involvement in the pathogenesis of psoriasis and the mechanism of action of biologics.

by increasing the elevated level of active, phosphorylated NF-κB, a crucial transcription factor involved in psoriatic pathogenesis [26]. TNF-α possesses proinflammatory properties; it activates the expression of C-reactive protein (which is a part of the acute phase response) and several cytokines such as IL-6 (which induces keratinocyte hyperproliferation and T-cell proliferation) and IL-23 (which is a potential mediator synthesized from DCs in psoriasis to stimulate IL-17 production). TNF-α also induces several chemokines including CXCL8/IL-8 (which recruits neutrophil infiltration) and CCL20 (which recruits myeloid DCs and Th17 cells). Therefore, TNF-α is an important regulator of the IL-23/Th17 axis in psoriasis. The multifaceted role of TNF-α has been evaluated in clinical trials of TNF-α antagonists in psoriasis patients, revealing their clinical efficacy [27].

TNF-α-targeting agents were approved for rheumatoid arthritis treatment years before being approved for psoriasis therapy. Inhibition of TNF-α signaling has been broadly used in targeted biological treatment of psoriasis. The three biologics currently approved for the treatment of moderate to severe psoriasis are infliximab, adalimumab, and etanercept (**Table 1**). Effective treatment with TNF antagonists downregulates T-cell and DC numbers and decreases their cytokine levels [27, 28]. Infliximab, a chimeric monoclonal antibody, suppresses TNF-α biologic activity by neutralizing both soluble and membrane-bound forms of TNF-α [29]. Blocking this cytokine activity with infliximab has been demonstrated to rapidly normalize keratinocyte differentiation and reduce the number of epidermal thickness, epidermal T-cell infiltration, and intracellular adhesion molecules of psoriatic plaques, such as e-selectin and VCAM [30–32]. Adalimumab is a fully humanized IgG1 monoclonal antibody [33] that binds with high specificity and affinity to human TNF-α. Adalimumab has been suggested as an effective treatment for moderate to severe chronic plaque psoriasis for up to 12 weeks of therapy [34]. Upon binding to this cytokine, adalimumab neutralizes biologic activities by blocking its interaction with the p55 and p75 cell-surface TNF receptors to inhibit TNF-involved biologic responses [35]. Etanercept, a fusion protein consisting of the extracellular ligand-binding domain of TNF-α receptors and Fc portion of human immunoglobulin G, performs its immune function by neutralizing soluble TNF-α and TNF-β (or known as lymphotoxin-α) [36], which also reduces IL-23, and by suppressing Th17 downstream molecules, including IL-17, IL-22, CC chemokine ligand (CCL) 20, and β-defensin 4 [27]. Particularly, successful treatment was found to be associated with the suppression of genes related to the differentiation and function of Th17 cells. Moreover, inhibition of the IL-23 and Th17 axis led to downregulation of IFN-γ-related genes associated with psoriasis resolution [27, 28]. Furthermore, etanercept can decrease lesional DC expression of co-stimulatory molecules in vitro, impairing DC-T-cell interactions and allogenic T-cell activation [27].

The clinical advantage of TNF-α suppression is related to blockage of the IL-23/Th17 axis. Furthermore, TNF-α and Th17 have been suggested to synergistically stimulate the production of several keratinocyte proinflammatory mediators involved in psoriasis [37]. Therefore, blocking either or both TNF-α and IL-23-Th17 pathways may affect immunopathogenic molecules involved in psoriasis.

Anti-TNF-α therapies for psoriasis are very effective. However, the diverse roles of this cytokine cause various drug-associated adverse effects. Patients treated with these biologic agents show an increased incidence of reactivating latent tuberculosis [38] and emerging serious infections (such as sepsis and opportunistic infections) [39]. Additionally, some studies have linked these anti-TNF drugs, particularly when used in combination with other drugs, to an increased risk of malignancies such as lymphoma [40–42].

Drug name	Drug target	Agent type	Administration	Efficacy (% with PASI 75)	References	Stage of development*
Infliximab (Remicade)	TNF-α	Chimeric TNF-α monoclonal antibody	2-h i.v. infusion (5 mg/kg) at weeks 0, 2, and 6 and then every 8 weeks	75–88 at 10 weeks	Gottlieb et al. [31]; Reich et al. [29]; Menter et al. [106]	Approved
Adalimumab (Humira)	TNF-α	Humanized TNF-α monoclonal antibody	s.c. 80 mg at week 0 and then 40 mg every 2 weeks	53–80 at 12 weeks	Gordon et al. [34]; Menter et al. [35]; Saurat et al. [107]	Approved
Etanercept (Enbrel)	TNF-α	Soluble TNF-α receptor-igg fusion protein	s.c 50 mg every 2 weeks for 3 months and then 50 mg weekly	47–49 at 12 weeks	Leonardi et al. [108]; Papp et al. [36]; Tyring et al. [109]	Approved
Ustekinumab (Stelara, CNTO1275)	p40 subunit of IL-12/IL-23	Humanized p40 monoclonal antibody	s.c. (1) 45 mg or (2) 90 mg weekly for 12 weeks	(1) 66.7–67.1 or (2) 66.4–75.7 at 12 weeks	Leonardi et al. [51]; Papp et al. [50]	Approved
Briakinumab (ABT-874)	p40 subunit of IL-12/IL-23	Humanized p40 monoclonal antibody	s.c. 200 mg at weeks 0 and 4 and then 100 mg at week 8	80.6–81.9 at 12 weeks	Gordon et al. [52]; Gottlieb et al. [53]; Strober et al. [54]	Terminated
Tildrakizumab (MK-3222)	p19 subunit of IL-23	Humanized p19 IgG1 monoclonal antibody	s.c (1) 5 mg or (2) 25 mg or (3) 100 or (4) 200 mg at weeks 0 and 4 and then every 12 weeks thereafter	(1) 33.3 or (2) 64.4 or (3) 66.3 or (4) 74.4 at 16 weeks	Papp et al. [58]	Phase III studies ongoing
Guselkumab (CNTO1959)	p19 subunit of IL-23	Humanized p19 IgG1 monoclonal antibody	s.c (1) 5 mg at weeks 0 and 4 and then every 12 weeks thereafter or (2) 15 mg every 8 weeks or (3) 50 at weeks 0 and 4 and then every 12 weeks thereafter or (4) 100 mg at weeks 0 and 4 and then every 12 weeks there after (5) 200 mg at weeks 0 and 4 and then every 12 weeks thereafter	(1) 44 or (2) 76 or (3) 81 or (4) 79 (5) 81 at 16 weeks	Gordon et al. [59]	Finished phase III trial
Secukinumab (Cosentyx, AIN457)	IL-17A	Humanized IL-17A IgG1 monoclonal antibody	s.c. (1) 150 mg or (2) 300 mg at weeks 0, 1, 2, 3, and 4 and every 4 weeks	(1) 67–71.6 or (2) 77.1–81.6 at 12 weeks	Langley et al. [68]	Approved

*State of development in the United States, as of January 2017.

Table 1. Biologic drugs for moderate to severe psoriasis at 10–16 weeks.

3.3. IL-12/IL-23

IL-12 and IL-23 are heterodimeric pleiotropic proteins that share a common p40 subunit (encoded by IL12B) and are thought to be essential for controlling the differentiation of Th1 and Th17 cells, respectively. The second distinct subunit of IL-12 is the p35 subunit, and the second unique subunit of IL-23 is the p19 subunit (encoded by IL23A). Expression of the p19 and p40 subunits was found to be significantly increased in psoriatic skin lesions, while the p35 subunit was not [43, 44], suggesting that IL-23 is important in the pathogenesis of psoriasis. Further support from clinical trials revealed that the expression of IL-12/IL-23 was decreased following psoriasis treatment [45–47]. IL-23 and IL-12 are primarily secreted by DCs and macrophages and play a crucial role in psoriatic pathogenesis by regulating Th17 and Th1 cells, including the activation and differentiation of effector T cells, stimulation of keratinocytes, and upregulation of TNF-α expression in psoriatic plaques [43, 48]. IL-23 binds to IL-23R, which is correlated with Jak2 and Tyk2. Binding of its receptor stimulates a signaling circuit via STAT3 activation.

Anti-IL-12/IL-23 and anti-IL-23 drugs are highly effective treatments for psoriasis (**Table 1**) [49]. Recently, the only published results from clinical trials describe two agents of the p40 subunit inhibitors, ustekinumab and briakinumab. Ustekinumab is a human IgG1 monoclonal antibody that neutralizes the shared p40 subunit of IL-12 and IL-23. The agent prevents the interaction of IL-23 and IL-12 with their cell-surface receptors, blocking the Th17 and Th1 signaling cascades. It has been demonstrated to be efficacious for moderate to severe psoriasis [50, 51]. Clinical trials showed that another fully human anti-IL-12/IL-23p40 monoclonal antibody, briakinumab, was also efficacious for the disease [52–54]. However, after phase III trials, safety results concerning a possible increased risk of major adverse cardiovascular events (myocardial infarction, cerebrovascular accident, and cardiac death) with the use of briakinumab let to cessation of its development and withdrawal of the application in 2011 [55, 56].

The structurally related p19 subunit of IL-23 has recently emerged as an attractive target for moderate to severe psoriasis treatment, although these drugs have not been FDA approved [57]. Several agents targeting the p19 subunit are under investigation in clinical trials. Tildrakizumab is a humanized IgG1κ that binds to the unique p19 subunit of IL-23 [58]. This agent was effective in treating moderate to severe plaque psoriasis in a phase IIb clinical trial. Phase III studies are currently underway. Similarly, phase III trials of another fully human IgG1λ monoclonal p19 antibody, guselkumab, are currently a success [59].

3.4. IL-17

IL-17, the main cytokine effector of Th17 cells, is an important cytokine in the pathogenesis of psoriasis. Neutrophils, mast cells, and natural killer (NK) cells also produce IL-17. It is thought to be a proximal regulator of psoriatic cutaneous inflammation and plays a key role in bridging the innate and adaptive immune responses. The IL-17 family comprises six subsets of homo- and heterodimeric cytokines: IL-17A, IL-17B, IL-17C, IL-D, IL-17E, and IL-17F. IL-17A and IL-17F are regarded as the most relevant subtypes in psoriasis. IL-17 is widely thought to be a direct regulator that stimulates keratinocyte proliferation and inhibits keratinocyte differentiation via the antimicrobial protein REG3A, a mediator with antimicrobial functions involved in wound repair [60]. IL-17 mRNA and protein levels are upregulated in lesional psoriatic plaques and/or blood samples from patients [61, 62]. Lowes et al. [63] demonstrated that psoriatic T cells generate large amounts of IL-17 ex vivo, but T cells from the normal healthy skin did not produce IL-17 under the same conditions.

Keratinocytes are the main target of IL-17A in psoriasis. The IL-17 receptor (IL-17R; consisting of two IL-17RA subunits complexed with one IL-17RC subunit) is expressed on the surface of keratinocytes throughout the epidermis and on scattered dermal cells (DCs, dermal fibroblasts, and endothelial cells) in the psoriatic skin [64]. The interaction between IL-17A and its receptor leads to the production of antimicrobial peptides (AMPs); proinflammatory cytokines such as IL-1, IL-6, IL-23, and IL-19; chemokines; and mediators of tissue injury [62].

IL-17A stimulates the expression of AMPs, including β-defensin and S100A family members, and thus activates the innate immune system [64]. A previous study demonstrated that IL-17A activates the production of multiple chemokines, including CCL20, CXCL1, CXCL2, CXCL3, CXCL5, and CXCL8/IL-8 [37, 64–66]. In addition to stimulating the recruitment and activation of neutrophils, IL-8 acts as a chemotactic factor for NK cells and T cells. CCL20 from human keratinocytes may direct the recruitment of CCR6-positive cells to the skin. Most Th17 cells express CCR6. Therefore, keratinocytes activate Th17-cell recruitment and increase the production of IL-17, promoting a positive feedback loop that maintains the inflammatory disease response [65, 67]. Moreover, CCL20 combined with ICAM-1 can facilitate the recruitment of DCs and T cells in psoriasis. IL-17A and TNF-α act synergistically on psoriatic keratinocytes, causing further production of TNF-α and other proinflammatory mediators.

Several drugs are available or under development that target IL-17 and its pathway. The potential role of the IL-17 pathway has been revealed in psoriatic clinical trials, which showed dramatic improvement. Secukinumab and ixekizumab are humanized IgG1κ and IgG4 monoclonal antibodies that bind and neutralize the IL-17A cytokine. [68, 69]. Secukinumab was approved by the FDA for moderate-to-severe treatment psoriasis in January 2015. In phase III studies, double-blind, 52-week trials, this agent achieved a PASI75 in 67.0–71.6% of patients at a 150-mg dose and 77.1–81.6% of patients with a 300-mg dose (**Table 1**) [68]. The common adverse effects associated with this agent are headache, nasopharyngitis, and upper respiratory tract infections, which are similar to those of other biologics. Ixekizumab, a monoclonal antibody specific for IL-17A, has been shown to be effective for treating psoriasis [70]. This biologic inhibits the expression of cytokines and chemokines involved in the IL-17 pathway [71]. Ixekizumab complete responses were observed in 30.8–35.0% of psoriasis patients and PASI90 in 59.7–65.3% after 12 weeks [69]. These results agree with recent findings that IL-17-producing cells are clearly present in the inflammatory infiltrate. Similar to prior biologic agents, the most commonly reported side effects were nasopharyngitis and injection site reactions. No serious adverse effects were observed [72]. Brodalumab, a unique fully human monoclonal antibody targeting the IL-17 receptor A (IL-17RA), is the newest biologic that has been FDA approved for psoriasis treatment. It binds with high affinity to IL-17RA and blocks the biological activity of IL-17A, IL-17F, and IL-25 (IL-17E), suppressing the downstream effect of IL-17 [73, 74]. In phase III trials to treat psoriasis, brodalumab achieved PASI75 in 83–86%

of patients with a 210-mg dose and 60–69% of patients with a 140-mg dose and PASI 90 in 69–70% after 12 weeks [75, 76]. The most common side effects were nasopharyngitis, upper respiratory infection, and injection site erythema [74]. Based on published results, drugs targeting IL-17 appear to have highly positive effects in moderate-to-severe psoriasis patients with no serious major side effects. Nevertheless, longer-term studies are needed.

3.5. IL-22

IL-22 belongs to the IL-10 family of cytokines, and its receptor (IL-22R) is a complex of two chains (IL-10R and IL-22RA1), which are exclusively expressed on epithelial cells such as keratinocytes [77]. Elevated levels of IL-22 mRNA in the lesional skin of psoriasis and serum IL-22 have been observed [78–80]. Its expression is also decreased after treatment with anti-psoriatic agents [80]. IL-22, produced from Th22 and Th17 cells, induces keratinocyte hyperproliferation, differentiation, migration, and dermal infiltration through STAT3 activation in vivo and in vitro [81]. It also mediates proinflammatory cytokine and AMP production [78, 82].

IL-22 in the human skin can stimulate keratinocytes in various ways. Combined with IL-17, IL-22 can induce AMP production by keratinocytes [83] and parakeratosis and acanthosis by increasing keratinocyte proliferation and inhibit keratinocyte differentiation during part of the tissue-remodeling phase of wound repair, which are observed in psoriasis [84].

Zheng et al. [81] reported that IL-23-induced epidermal hyperplasia in a murine model of psoriasis was dependent on IL-22, and blocking IL-22 in vivo or genetic deletion resulted in downregulation of IL-23-mediated epidermal hyperplasia. Therefore, the important association between the IL-23/Th17 axis and IL-22/Th22 is supported by these studies. However, trials of a human monoclonal antibody targeted against IL-22, fezakinumab, were discontinued because initial processes revealed that the efficacy endpoint could not be achieved [85]. The negative data from these studies suggest that this cytokine is not as critical to psoriasis immunopathogenesis as had initially been considered in earlier studies.

3.6. IL-9

IL-9 is a member of the IL-2 cytokine family. Singh et al. demonstrated markedly elevated expression of IL-9 in the lesional skin of psoriasis patients compared to control subjects. They found increased IL-9R and IL-9 expression in the psoriatic skin and observed a Th17-related inflammatory response after intradermal IL-9 injection in a mouse model [86]. IL-9 is a proinflammatory cytokine that stimulates the production of IL-17, IL-13, IFN-γ, and TNF-α in psoriasis. Both Th9 and Th17 cells are sources of IL-9.

3.7. IL-33

Interleukin-33 is a recently discovered mediator of the IL-1 family [87]. IL-33 mRNA is constitutively expressed in several tissues but is predominantly distributed in epithelial cells, keratinocytes, fibroblasts, DCs, smooth muscle cells, and macrophages. Interestingly, IL-33 specifically localizes to the nucleus of endothelial cells along the vessels and epithelial cells of tissue exposed to the environment [88–90].

The IL-33 receptor is selectively expressed on various cell types, including T-helper-cell (Th) type 2, mast cells, eosinophils, basophils, dendritic cells, group 2 innate lymphoid cells, keratinocytes, and invariant NKT cells [87, 91–94].

IL-33 can act both as a released cytokine, activating ST2L, and as a nuclear-binding factor, regulating gene transcription [95, 96]. Balato et al. [97] showed that IL-33 is present in both the nucleus and cytoplasm of psoriatic keratinocytes. The structure of IL-33 has been determined, and it exhibits the ability to act both as an extracellular cytokine stimulating the ST2L receptor and an intracellular factor controlling gene transcription. However, the role of IL-33 in psoriasis remains unclear.

Many recent studies have shown that IL-33 expression is increased in the lesional skin of psoriasis compared to the normal skin [91, 97, 98]. Hueber et al. [99] demonstrated that IL-33 and ST2 expression are upregulated in human lesional psoriatic plaques compared to the perilesional and normal healthy skin. Moreover, IL-33 is strongly expressed in the nuclei of keratinocytes in psoriasis, which is considered to be a Th1- and Th17-mediated disease, compared with atopic dermatitis which is a Th2-related disease and lichen planus which is related to Th1 cells [96]. We previously demonstrated that IL-17A induces IL-33 expression in normal human epidermal keratinocytes, suggesting that IL-17 in the lesional skin of psoriasis can induce IL-33 expression in the epidermis [91].

Relatively few studies have demonstrated the pathogenic association between IL-33 and psoriasis. Suttle et al. [100] reported decreased IL-33 immunostaining in biopsies in Koebner-positive psoriasis patients, which can reflect the release of IL-33 after skin injury by tape stripping. Interestingly, the proinflammatory cytokine TNF-α dose- and time-dependently activated IL-33 mRNA expression in normal skin cultures ex vivo. Similarly, TNF-α may stimulate the gene expression of IL-33 in normal human epidermal sheets and psoriatic skin [101]. Moreover, the levels of IL-33 were significantly reduced after TNF-α inhibitor therapy [101, 102].

Furthermore, Mitsui et al. [103] recently found that serum IL-33 levels are significantly elevated in patients with psoriasis and are particularly correlated with serum TNF-α levels; this elevation was decreased after anti-TNF-α treatment. They suggested that IL-33 is a general indicator of inflammation in psoriasis. In contrast, Tamagawa-Mineoka et al. [104], Balato et al. [97], and Talabot-Ayer et al. [105] did not detect serum IL-33 expression in psoriasis patients.

Author details

Jitlada Meephansan[1], Urairack Subpayasarn[1], Mayumi Komine[2*] and Mamitaro Ohtsuki[2]

*Address all correspondence to: mkomine12@jichi.ac.jp

1 Division of Dermatology, Chulabhorn International College of Medicine, Thammasat University, Pathum Thani, Thailand

2 Department of Dermatology, Jichi Medical University, Tochigi, Japan

References

[1] Nestle FO, Kaplan DH, Barker J. Psoriasis. New England Journal of Medicine. 2009;**361**(5):496–509

[2] Perera GK, Di Meglio P, Nestle FO. Psoriasis. Annual Review of Pathology. 2012;**7**:385–422

[3] Griffiths CE, Barker JN. Pathogenesis and clinical features of psoriasis. Lancet. 2007;**370**(9583):263–271

[4] Sabat R, Philipp S, Hoflich C, Kreutzer S, Wallace E, Asadullah K, et al. Immunopathogenesis of psoriasis. Experimental Dermatology. 2007;**16**(10):779–798

[5] Kim J, Krueger JG. The immunopathogenesis of psoriasis. Dermatologic Clinics. 2015;**33**(1):13–23

[6] Schon MP, Boehncke WH. Psoriasis. New England Journal of Medicine. 2005;**352**(18): 1899–1912

[7] Ganguly D, Chamilos G, Lande R, Gregorio J, Meller S, Facchinetti V, et al. Self-RNA-antimicrobial peptide complexes activate human dendritic cells through TLR7 and TLR8. Journal of Experimental Medicine. 2009;**206**(9):1983–1994

[8] Lande R, Gregorio J, Facchinetti V, Chatterjee B, Wang YH, Homey B, et al. Plasmacytoid dendritic cells sense self-DNA coupled with antimicrobial peptide. Nature. 2007;**449**(7162):564–569

[9] Nestle FO, Conrad C, Tun-Kyi A, Homey B, Gombert M, Boyman O, et al. Plasmacytoid predendritic cells initiate psoriasis through interferon-alpha production. Journal of Experimental Medicine. 2005;**202**(1):135–143

[10] Albanesi C, Scarponi C, Bosisio D, Sozzani S, Girolomoni G. Immune functions and recruitment of plasmacytoid dendritic cells in psoriasis. Autoimmunity. 2010;**43**(3):215–219

[11] Gregorio J, Meller S, Conrad C, Di Nardo A, Homey B, Lauerma A, et al. Plasmacytoid dendritic cells sense skin injury and promote wound healing through type I interferons. Journal of Experimental Medicine. 2010;**207**(13):2921–2930

[12] Lew W, Bowcock AM, Krueger JG. Psoriasis vulgaris: Cutaneous lymphoid tissue supports T-cell activation and "Type 1" inflammatory gene expression. Trends in Immunology. 2004;**25**(6):295–305

[13] Lowes MA, Russell CB, Martin DA, Towne JE, Krueger JG. The IL-23/T17 pathogenic axis in psoriasis is amplified by keratinocyte responses. Trends in Immunology. 2013;**34**(4):174–181

[14] Sofen H, Smith S, Matheson RT, Leonardi CL, Calderon C, Brodmerkel C, et al. Guselkumab (an IL-23-specific mAb) demonstrates clinical and molecular response in patients with moderate-to-severe psoriasis. Journal of Allergy and Clinical Immunology. 2014;**133**(4):1032–1040

[15] Johnson-Huang LM, Suarez-Farinas M, Pierson KC, Fuentes-Duculan J, Cueto I, Lentini T, et al. A single intradermal injection of IFN-gamma induces an inflammatory state in both non-lesional psoriatic and healthy skin. Journal of Investigative Dermatology. 2012;**132**(4):1177–1187

[16] Madonna S, Scarponi C, Sestito R, Pallotta S, Cavani A, Albanesi C. The IFN-gamma-dependent suppressor of cytokine signaling 1 promoter activity is positively regulated by IFN regulatory factor-1 and Sp1 but repressed by growth factor independence-1b and Kruppel-like factor-4, and it is dysregulated in psoriatic keratinocytes. Journal of Immunology. 2010;**185**(4):2467–2481

[17] Abdallah MA, Abdel-Hamid MF, Kotb AM, Mabrouk EA. Serum interferon-gamma is a psoriasis severity and prognostic marker. Cutis. 2009;**84**(3):163–168

[18] Harden JL, Johnson-Huang LM, Chamian MF, Lee E, Pearce T, Leonardi CL, et al. Humanized anti-IFN-gamma (HuZAF) in the treatment of psoriasis. Journal of Allergy and Clinical Immunology. 2015;**135**(2):553–556

[19] Zhang J. Yin and yang interplay of IFN-gamma in inflammation and autoimmune disease. Journal of Clinical Investigation. 2007;**117**(4):871–873

[20] Cua DJ, Sherlock J, Chen Y, Murphy CA, Joyce B, Seymour B, et al. Interleukin-23 rather than interleukin-12 is the critical cytokine for autoimmune inflammation of the brain. Nature. 2003;**421**(6924):744–748

[21] Zaba LC, Fuentes-Duculan J, Eungdamrong NJ, Johnson-Huang LM, Nograles KE, White TR, et al. Identification of TNF-related apoptosis-inducing ligand and other molecules that distinguish inflammatory from resident dendritic cells in patients with psoriasis. Journal of Allergy and Clinical Immunology. 2010;**125**(6):1261–1268. e9

[22] Lowes MA, Chamian F, Abello MV, Fuentes-Duculan J, Lin SL, Nussbaum R, et al. Increase in TNF-alpha and inducible nitric oxide synthase-expressing dendritic cells in psoriasis and reduction with efalizumab (anti-CD11a). Proceedings of the National Academy of Sciences of the United States of America. 2005;**102**(52):19057–19062

[23] Arican O, Aral M, Sasmaz S, Ciragil P. Serum levels of TNF-alpha, IFN-gamma, IL-6, IL-8, IL-12, IL-17, and IL-18 in patients with active psoriasis and correlation with disease severity. Mediators of Inflammation. 2005;**2005**(5):273–279

[24] Abanmi A, Al Harthi F, Al Agla R, Khan HA, Tariq M. Serum levels of proinflammatory cytokines in psoriasis patients from Saudi Arabia. International Journal of Dermatology. 2005;**44**(1):82–83

[25] Jacob SE, Nassiri M, Kerdel FA, Vincek V. Simultaneous measurement of multiple Th1 and Th2 serum cytokines in psoriasis and correlation with disease severity. Mediators of Inflammation. 2003;**12**(5):309–313

[26] Goldminz AM, Au SC, Kim N, Gottlieb AB, Lizzul PF. NF-kappaB: An essential transcription factor in psoriasis. Journal of Dermatological Science. 2013;**69**(2):89–94

[27] Zaba LC, Cardinale I, Gilleaudeau P, Sullivan-Whalen M, Suarez-Farinas M, Fuentes-Duculan J, et al. Amelioration of epidermal hyperplasia by TNF inhibition is associated with reduced Th17 responses. Journal of Experimental Medicine. 2007;**204**(13):3183–3194

[28] Zaba LC, Suarez-Farinas M, Fuentes-Duculan J, Nograles KE, Guttman-Yassky E, Cardinale I, et al. Effective treatment of psoriasis with etanercept is linked to suppression of IL-17 signaling, not immediate response TNF genes. Journal of Allergy and Clinical Immunology. 2009;**124**(5):1022–1030.e1–395

[29] Reich K, Nestle FO, Papp K, Ortonne JP, Evans R, Guzzo C, et al. Infliximab induction and maintenance therapy for moderate-to-severe psoriasis: A phase III, multicentre, double-blind trial. Lancet. 2005;**366**(9494):1367–1374

[30] Gottlieb AB, Masud S, Ramamurthi R, Abdulghani A, Romano P, Chaudhari U, et al. Pharmacodynamic and pharmacokinetic response to anti-tumor necrosis factor-alpha monoclonal antibody (infliximab) treatment of moderate to severe psoriasis vulgaris. Journal of the American Academy of Dermatology. 2003;**48**(1):68–75

[31] Gottlieb AB, Evans R, Li S, Dooley LT, Guzzo CA, Baker D, et al. Infliximab induction therapy for patients with severe plaque-type psoriasis: A randomized, double-blind, placebo-controlled trial. Journal of the American Academy of Dermatology. 2004;**51**(4):534–542

[32] Chaudhari U, Romano P, Mulcahy LD, Dooley LT, Baker DG, Gottlieb AB. Efficacy and safety of infliximab monotherapy for plaque-type psoriasis: A randomised trial. Lancet. 2001;**357**(9271):1842–1847

[33] Calabrese LH. Molecular differences in anticytokine therapies. Clinical and Experimental Rheumatology. 2003;**21**(2):241–248

[34] Gordon KB, Langley RG, Leonardi C, Toth D, Menter MA, Kang S, et al. Clinical response to adalimumab treatment in patients with moderate to severe psoriasis: Double-blind, randomized controlled trial and open-label extension study. Journal of the American Academy of Dermatology. 2006;**55**(4):598–606

[35] Menter A, Tyring SK, Gordon K, Kimball AB, Leonardi CL, Langley RG, et al. Adalimumab therapy for moderate to severe psoriasis: A randomized, controlled phase III trial. Journal of the American Academy of Dermatology. 2008;**58**(1):106–115

[36] Papp KA, Tyring S, Lahfa M, Prinz J, Griffiths CE, Nakanishi AM, et al. A global phase III randomized controlled trial of etanercept in psoriasis: Safety, efficacy, and effect of dose reduction. British Journal of Dermatology. 2005;**152**(6):1304–1312

[37] Chiricozzi A, Guttman-Yassky E, Suárez-Fariñas M, Nograles KE, Tian S, Cardinale I, et al. Integrative responses to IL-17 and TNF-&α in human keratinocytes account for key inflammatory pathogenic circuits in psoriasis. Journal of Investigative Dermatology. 2011;**131**(3):677–687

[38] Mankia S, Peters JE, Kang S, Moore S, Ehrenstein MR. Tuberculosis and anti-TNF treatment: Experience of a central London hospital. Clinical Rheumatology. 2011;**30**(3):399–401

[39] Galloway JB, Hyrich KL, Mercer LK, Dixon WG, Fu B, Ustianowski AP, et al. Anti-TNF therapy is associated with an increased risk of serious infections in patients with rheumatoid arthritis especially in the first 6 months of treatment: Updated results from the British Society for Rheumatology Biologics Register with special emphasis on risks in the elderly. Rheumatology (Oxford). 2011;**50**(1):124–131

[40] Mariette X, Tubach F, Bagheri H, Bardet M, Berthelot JM, Gaudin P, et al. Lymphoma in patients treated with anti-TNF: Results of the 3-year prospective French RATIO registry. Annals of the Rheumatic Diseases. 2010;**69**(2):400–408

[41] Lakatos PL, Miheller P. Is there an increased risk of lymphoma and malignancies under anti-TNF therapy in IBD? Current Drug Targets. 2010;**11**(2):179–186

[42] Herrinton LJ, Liu L, Weng X, Lewis JD, Hutfless S, Allison JE. Role of thiopurine and anti-TNF therapy in lymphoma in inflammatory bowel disease. American Journal of Gastroenterology. 2011;**106**(12):2146–2153

[43] Lee E, Trepicchio WL, Oestreicher JL, Pittman D, Wang F, Chamian F, et al. Increased expression of interleukin 23 p19 and p40 in lesional skin of patients with psoriasis vulgaris. Journal of Experimental Medicine. 2004;**199**(1):125–130

[44] Tonel G, Conrad C, Laggner U, Di Meglio P, Grys K, McClanahan TK, et al. Cutting edge: A critical functional role for IL-23 in psoriasis. Journal of Immunology. 2010;**185**(10):5688–5691

[45] Chamian F, Lowes MA, Lin SL, Lee E, Kikuchi T, Gilleaudeau P, et al. Alefacept reduces infiltrating T cells, activated dendritic cells, and inflammatory genes in psoriasis vulgaris. Proceedings of the National Academy of Sciences of the United States of America. 2005;**102**(6):2075–2080

[46] Gottlieb AB, Chamian F, Masud S, Cardinale I, Abello MV, Lowes MA, et al. TNF inhibition rapidly down-regulates multiple proinflammatory pathways in psoriasis plaques. Journal of Immunology. 2005;**175**(4):2721–2729

[47] Piskin G, Tursen U, Sylva-Steenland RM, Bos JD, Teunissen MB. Clinical improvement in chronic plaque-type psoriasis lesions after narrow-band UVB therapy is accompanied by a decrease in the expression of IFN-gamma inducers – IL-12, IL-18 and IL-23. Experimental Dermatology. 2004;**13**(12):764–772

[48] Zhou L, Ivanov, II, Spolski R, Min R, Shenderov K, Egawa T, et al. IL-6 programs T(H)-17 cell differentiation by promoting sequential engagement of the IL-21 and IL-23 pathways. Nature Immunology. 2007;**8**(9):967–974

[49] Gandhi M, Alwawi E, Gordon KB. Anti-p40 antibodies ustekinumab and briakinumab: Blockade of interleukin-12 and interleukin-23 in the treatment of psoriasis. Seminars in Cutaneous Medicine and Surgery. 2010;**29**(1):48–52

[50] Papp KA, Langley RG, Lebwohl M, Krueger GG, Szapary P, Yeilding N, et al. Efficacy and safety of ustekinumab, a human interleukin-12/23 monoclonal antibody, in patients

with psoriasis: 52-week results from a randomised, double-blind, placebo-controlled trial (PHOENIX 2). Lancet. 2008;**371**(9625):1675–1684

[51] Leonardi CL, Kimball AB, Papp KA, Yeilding N, Guzzo C, Wang Y, et al. Efficacy and safety of ustekinumab, a human interleukin-12/23 monoclonal antibody, in patients with psoriasis: 76-week results from a randomised, double-blind, placebo-controlled trial (PHOENIX 1). Lancet. 2008;**371**(9625):1665–1674

[52] Gordon KB, Langley RG, Gottlieb AB, Papp KA, Krueger GG, Strober BE, et al. A phase III, randomized, controlled trial of the fully human IL-12/23 mAb briakinumab in moderate-to-severe psoriasis. Journal of Investigative Dermatology. 2012;**132**(2):304–314

[53] Gottlieb AB, Leonardi C, Kerdel F, Mehlis S, Olds M, Williams DA. Efficacy and safety of briakinumab vs. etanercept and placebo in patients with moderate to severe chronic plaque psoriasis. British Journal of Dermatology. 2011;**165**(3):652–660

[54] Strober BE, Crowley JJ, Yamauchi PS, Olds M, Williams DA. Efficacy and safety results from a phase III, randomized controlled trial comparing the safety and efficacy of briakinumab with etanercept and placebo in patients with moderate to severe chronic plaque psoriasis. British Journal of Dermatology. 2011;**165**(3):661–668

[55] Langley RG, Papp K, Gottlieb AB, Krueger GG, Gordon KB, Williams D, et al. Safety results from a pooled analysis of randomized, controlled phase II and III clinical trials and interim data from an open-label extension trial of the interleukin-12/23 monoclonal antibody, briakinumab, in moderate to severe psoriasis. Journal of the European Academy of Dermatology and Venereology. 2013;**27**(10):1252–1261

[56] Ryan C, Leonardi CL, Krueger JG, Kimball AB, Strober BE, Gordon KB, et al. Association between biologic therapies for chronic plaque psoriasis and cardiovascular events: A meta-analysis of randomized controlled trials. The Journal of the American Medical Association. 2011;**306**(8):864–871

[57] Kofoed K, Skov L, Zachariae C. New drugs and treatment targets in psoriasis. Acta Dermato-Venereologica. 2015;**95**(2):133–139

[58] Papp K, Thaci D, Reich K, Riedl E, Langley RG, Krueger JG, et al. Tildrakizumab (MK-3222), an anti-interleukin-23p19 monoclonal antibody, improves psoriasis in a phase IIb randomized placebo-controlled trial. British Journal of Dermatology. 2015;**173**(4):930–939

[59] Gordon KB, Duffin KC, Bissonnette R, Prinz JC, Wasfi Y, Li S, et al. A phase 2 trial of guselkumab versus adalimumab for plaque psoriasis. New England Journal of Medicine. 2015;**373**(2):136–144

[60] Lai Y, Li D, Li C, Muehleisen B, Radek KA, Park HJ, et al. The antimicrobial protein REG3A regulates keratinocyte proliferation and differentiation after skin injury. Immunity. 2012;**37**(1):74–84

[61] Johansen C, Usher PA, Kjellerup RB, Lundsgaard D, Iversen L, Kragballe K. Characterization of the interleukin-17 isoforms and receptors in lesional psoriatic skin. British Journal of Dermatology. 2009;**160**(2):319–324

[62] Lynde CW, Poulin Y, Vender R, Bourcier M, Khalil S. Interleukin 17A: Toward a new understanding of psoriasis pathogenesis. Journal of the American Academy of Dermatology. 2014;**71**(1):141–150

[63] Lowes MA, Kikuchi T, Fuentes-Duculan J, Cardinale I, Zaba LC, Haider AS, et al. Psoriasis vulgaris lesions contain discrete populations of Th1 and Th17 T cells. Journal of Investigative Dermatology. 2008;**128**(5):1207–1211

[64] Nograles KE, Zaba LC, Guttman-Yassky E, Fuentes-Duculan J, Suarez-Farinas M, Cardinale I, et al. Th17 cytokines interleukin (IL)-17 and IL-22 modulate distinct inflammatory and keratinocyte-response pathways. British Journal of Dermatology. 2008;**159**(5):1092–1102

[65] Harper EG, Guo C, Rizzo H, Lillis JV, Kurtz SE, Skorcheva I, et al. Th17 cytokines stimulate CCL20 expression in keratinocytes in vitro and in vivo: Implications for psoriasis pathogenesis. Journal of Investigative Dermatology. 2009;**129**(9):2175–2183

[66] Homey B, Dieu-Nosjean MC, Wiesenborn A, Massacrier C, Pin JJ, Oldham E, et al. Up-regulation of macrophage inflammatory protein-3 alpha/CCL20 and CC chemokine receptor 6 in psoriasis. Journal of Immunology. 2000;**164**(12):6621–6632

[67] Ramirez-Carrozzi V, Sambandam A, Luis E, Lin Z, Jeet S, Lesch J, et al. IL-17C regulates the innate immune function of epithelial cells in an autocrine manner. Nature Immunology. 2011;**12**(12):1159–1166

[68] Langley RG, Elewski BE, Lebwohl M, Reich K, Griffiths CE, Papp K, et al. Secukinumab in plaque psoriasis – results of two phase 3 trials. New England Journal of Medicine. 2014;**371**(4):326–338

[69] Griffiths CE, Reich K, Lebwohl M, van de Kerkhof P, Paul C, Menter A, et al. Comparison of ixekizumab with etanercept or placebo in moderate-to-severe psoriasis (UNCOVER-2 and UNCOVER-3): Results from two phase 3 randomised trials. Lancet. 2015;**386**(9993):541–551

[70] Gordon KB, Blauvelt A, Papp KA, Langley RG, Luger T, Ohtsuki M, et al. Phase 3 trials of ixekizumab in moderate-to-severe plaque psoriasis. New England Journal of Medicine. 2016;**375**(4):345–356

[71] Krueger JG, Fretzin S, Suarez-Farinas M, Haslett PA, Phipps KM, Cameron GS, et al. IL-17A is essential for cell activation and inflammatory gene circuits in subjects with psoriasis. Journal of Allergy and Clinical Immunology. 2012;**130**(1):145–154.e9

[72] Leonardi C, Matheson R, Zachariae C, Cameron G, Li L, Edson-Heredia E, et al. Anti-interleukin-17 monoclonal antibody ixekizumab in chronic plaque psoriasis. New England Journal of Medicine. 2012;**366**(13):1190–1199

[73] Farahnik B, Beroukhim K, Abrouk M, Nakamura M, Zhu TH, Singh R, et al. Brodalumab for the treatment of psoriasis: A review of phase III trials. Dermatology and Therapy (Heidelb). 2016;**6**(2):111–124

[74] Papp KA, Leonardi C, Menter A, Ortonne JP, Krueger JG, Kricorian G, et al. Brodalumab, an anti-interleukin-17-receptor antibody for psoriasis. New England Journal of Medicine. 2012;**366**(13):1181–1189

[75] Lebwohl M, Strober B, Menter A, Gordon K, Weglowska J, Puig L, et al. Phase 3 studies comparing brodalumab with ustekinumab in psoriasis. New England Journal of Medicine. 2015;**373**(14):1318–1328

[76] Papp K, Menter A, Strober B, Kricorian G, Thompson EH, Milmont CE, et al. Efficacy and safety of brodalumab in subpopulations of patients with difficult-to-treat moderate-to-severe plaque psoriasis. Journal of the American Academy of Dermatology. 2015;**72**(3):436–439.e1

[77] Mashiko S, Bouguermouh S, Rubio M, Baba N, Bissonnette R, Sarfati M. Human mast cells are major IL-22 producers in patients with psoriasis and atopic dermatitis. Journal of Allergy and Clinical Immunology. 2015;**136**(2):351–359.e1

[78] Wolk K, Witte E, Wallace E, Docke WD, Kunz S, Asadullah K, et al. IL-22 regulates the expression of genes responsible for antimicrobial defense, cellular differentiation, and mobility in keratinocytes: A potential role in psoriasis. European Journal of Immunology. 2006;**36**(5):1309–1323

[79] Coimbra S, Oliveira H, Reis F, Belo L, Rocha S, Quintanilha A, et al. Interleukin (IL)-22, IL-17, IL-23, IL-8, vascular endothelial growth factor and tumour necrosis factor-alpha levels in patients with psoriasis before, during and after psoralen-ultraviolet A and narrowband ultraviolet B therapy. British Journal of Dermatology. 2010;**163**(6):1282–1290

[80] Boniface K, Lecron JC, Bernard FX, Dagregorio G, Guillet G, Nau F, et al. Keratinocytes as targets for interleukin-10-related cytokines: A putative role in the pathogenesis of psoriasis. European Cytokine Network. 2005;**16**(4):309–319

[81] Zheng Y, Danilenko DM, Valdez P, Kasman I, Eastham-Anderson J, Wu J, et al. Interleukin-22, a T(H)17 cytokine, mediates IL-23-induced dermal inflammation and acanthosis. Nature. 2007;**445**(7128):648–651

[82] Eyerich S, Eyerich K, Pennino D, Carbone T, Nasorri F, Pallotta S, et al. Th22 cells represent a distinct human T cell subset involved in epidermal immunity and remodeling. Journal of Clinical Investigation. 2009;**119**(12):3573–3585

[83] Liang SC, Tan XY, Luxenberg DP, Karim R, Dunussi-Joannopoulos K, Collins M, et al. Interleukin (IL)-22 and IL-17 are coexpressed by Th17 cells and cooperatively enhance expression of antimicrobial peptides. Journal of Experimental Medicine. 2006;**203**(10):2271–2279

[84] Boniface K, Bernard FX, Garcia M, Gurney AL, Lecron JC, Morel F. IL-22 inhibits epidermal differentiation and induces proinflammatory gene expression and migration of human keratinocytes. Journal of Immunology. 2005;**174**(6):3695–3702

[85] Gudjonsson JE, Johnston A, Ellis CN. Novel systemic drugs under investigation for the treatment of psoriasis. Journal of the American Academy of Dermatology. 2012;**67**(1):139–147

[86] Singh TP, Schon MP, Wallbrecht K, Gruber-Wackernagel A, Wang XJ, Wolf P. Involvement of IL-9 in Th17-associated inflammation and angiogenesis of psoriasis. PLoS One. 2013;**8**(1):e51752

[87] Schmitz J, Owyang A, Oldham E, Song Y, Murphy E, McClanahan TK, et al. IL-33, an interleukin-1-like cytokine that signals via the IL-1 receptor-related protein ST2 and induces T helper type 2-associated cytokines. Immunity. 2005;**23**(5):479–490

[88] Carriere V, Roussel L, Ortega N, Lacorre DA, Americh L, Aguilar L, et al. IL-33, the IL-1-like cytokine ligand for ST2 receptor, is a chromatin-associated nuclear factor in vivo. Proceedings of the National Academy of Sciences of the United States of America. 2007;**104**(1):282–287

[89] Moussion C, Ortega N, Girard JP. The IL-1-like cytokine IL-33 is constitutively expressed in the nucleus of endothelial cells and epithelial cells in vivo: A novel 'alarmin'? PLoS One. 2008;**3**(10):e3331

[90] Kuchler AM, Pollheimer J, Balogh J, Sponheim J, Manley L, Sorensen DR, et al. Nuclear interleukin-33 is generally expressed in resting endothelium but rapidly lost upon angiogenic or proinflammatory activation. American Journal of Pathology. 2008;**173**(4):1229–1242

[91] Meephansan J, Komine M, Tsuda H, Karakawa M, Tominaga S, Ohtsuki M. Expression of IL-33 in the epidermis: The mechanism of induction by IL-17. Journal of Dermatological Science. 2013;**71**(2):107–114

[92] Suzukawa M, Iikura M, Koketsu R, Nagase H, Tamura C, Komiya A, et al. An IL-1 cytokine member, IL-33, induces human basophil activation via its ST2 receptor. The Journal of Immunology. 2008;**181**(9):5981–5989

[93] Cherry WB, Yoon J, Bartemes KR, Iijima K, Kita H. A novel IL-1 family cytokine, IL-33, potently activates human eosinophils. Journal of Allergy and Clinical Immunology. 2008;**121**(6):1484–1490

[94] Smithgall MD, Comeau MR, Yoon BR, Kaufman D, Armitage R, Smith DE. IL-33 amplifies both Th1- and Th2-type responses through its activity on human basophils, allergen-reactive Th2 cells, iNKT and NK cells. International Immunology. 2008;**20**(8):1019–1030

[95] Ali S, Mohs A, Thomas M, Klare J, Ross R, Schmitz ML, et al. The dual function cytokine IL-33 interacts with the transcription factor NF-kappaB to dampen NF-kappaB-stimulated gene transcription. Journal of Immunology. 2011;**187**(4):1609–1616

[96] Meephansan J, Tsuda H, Komine M, Tominaga S, Ohtsuki M. Regulation of IL-33 expression by IFN-gamma and tumor necrosis factor-alpha in normal human epidermal keratinocytes. Journal of Investigative Dermatology. 2012;**132**(11):2593–2600

[97] Balato A, Lembo S, Mattii M, Schiattarella M, Marino R, De Paulis A, et al. IL-33 is secreted by psoriatic keratinocytes and induces pro-inflammatory cytokines via keratinocyte and mast cell activation. Experimental Dermatology. 2012;21(11):892–894

[98] Theoharides TC, Zhang B, Kempuraj D, Tagen M, Vasiadi M, Angelidou A, et al. IL-33 augments substance P-induced VEGF secretion from human mast cells and is increased in psoriatic skin. Proceedings of the National Academy of Sciences of the United States of America. 2010;**107**(9):4448–4453

[99] Hueber AJ, Alves-Filho JC, Asquith DL, Michels C, Millar NL, Reilly JH, et al. IL-33 induces skin inflammation with mast cell and neutrophil activation. European Journal of Immunology. 2011;**41**(8):2229–2237

[100] Suttle MM, Enoksson M, Zoltowska A, Chatterjee M, Nilsson G, Harvima IT. Experimentally induced psoriatic lesions associate with rapid but transient decrease in interleukin-33 immunostaining in epidermis. Acta Dermato-Venereologica. 2015;**95**(5): 536–541

[101] Balato A, Di Caprio R, Canta L, Mattii M, Lembo S, Raimondo A, et al. IL-33 is regulated by TNF-alpha in normal and psoriatic skin. Archives of Dermatological Research. 2014;**306**(3):299–304

[102] Vageli DP, Exarchou A, Zafiriou E, Doukas PG, Doukas S, Roussaki-Schulze A. Effect of TNF-alpha inhibitors on transcriptional levels of pro-inflammatory interleukin-33 and Toll-like receptors-2 and -9 in psoriatic plaques. Experimental and Therapeutic Medicine. 2015;**10**(4):1573–1577

[103] Mitsui A, Tada Y, Takahashi T, Shibata S, Kamata M, Miyagaki T, et al. Serum IL-33 levels are increased in patients with psoriasis. Clinical and Experimental Dermatology. 2016;**41**(2):183–189

[104] Tamagawa-Mineoka R, Okuzawa Y, Masuda K, Katoh N. Increased serum levels of interleukin 33 in patients with atopic dermatitis. Journal of the American Academy of Dermatology. 2014;**70**(5):882–888

[105] Talabot-Ayer D, McKee T, Gindre P, Bas S, Baeten DL, Gabay C, et al. Distinct serum and synovial fluid interleukin (IL)-33 levels in rheumatoid arthritis, psoriatic arthritis and osteoarthritis. Joint, Bone, Spine. 2012;**79**(1):32–37

[106] Menter A, Feldman SR, Weinstein GD, Papp K, Evans R, Guzzo C, et al. A randomized comparison of continuous vs. intermittent infliximab maintenance regimens over 1 year in the treatment of moderate-to-severe plaque psoriasis. J Am Acad Dermatol. 2007;**56**(1):31.e1–15.

[107] Saurat JH, Stingl G, Dubertret L, Papp K, Langley RG, Ortonne JP, et al. Efficacy and safety results from the randomized controlled comparative study of adalimumab vs. methotrexate vs. placebo in patients with psoriasis (CHAMPION). Br J Dermatol. 2008;**158**(3):558–66.

[108] Leonardi CL, Powers JL, Matheson RT, Goffe BS, Zitnik R, Wang A, et al. Etanercept as monotherapy in patients with psoriasis. N Engl J Med. 2003;**349**(21):2014–22.

[109] Tyring S, Gottlieb A, Papp K, Gordon K, Leonardi C, Wang A, et al. Etanercept and clinical outcomes, fatigue, and depression in psoriasis: double-blind placebo-controlled randomised phase III trial. Lancet. 2006;**367**(9504):29–35.

Chapter 4

Human Translational Research in Psoriasis Using CLA+ T Cells

Ester Ruiz-Romeu and Luis F. Santamaria-Babi

Additional information is available at the end of the chapter

http://dx.doi.org/10.5772/67815

Abstract

Focusing on the study of human memory CLA+ T cells to understand psoriasis pathology constitutes an innovative approach to explore the pathological mechanism of this chronic cutaneous inflammatory disease. CLA+ T cells can be considered peripheral cell biomarkers in the study of T-cell mediated human skin diseases. During the last few years, new evidences have been found that link streptococcal infection with IL-17 response in psoriasis by studying the interaction between *Streptococcus pyogenes* with CLA+ T cells and autologous epidermal cells. *S. pyogenes* constitutes the best clinically characterized trigger of psoriasis and by exploring its effect on CLA+ T cells and epidermal cells in psoriasis may allow understanding psoriasis by using patient's clinical samples *ex vivo*.

Keywords: psoriasis, CLA+ T cells, translational research, *Streptococcus pyogenes*, IL17

1. CLA+ T cells and the regional cutaneous immune system

The adaptive immune responses taking place during cutaneous chronic inflammation in psoriasis preferentially involve a subset of memory T lymphocytes, which are related to the skin and that belong to the cutaneous immune system, and constitute one of the best characterized regional immune systems of the body and known for decades [1]. In the humans, the cutaneous lymphocyte-associated antigen (CLA) is a surface cell marker that allows identifying T cells that belong to the cutaneous immune system. The CLA antigen is a carbohydrate expressed by 15% of human circulating T cells, and on most (>90%) skin-infiltrating T cells, contrary to other inflamed organs [2]. CLA is expressed preferentially on memory antigen-experienced T cells.

The CLA is one of the adhesion molecule that, together with chemokine receptors, allows T cells to selectively migrate to the skin, in either homeostatic or inflammatory conditions, by binding to endothelial cell wall via adhesion molecules or ligands. The molecular interactions between CLA/E-selectin, very late antigen-4 (VLA-4)/vascular cell adhesion protein-1 (VCAM-1), lymphocyte function-associated antigen-1 (LFA-1)/intercellular adhesion molecule-1 (ICAM-1), and chemokine ligands for chemokine, C-C motif receptor (CCR) 10, CCR4, CCR6, and CCR8 constitute a code bar system enabling skin infiltration [3].

The importance of circulating CLA+ T cells for understanding the skin immune system is not only based on their capacity to selectively migrate to skin, but also on the fact that these circulating memory T cells are functionally related to the immune response taking place in the cutaneous inflamed lesions. This feature is based on the recirculating capacity of those cells between lesional skin and blood during cutaneous inflammation in psoriasis [3]. The adhesive interaction between LFA-1 and ICAM-1 is one of the mechanisms involved in the transendothelial migration of CLA+ T cells [4]. Interestingly, the blockade of LFA-1/ICAM-1 interaction in psoriasis patients with anti-LFA-1 in patients blocks extravasation and leads to CLA+ T cell lymphocytosis. Such accumulation of CLA+ T cells in the blood has clinical relevance since skin relapse may develop after stopping the anti-LFA-1 treatment [3].

The function and phenotype of circulating CLA+ T cells in T-cell mediated skin disease have been studied in many different human skin conditions. Those skin-seeking memory T cells respond to antigens, allergens, or superantigens that play a key role in disease triggering of different human T-cell mediated skin diseases, see **Table 1**. In addition, their phenotype and function are related to clinical status of the patient. For these reasons, those cells are considered peripheral cell biomarkers of T-cell mediated human cutaneous diseases [3, 5, 6].

Disease	Antigen involved in disease triggering
Atopic dermatitis	House dust mite [59] Casein [60] TCRVβ for SEB [61]
Contact dermatitis	Nickel [59]
Drug-induced allergic reaction	Betalactams [62]
Herpex simplex	HSV-2 [63]
Vitiligo	Melan-A [64]

Table 1. Selective response of circulating CLA+ T cells to antigens involved in cutaneous disease triggering.

2. Translational research and clinically relevant pathological mechanism of psoriasis

The innovation in psoriasis treatment has benefited from the continuous bidirectional flow of information from the bedside of clinic to the laboratory and vice versa [7]. Innovative pathogenic concepts have been tested in patients through the use of targeted therapeutics leading to clinically validated mechanism of disease. Those mechanisms that started as a merely scientific hypothesis of disease that can be proven to be relevant in the clinic by specific biological treatments allow improvement in the therapeutic arsenal for patients. At present, it is possible to understand psoriasis from several of its clinically relevant mechanism/targets that has been validated in the clinic since that has provided clinical benefit in patient. The current clinically validated concept of psoriasis is summarized in **Tables 2** and **3**. During the last two decades approximately, it has been demonstrated the key role of the IL-23/Th17 axis in psoriasis [8]. The journey to the current situation in psoriasis treatment started by evidencing that T-cell activity in psoriasis had real implications for the patients. Thus, depletion of T cells [9, 10], costimulation [11], and inhibition of their migration from blood to skin demonstrated improvement in the clinical severity [12]. Not only memory T cells are of translational relevance in psoriasis, but also TNF-α is a key cytokine for this disease. Although originally thought not to be associated to T-cell function, lately it was demonstrated that TNF-α neutralization affects Th17 function [13]. The introduction of ustekinumab, a monoclonal antibody that neutralizes both IL-12 and IL-23, cytokines involved in differentiation of Th1 and Th17 cells, respectively, marked the initiation of the IL-23/Th17 axis era [14]. In contrast to the increased amounts of IL-23, there is no marked increase of IL-12 in psoriatic lesion in comparison to nonlesional or healthy [15]. It became evident that the ustekinumab clinical efficacy was related to inhibition of the IL-23 biological effect.

The next step was to translate the consequence of blocking the IL-23, a cytokine involved in the differentiation of T cells producing IL-17, into the clinic. The selective inhibition of the biological activity of IL-17A, or its receptor IL-17RA, has demonstrated an impressive clinical efficacy in patients in the clinical trials. The most innovative approach currently is to block

Biological treatment	Mechanism action	Target	Relevance
DAB389-IL-2	Toxin acting on cells expressing IL-2 receptor	CD25	T-cells are important in psoriasis [9]
CTLA4-Ig	T cell costimulation blockade	CD80, CD86	Blocking T cell activation improve psoriasis [11]
LFA-3-Ig	Memory T cell depletion	CD2	Memory T cells are relevant in psoriasis [10]
Anti-LFA-1	T cell migration and T-cell costimulation inhibitor	LFA-1	Migration of T cells to psoriasis lesion is involved in disease [12]
Anti-TNF-α	Neutralization of biological activity	TNF-α	Biological activity of TNF-α is involved in psoriasis [65]
Anti-p40 (IL-12/ IL-23)	Neutralization of biological activity	p40 (IL-12/IL-23)	Cytokines involved in generating Th1 and Th17 are relevant in psoriasis [14]
Anti-IL-17A	Neutralization of I biological activity	IL-17A	Other cytokines besides TNF play a role in psoriasis [66]
Anti-IL-17RA	Blockade of receptor	IL-17RA	IL-17 signaling plays a relevant role in psoriasis [67]
Anti-IL-23p19	Neutralization of biological activity	IL-23p19	IL-23/Th17 axis play essential role in psoriasis [16]

Table 2. Targeted therapeutics that have evidenced clinically relevant mechanisms of psoriasis.

Biological treatment	Mechanism of action	Target	Relevance
IL-8	Neutralization of biological activity	IL-8	IL-8 is not clinically validated in psoriasis [68]
IFN-γ	Neutralization of biological activity	IFN-γ	IFN-γ is not clinically validated in psoriasis [69]
IFN-α	Neutralization of biological activity	IFN-α	IFN-α is not clinically validated in psoriasis [70]
IL-22	Neutralization of biological activity	IL-22	IL-22 is not clinically validated in psoriasis [71]

Table 3. Lack of efficacy by targeted therapeutics evidenced nonclinically validated mechanisms of psoriasis.

selectively IL-23, which also has confirmed the clinical relevance of specifically blocking the IL-23/Th17 in psoriasis [16].

In contrast to the mediators or cells that have confirmed its relevance in psoriasis due to its clinical importance in reducing disease severity, there are several well-known mechanisms present in psoriasis that have not been validated in the clinic, since their biological neutralization in the patient has not brought clinical benefit, see **Table 3**. Mediators such us IFN-γ, IFN-α, IL-8, and IL-22 have been neutralized in patients without significant clinical improvement.

When studying psoriasis triggering factors from the translational point of view, perhaps the best characterized environmental factor is throat infection by β-hemolytic streptococci. As it is commented below, there is a great body of evidences that associate streptococcal infection with psoriasis flares or exacerbations in both guttate and plaque psoriasis. This can be considered a translational opportunity of studying psoriasis immune response from a different and innovative perspective.

3. *Streptococcal pyogenes* infection and psoriasis

Throat infection by β-hemolytic streptococci has been associated with both the flare and exacerbation of psoriasis [17–19]. In guttate psoriasis, this infection precedes clinical cutaneous symptoms in 56–97% of the cases [20]. Interestingly, chronic plaque psoriasis patients are more susceptible to throat infections by *Streptococcus pyogenes* (*Sp*) than healthy controls [19], present increased levels of IgG for *S. pyogenes* in comparison to healthy controls [21], and a substantial proportion of patients suffer from disease exacerbations by streptococcal throat infections [22]. The association of *S. pyogenes* infection and psoriasis, besides being clinically evidenced for many years, may also open opportunities to treat psoriasis since several studies have shown that tonsillectomy can bring clinical benefits [23–26] and also improvement in the quality of life of the patients [26].

An immunological model has been proposed to explain how an infection taking place in the throat can lead to a chronic inflammation in a distant tissue such as the skin. One interesting observation is to note that dendritic cells from tonsils and upper respiratory truck are capable of generating some skin-tropic CLA+ T cells [27], thus indicating that those cells can acquire antigen-specificity for microbes infecting noncutaneous sites. In this regard, streptococcal superantigens promote the expression of CLA on T cells [28], as well as the activation and expansion of CLA+ T cells, at least from guttate psoriasis. Guttate psoriasis is an acute form of psoriasis, which erupts as small drop-shaped papules, and is frequently associated with streptococcal throat infection. In particular, accumulation of $V_{\beta}2^{+}$ T cells in acute guttate lesions has been reported, a variable β chain expressed on T cells that are preferentially expanded through the streptococcal pyrogenic exotoxin (SPE)-C [29], which contained T cells with different junctional sequences in the CDR3 region, thus supporting a superantigen-driven expansion. However, as psoriasis progresses, such superantigen hypothesis does not seem to explain the presence of identical TCR rearrangements in plaque psoriasis patients, probably indicating that a stable antigen-specific T-cell response is involved for longer stages of the disease [30, 31]. Interestingly, T-cell lines isolated from psoriatic lesions have shown strong cross-reactivity to streptococcal antigens [32]. Furthermore, restricted TCRVβ spectratypes shared by CLA+ T cells in streptococcal angina, but not by CLA− T cells, with T cells in psoriasis skin lesions supports the idea of the existence of a tonsillar source of antigen-driven T-cell expansion that then migrate to the skin [33]. Altogether, streptococcal superantigens could facilitate at least early migration of tonsillar T cells to the skin by upregulating CLA expression and could be especially involved in guttate-type flares.

S. pyogenes-primed T cells that reach the skin under postinfection circumstances are, however, unlikely to be maintained by the intracutaneous presence of streptococcal antigens in the skin for long periods of time. Therefore, other antigens would be responsible for the activation of those T cells. The hypothesis of molecular mimicry between streptococcal and skin peptides has been proposed by some authors. This view supports that CD8+ T cells could be cross-reacting to auto-epitopes presented through the context of MHC-I molecules on the surface of activated keratinocytes or cross-presenting dendritic cells [32, 34]. Actually, common determinants have been identified between streptococcal M-protein and skin keratins. Interestingly, the expression of M-protein is only associated with the three groups of β-hemolytic streptococci (A, C and G) that more often cause throat infections that precede the onset or exacerbations of psoriasis lesions [19]. In fact, circulating CLA+ T cells that cross-react with M-protein and human keratin 17, which is upregulated in psoriatic lesions, decrease after tonsillectomy and correlate with clinical improvement [35].

Despite the evidence of streptococcal involvement in psoriasis course, the use of antibiotics has not proven effectiveness in psoriasis [36]. However, it might be explained by the fact that streptococci can exist in intracellular reservoirs in the tonsillar epithelia and macrophages, and that could not be affected by the use of antibiotics. Then, this quiescent load could be reactivated and cause disease symptoms again, whereas tonsillectomy, which has been associated to clinical improvement, might remove this hidden pool of streptococci [22, 37].

Other entry routes for *S. pyogenes* can be considered, such as through the skin barrier itself, and could play a role as instigators of psoriasis disease. In fact, it has been detected in the skin but not in the throats of some guttate psoriasis patients [38]. Such presence, although transitory, might be enough to generate an antibacterial immune response that could lead to autoimmune reactions against local skin-derived peptides [39]. Overall, there is a strong relationship between streptococcal infections and subsequent clinical events in psoriasis that needs further attention.

4. *Streptococcus pyogenes*: an innate trigger that induces IL-17 production through skin-related memory CLA+ T cells in psoriasis

Analyzing the antigen-specific immune responses with clinically relevant stimuli in responding patients allows identifying pathologic translational mechanisms of several immunologic diseases, including psoriasis. This experimental approach can be reproduced *ex vivo* by coculturing circulating memory CLA+ T cells together with autologous epidermal cells from psoriasis patients and are activated by the *S. pyogenes* extract [40]. In this study, it was demonstrated that in psoriasis *S. pyogenes* preferentially activates cocultures of CLA+ T cells and epidermal cells, but not with CLA− T cells from the same patient, nor in cultures using CLA+/CLA− cells from healthy controls. The activation of CLA+ T cells showed at the transcript and protein level a response to the *S. pyogenes* extract with a mixed Th17/Th1/Th22 profile, since IL-17A, IFN-γ, and IL-22 were already upregulated in the coculture at 24 hours after activation and secreted as early as 48 hours. The CLA-dependent immune reaction in the coculture also included several other psoriasis-associated mediators such as the immune cell-chemoattractants CXCL8 (also known as IL-8), CXCL9, CXCL10, and CXCL11, which are expressed in psoriasis lesions [41], and when such enriched media were intradermally injected in mice, an epidermal hyperplasia was found. Furthermore, the presence of epidermal cells in the *ex vivo* model seems crucial for cytokine production through the activation with *S. pyogenes*, proving an intercellular interaction which may imply both CD4+ and CD8+ T cells. This conclusion was based on the observation that cytokine levels were highly impaired after blocking HLA class I and class II molecules. Interestingly, if circulating CLA+ T cells were cocultured with nonlesional epidermal cells, levels of several inflammatory mediators were upregulated when cells were activated with *S. pyogenes*, thus supporting the initial role of CLA+ T cells in driving nonlesional skin to the plaque formation [42, 43]. Overall, this novel model provided first evidence of a direct implication of CLA+ T cells and *S. pyogenes* in psoriasis samples treated *ex vivo*, while no such response was reproduced with healthy samples. These first results shed new light on the study of psoriasis, providing a tool for further valuable translational studies.

Since the closest and clearest relationship between streptococcal infection and subsequent onset of lesions has been described for guttate-type psoriasis, the evaluation of immune responses in the context of *S. pyogenes*-activation of key cellular components of psoriasis lesions from guttate psoriasis patients may generate more faithful results regarding the clinical status of such patients. Moreover, guttate psoriasis represents an important form of psoriasis since it contributes to its natural history. Actually, almost 40% of guttate psoriasis cases develop chronic plaque psoriasis in the future, and guttate-type eruptions are seen in plaque-affected patients [44]. Therefore, early events of psoriasis development can be studied in guttate psoriasis under the abovementioned microbial trigger [45].

A second study based on this *ex vivo* model focused on guttate psoriasis and revealed the importance of the Th17 immune response over other T cell-dependent responses, such as Th1, since IL-17A and IL-17F levels produced by CLA+ T cells in the cocultures in the presence of *S. pyogenes* extract were significantly higher than those of IFN-γ [46].

The importance of Th17 role in initial steps of psoriasis development is also supported by other findings, such as the high levels in serum of IL-17 found in patients with early spreading guttate form [47]. Even a bimodal immunopathology theory proposes that psoriasis is initiated by IL-1/Th17-dominated responses [48]. In addition to the well-known association of preceding pharyngitis episode, guttate psoriasis onset is mostly confined to individuals carrying the HLA-Cw6 allele [49], a genetic risk factor for early psoriasis. Interestingly, when immune responses from guttate psoriasis samples were classified according with the simultaneous presence of both genetic and environmental factors, that is HLA-Cw6 allele and a prior pharyngitis episode, respectively, the Th17-associated response was higher than that exerted by samples from the other "nonpredisposed" guttate psoriatic individuals. In fact, significant higher levels of IL-17A, IL-17F, and even IL-6, which participates in Th17-differentiation, were found in those "predisposed" guttate psoriasis patients. Furthermore, the treatment of *in vitro* cultured normal keratinocytes with those Th17-predominant supernatants produced by CLA+ T cells in the cocultures, resulted in the upregulation of the IL-17-targeted transcripts *DEFB4, S100A7, LCN2, IL36G*, and *IL8*, which are all overexpressed in psoriasis lesions [50]. Interestingly, filaggrin and loricrin, encoded by *FLG* and *LOR* genes, respectively, which are important skin barrier proteins whose expression is impaired in psoriatic lesions [51, 52], were downregulated in those same treated keratinocytes. Therefore, *S. pyogenes* selective-activation of CLA+ T cells in the presence of epidermal cells from high-responders guttate psoriasis samples recreates a psoriasis-like inflammatory milieu, thus supporting the high translational value of this *ex vivo* model.

Therapies targeting the IL-23/Th17-axis are showing the best efficacy rates in terms of percentage of patients reaching PASI improvement. The observation of rapid normalization of hundreds of psoriasis-related genes as soon as 2 weeks after the use of IL-17A or IL-17RA-blocking antibodies [53, 54] may partly explain the importance of IL-17A effects in psoriasis pathology, and why its blockade provides such impressive clinical improvement. Therefore, the characterization of IL-17-targeted transcripts that are rapidly normalized after these therapies could reveal relevant information regarding to the development of skin lesions.

In this regard, Ruiz-Romeu et al. [55] have taken advantage of the use of CLA+ T cell and epidermal cells activated by SE conditioned supernatants to activate normal keratinocytes and to evaluate gene expression of noncharacterized IL-17A targets. In their study, they characterize the expression of *ZC3H12A*, a gene whose rapid normalization was found in gene arrays of biopsies taken from psoriasis patients treated with the anti-IL-17A monoclonal antibody [53]. *ZC3H12A* encodes for the ribonuclease MCPIP1, and it was upregulated in keratinocytes treated with enriched supernatants in an IL-17A-dependent manner. The fact that lack of upregulation in *Zc3h12a* expression in the skin of an innate psoriasis model induced in *Il17ra*$^{-/-}$ mice supports the key dependence on IL-17 for its increased expression in psoriasis. MCPIP1 activity has been linked to many different biological processes within various cell types, such as inhibition of inflammation, angiogenesis, cell migration, or cell differentiation [56], but no prior evidence of MCPIP1 expression and function in the skin had been reported. In this study, MCPIP1 expression was found to be aberrantly expressed by suprabasal keratinocytes of psoriasis lesions, which is consistent with the distribution of that described for IL-17RA in the psoriatic epidermis [57, 58]. In this regard, only differentiating keratinocytes isolated from psoriatic lesional skin, but not from healthy skin, were susceptible to undergo an increased expression of MCPIP1 to exogenous IL-17A. Regarding to the potential role of MCPIP1 ribonuclease activity, genes involved in epidermal differentiation, or other altered transcripts in psoriasis lesions, are modified after a *ZC3H12A* knockdown in keratinocytes.

5. Conclusions

The translational approach of developing an *ex vivo* model using peripheral CLA+ T cells and epidermal cells, activated by a clinically relevant innate trigger, such as *S. pyogenes*, can be useful in the characterization of immune responses and new molecular mechanisms that could be involved in the psoriasis pathogenesis.

Acknowledgements

The study was funded by FIS/ISCIII 2013 (Ministerio de Economía y Competitividad e Instituto de Salud Carlos III; PI09/2222, PI13/01845 and PI13/01716) and FIS/ISCIII 2016 (PI16/01573 and PI016/99532). This work was supported by European Regional Development Fund grants. E. R. R was granted by a PhD fellowship by the Ministerio de Educación, Cultura y Deporte of the Spanish Government (FPU13/02308).

Author details

Ester Ruiz-Romeu and Luis F. Santamaria-Babi*

*Address all correspondence to: luis.santamaria@ub.edu

Translational Immunology, Department of Cellular Biology, Physiology and Immunology, Faculty of Biology, University of Barcelona, Barcelona, Spain

References

[1] Picker L, and Butcher E. Physiological and molecular mechanisms of lymphocyte homing. Annu Rev Immunol. 1992; 10: 561-591. 10.1146/annurev.iy.10.040192.003021

[2] Picker L, Michie S, Rott L, Butcher E. A unique phenotype of skin-associated lymphocytes in humans. Preferential expression of the HECA-452 epitope by benign and malignant T cells at cutaneous sites. Am J Pathol. 1990; 136: 1053-1068.

[3] Ferran M, Romeu E, Rincon C, Sagrista M, Gimenez Arnau A, Celada A, Pujol R, Hollo P, Jokai H, Santamaria-Babi L. Circulating CLA+ T lymphocytes as peripheral cell biomarkers in T-cell-mediated skin diseases. Exp Dermatol. 2013; 22: 439-442. 10.1111/exd.12154

[4] Santamaria Babi L, Moser R, Perez Soler M, Picker L, Blaser K, Hauser C. Migration of skin-homing T cells across cytokine-activated human endothelial cell layers involves interaction of the cutaneous lymphocyte-associated antigen (CLA), the very late antigen-4 (VLA-4), and the lymphocyte function-associated antigen-1 (LFA-1). J Immunol. 1995; 154: 1543-1550.

[5] Czarnowicki T, Santamaria-Babi L, Guttman-Yassky E. Circulating CLA+ T cells in atopic dermatitis and their possible role as peripheral biomarkers. Allergy. 2016; 72: 366-372

[6] Santamaria Babi L, Perez Soler M, Hauser C, Blaser K. Skin-homing T cells in human cutaneous allergic inflammation. Immunol Res. 1995; 14: 317-324. 90232 [pii];10.1159/000090232

[7] Guttman-Yassky, Krueger J. Psoriasis: evolution of pathogenic concepts and new therapies through phases of translational research. Br J Dermatol. 2007; 157: 1103-1115. BJD8135 [pii];10.1111/j.1365-2133.2007.08135.x

[8] Kim J, Krueger JG. Highly effective new treatments for psoriasis target the IL-23/Type 17 T Cell autoimmune axis. Annu Rev Med. 2017; 68: 255-269. 10.1056/NEJM200107263450403

[9] Gottlieb SL, Gilleaudeau P, Johnson R, Estes L, Woodworth TG, Gottlieb AB, Krueger JG: 1995. Response of psoriasis to a lymphocyte-selective toxin (DAB389IL-2) suggests a primary immune, but not keratinocyte, pathogenic basis. Nat Med. 1995; 1: 442-447.

[10] Ellis CN, Krueger GC. Treatment of chronic plaque psoriasis by selective targeting of memory effector T lymphocytes. N Engl J Med. 2001; 345: 248-255. 10.1056/NEJM200107263450403

[11] Abrams JR, Kelley SL, Hayes E, Kikuchi T, Brown MJ, Kang S, Lebwohl MG, Guzzo CA, Jegasothy BV, Linsley PS, Krueger JG. Blockade of T lymphocyte costimulation with cytotoxic T lymphocyte-associated antigen 4-immunoglobulin (CTLA4Ig) reverses the cellular pathology of psoriatic plaques, including the activation of keratinocytes, dendritic cells, and endothelial cells. J Exp Med. 2000; 192: 681-694.

[12] Gottlieb AB, Miller B, Lowe N, Shapiro W, Hudson C, Bright R, Ling M, Magee A, McCall CO, Rist T, Dummer W, Walicke P, Bauer RJ, White M, Garovoy M. Subcutaneously administered efalizumab (anti-CD11a) improves signs and symptoms of moderate to severe plaque psoriasis. J Cutan Med Surg. 2003; 7: 198-207. 10.1007/s10227-002-0118-1

[13] Zaba LC, Cardinale I, Gilleaudeau P, Sullivan-Whalen M, Suarez-Farinas M, Fuentes-Duculan J, Novitskaya I, Khatcherian A, Bluth MJ, Lowes MA, Krueger JG. Amelioration of epidermal hyperplasia by TNF inhibition is associated with reduced Th17 responses. J Exp Med. 2007; 204: 3183-3194. jem.20071094 [pii];10.1084/jem.20071094

[14] Leonardi CL, Kimball AB, Papp KA, Yeilding N, Guzzo C, Wang Y, Li S, Dooley LT, and Gordon KB. Efficacy and safety of ustekinumab, a human interleukin-12/23 monoclonal antibody, in patients with psoriasis: 76-week results from a randomised, double-blind, placebo-controlled trial (PHOENIX 1). Lancet. 2008; 371: 1665-1674. S0140-6736(08)60725-4 [pii];10.1016/S0140 6736(08)60725-4.

[15] Lee E, Trepicchio WL, Oestreicher JL, Pittman D, Wang F, Chamian F, Dhodapkar M, Krueger JG. Increased expression of interleukin 23 p19 and p40 in lesional skin of patients with psoriasis vulgaris. J Exp Med. 2004; 199: 125-130. 10.1084/jem.20030451 [doi];199/1/125

[16] Sofen H, Smith S, Matheson RT, Leonardi CL, Calderon C, Brodmerkel C, Li K, Campbell K, Marciniak SJ, Wasfi Y, Wang Y, Szapary P, Krueger JG. Guselkumab (an IL-23-specific mAb) demonstrates clinical and molecular response in patients with moderate-to-severe psoriasis. J Allergy Clin Immunol. 2014; 133: 1032-1040. S0091-6749(14)00181-X [pii];10.1016/j.jaci.2014.01.025

[17] Telfer NR, Chalmers RJ, Whale J, Colman G. The role of streptococcal infection in the initiation of guttate psoriasis. Arch Dermatol. 1992; 128: 39-42.

[18] Wardrop P, Weller R, Marais J, Kavanagh G. Tonsillitis and chronic psoriasis. Clin Otolaryngol Allied Sci.1998; 23: 67-68.

[19] Gudjonsson JE, Thorarinsson AM, Sigurgeirsson S, Kristinsson KG, Valdimarsson H. Streptococcal throat infections and exacerbation of chronic plaque psoriasis: a prospective study. Br J Dermatol. 2003; 149: 530-534. 5552 [pii]

[20] Prin JC. Psoriasis vulgaris—a sterile antibacterial skin reaction mediated by cross-reactive T cells? An immunological view of the pathophysiology of psoriasis. Clin Exp Dermatol. 2001; 26: 326-332. ced831 [pii]

[21] El-Rachkidy RG, Hales JM, Freestone PP, Young HS, Griffiths CE, Camp RD Increased blood levels of IgG reactive with secreted *Streptococcus pyogenes* proteins in chronic plaque psoriasis. J Invest Dermatol. 2007; 127: 1337-1342. S0022-202X(15)33401-1 [pii];10.1038/sj.jid.5700744

[22] Thorleifsdottir RH, Eysteinsdottir JH, J. Olafsson JH, Sigurdsson MI, Johnston A, Valdimarsson H, Sigurgeirsson. Throat infections are associated with exacerbation in a substantial proportion of patients with chronic plaque psoriasis. Acta Derm Venereol. 2016; 96: 788-791. 10.2340/00015555-2408

[23] Thorleifsdottir RH, Sigurdardottir SL, Sigurgeirsson B, Olafsson JH, Sigurdsson MI, Petersen H, Arnadottir S, Gudjonsson JE, Johnston A, Valdimarsson H. Improvement of psoriasis after tonsillectomy is associated with a decrease in the frequency of circulating T cells that recognize streptococcal determinants and homologous skin determinants. J Immunol. 2012; 188: 5160-5165. jimmunol.1102834 [pii];10.4049/jimmunol.1102834

[24] Hone SW, Donnelly MJ, Powell F, Blayney AW. Clearance of recalcitrant psoriasis after tonsillectomy. Clin Otolaryngol Allied Sci. 1996; 21: 546-547.

[25] Nyfors A, Rasmussen PA, Lemholt K, Eriksen B. Improvement of recalcitrant psoriasis vulgaris after tonsillectomy. J Laryngol Otol. 1976; 90: 789-794.

[26] Thorleifsdottir RH, Sigurdardottir SL, Sigurgeirsson B, Olafsson JH, Sigurdsson MI, Petersen H, Gudjonsson JE, Johnston A, Valdimarsson H. Patient-reported outcomes and clinical response in patients with moderate-to-severe plaque psoriasis treated with tonsillectomy: a randomized controlled trial. Acta Derm Venereol. 2017; 97: 340-345.

[27] Sabat R, Philipp S, Hoflich C, Kreutzer S, Wallace E, Asadullah K, Volk HD, Sterry W, Wolk K. Immunopathogenesis of psoriasis. Exp Dermatol. 2007; 16: 779-798. EXD629 [pii];10.1111/j.1600-0625.2007.00629.x

[28] Leung DY, Gately M, Trumble A, Ferguson-Darnell B, Schlievert PM, Picker LJ. Bacterial superantigens induce T cell expression of the skin-selective homing receptor, the cutaneous lymphocyte-associated antigen, via stimulation of interleukin 12 production. J Exp Med. 1995; 181: 747-753.

[29] Leung DY, Travers JB, Giorno R, Norris DA, Skinner R, Aelion J, Kazemi LV, Kim MH, Trumble AE, Kotb M. Evidence for a streptococcal superantigen-driven process in acute guttate psoriasis. J Clin Invest. 1995; 96: 2106-2112. 10.1172/JCI118263

[30] Prinz JC, Vollmer S, Boehncke WH, Menssen A, Laisney I, Trommler P. Selection of conserved TCR VDJ rearrangements in chronic psoriatic plaques indicates a common antigen in psoriasis vulgaris. Eur J Immunol. 1999; 29: 3360-3368. 10.1002/(SICI)1521-4141(199910)29:10<3360::AID-IMMU3360>3.0.CO;2-G[pii];10.1002/(SICI)1521-4141(199910) 29:10<3360::AID-IMMU3360>3.0.CO;2-G

[31] Vollmer S, Menssen A, Prinz JC. Dominant lesional T cell receptor rearrangements persist in relapsing psoriasis but are absent from nonlesional skin: evidence for a stable antigen-specific pathogenic T cell response in psoriasis vulgaris. J Invest Dermatol. 2001; 117: 1296-1301. S0022-202X(15)41455-1 [pii];10.1046/j.0022-202x.2001.01494.x

[32] Valdimarsson H, Thorleifsdottir RH, Sigurdardottir SL, Gudjonsson JE, Johnston A. Psoriasis—as an autoimmune disease caused by molecular mimicry. Trends Immunol. 2009; 30: 494-501. S1471-4906(09)00153-7 [pii];10.1016/j.it.2009.07.008

[33] Diluvio L, Vollmer S, Besgen P, Ellwart JW, Chimenti S, Prinz JC. Identical TCR beta-chain rearrangements in streptococcal angina and skin lesions of patients with psoriasis vulgaris. J Immunol. 2006; 176: 7104-7111. 176/11/7104

[34] Gudjonsson JE, Johnston A, Sigmundsdottir H, Valdimarsson H. Immunopathogenic mechanisms in psoriasis. Clin Exp Immunol. 2004; 135: 1-8. 2310 [pii]

[35] Thorleifsdottir RH, Sigurdardottir SL, Sigurgeirsson B, Olafsson JH, Sigurdsson ML, Petersen H, Arnadottir S, Gudjonsson JE, Johnston A, Valdimarsson H. Improvement of psoriasis after tonsillectomy is associated with a decrease in the frequency of circulating T cells that recognize streptococcal determinants and homologous skin determinants. J Immunol. 2012; 188: 5160-5165. jimmunol.1102834 [pii];10.4049/jimmunol. 1102834

[36] Owen CM, Chalmers RJ, O'Sullivan T, Griffiths CE. A systematic review of antistreptococcal interventions for guttate and chronic plaque psoriasis. Br J Dermatol. 2001 145: 886-890.

[37] Osterlund A, Popa R, Nikkila T, Scheynius A, Engstrand L. Intracellular reservoir of *Streptococcus pyogenes* in vivo: a possible explanation for recurrent pharyngotonsillitis. Laryngoscope. 1997; 107: 640-647.

[38] Fahlen A, Engstrand L, Baker BS, Powles A, Fry L. Comparison of bacterial microbiota in skin biopsies from normal and psoriatic skin. Arch Dermatol Res. 2012; 304: 15-22. 10.1007/s00403-011-1189-x

[39] Mallbris L, Larsson P, Bergqvist S, Vingard E, Granath F, Stahle M. Psoriasis phenotype at disease onset: clinical characterization of 400 adult cases. J Invest Dermatol. 2005; 124: 499-504. S0022-202X(15)32215-6 [pii];10.1111/j.0022-202X.2004.23611.x

[40] Ferran M, Galvan AB, Rincon C, Romeu ER, Sacrista M, Barboza E, Gimenez-Arnau A, Celada A, Pujol RM, Santamaria-Babi LF. Streptococcus induces circulating CLA(+) memory T-cell-dependent epidermal cell activation in psoriasis. J. Invest Dermatol. 2013; 133: 999-1007. S0022-202X(15)36179-0 [pii];10.1038/jid.2012.418

[41] Nograles KE, Zaba LC, Guttman-Yassky E, Fuentes-Duculan J, Suarez-Farinas M, Cardinale I, Khatcherian A, Gonzalez J, Pierson JC, White TR, Pensabene C, Coats I, Novitskaya I, Lowes MA, Krueger JG. Th17 cytokines interleukin (IL)-17 and IL-22 modulate distinct inflammatory and keratinocyte-response pathways. Br J Dermatol. 2008; 159: 1092-1102. BJD8769 [pii];10.1111/j.1365-2133.2008.08769.x

[42] Vissers, WH, Arndtz CH, Muys L, Van Erp PE,. de Jong E M, and van de Kerkhof PC. 2004. Memory effector (CD45RO+) and cytotoxic (CD8+) T cells appear early in the margin zone of spreading psoriatic lesions in contrast to cells expressing natural killer receptors, which appear late. Br J Dermatol. 150: 852-859. 10.1111/j.1365-2133.2004.05863.x [doi];BJD5863

[43] Davison SC, Ballsdon A, Allen MH, Barker JN. Early migration of cutaneous lymphocyte-associated antigen (CLA) positive T cells into evolving psoriatic plaques. Exp Dermatol. 2001; 10: 280-285. exd100408

[44] Langley RG, Krueger GK, Griffiths CE. Psoriasis: epidemiology, clinical features, and quality of life. Ann Rheum Dis. 2005; 64(Suppl 2): ii18–ii23. 64/suppl_2/ii18 [pii];10.1136/ard.2004.033217

[45] Weisenseel P, Laumbacher B, Besgen P, Ludolph-Hauser D, Herzinger T, Roecken M, Wank R, Prinz JC. Streptococcal infection distinguishes different types of psoriasis. J. Med. Genet. 2002; 39: 767-768.

[46] Ruiz-Romeu E, Ferran M, Sagrista M, Gomez J, Gimenez-Arnau A, Herszenyi K, Hollo P, Celada A, Pujol R, Santamaria-Babi LF. *Streptococcus pyogenes*-induced cutaneous lymphocyte antigen-positive T cell-dependent epidermal cell activation triggers TH17 responses in patients with guttate psoriasis. J Allergy Clin Immunol. 2016; 138: 491-499. S0091-6749(16)00360-2 [pii];10.1016/j.jaci.2016.02.008

[47] Choe YB, Hwang YJ, Hahn HJ, Jung JW, Jung HJ, Lee YW, Ahn KJ, Youn JI. A comparison of serum inflammatory cytokines according to phenotype in patients with psoriasis. Br J Dermatol. 2012; 167: 762-767. 10.1111/j.1365-2133.2012.11038.x

[48] Christophers E, Metzler G, Rocken M. Bimodal immune activation in psoriasis. Br J Dermatol. 2014;170: 59-65. 10.1111/bjd.12631

[49] Asumalahti K, Ameen M, Suomela S, Hagforsen E, Michaelsson G, Evans J, Munro M, Veal C, Allen M, Leman J, David BA, Kirby B, Connolly M, Griffiths CE, Trembath RC, Kere J, Saarialho-Kere U, Barker JN. Genetic analysis of PSORS1 distinguishes guttate psoriasis and palmoplantar pustulosis. J Invest Dermatol. 2003; 120: 627-632. S0022-202X(15)30213-X [pii];10.1046/j.1523-1747.2003.12094.x

[50] Chiricozzi A,Guttman-Yassky E, Suarez-Farinas M, Nograles K E, Tian S, Cardinale I, Chimenti S, Krueger JG. Integrative responses to IL-17 and TNF-alpha in human keratinocytes account for key inflammatory pathogenic circuits in psoriasis. J Invest Dermatol. 2011; 131: 677-687. S0022-202X(15)35175-7 [pii];10.1038/jid.2010.340

[51] Kim BE, Howell MD, Guttman-Yassky E, Gilleaudeau PM, Cardinale IR, Boguniewicz M, Krueger JG, Leung DY. TNF-alpha downregulates filaggrin and loricrin through c-Jun N-terminal kinase: role for TNF-alpha antagonists to improve skin barrier. J Invest Dermatol. 2011; 131: 1272-1279. S0022-202X(15)35315-X [pii];10.1038/jid.2011.24

[52] Roberson ED, Bowcock AM. Psoriasis genetics: breaking the barrier. Trends Genet. 2010; 26: 415-423. S0168-9525(10)00129-0 [pii];10.1016/j.tig.2010.06.006

[53] Krueger JG, Fretzin S, Suarez-Farinas M, Haslett PA, Phipps KM, Cameron GS, McColm J, Katcherian A, Cueto I, White T, Banerjee S, Hoffman RW. IL-17A is essential for cell activation and inflammatory gene circuits in subjects with psoriasis. J Allergy Clin Immunol. 2012; 130: 145-154. S0091-6749(12)00695-1 [pii];10.1016/j.jaci.2012.04.024

[54] Russell CB, Rand H, Bigler J, Kerkof K, Timour M, Bautista E, Krueger JG, Salinger DH, Welcher AA, Martin DA. Gene expression profiles normalized in psoriatic skin by treatment with brodalumab, a human anti-IL-17 receptor monoclonal antibody. J Immunol. 2014; 192: 3828-3836. jimmunol.1301737 [pii];10.4049/jimmunol.1301737

[55] Ruiz-Romeu E, Ferran M, Gimenez-Arnau A, Bugara B, Lipert B, Jura J, Florencia EF, Prens EP, Celada A, Pujol RM, Santamaria-Babi LF. MCPIP1 RNase Is Aberrantly Distributed in Psoriatic Epidermis and Rapidly Induced by IL-17A. J Invest Dermatol. 2016; 136: 1599-1607. S0022-202X(16)31153-8 [pii];10.1016/j.jid.2016.04.030

[56] Chao J, Dai X, Pena T, Doyle DA, Guenther TM, Carlson MA. MCPIP1 Regulates Fibroblast Migration in 3-D Collagen Matrices Downstream of MAP Kinases and NF-kappaB. J Invest Dermatol. 2015; 135: 2944-2954. S0022-202X(15)60179-8 [pii];10.1038/jid.2015.334

[57] Chiricozzi A, Nograles KE, Johnson-Huang LM, Fuentes-Duculan J, Cardinale I, Bonifacio KM, Gulati N, Mitsui H, Guttman-Yassky E, Suarez-Farinas M, Krueger JG. IL-17 induces an expanded range of downstream genes in reconstituted human epidermis model. PLoS One. 2014; 9: e90284. 10.1371/journal.pone.0090284 [doi];PONE-D-13-37082

[58] Peric M, Koglin S, Kim SM, Morizane S, Besch R, Prinz JC, Ruzicka T, Gallo RL, Schauber J. IL-17A enhances vitamin D3-induced expression of cathelicidin antimicrobial peptide in human keratinocytes. J. Immunol. 2008; 181: 8504-8512. 181/12/8504

[59] Santamaria Babi LF, Picker LJ, Perez Soler MT, Drzimalla K, Flohr P, Blaser K, Hauser C. Circulating allergen-reactive T cells from patients with atopic dermatitis and allergic

contact dermatitis express the skin-selective homing receptor, the cutaneous lymphocyte-associated antigen. J Exp Med. 1995; 181: 1935-1940.

[60] Abernathy-Carver KJ, Sampson HA, Picker LJ, Leung DY. Milk-induced eczema is associated with the expansion of T cells expressing cutaneous lymphocyte antigen. J Clin Invest. 1995. 95: 913-918. 10.1172/JCI117743

[61] Torres MJ, Gonzalez FJ, Corzo JL, Giron MD, Carvajal MJ, Garcia V, Pinedo A, Martinez-Valverde A, Blanca M, Santamaria LF. Circulating CLA+ lymphocytes from children with atopic dermatitis contain an increased percentage of cells bearing staphylococcal-related T-cell receptor variable segments. Clin Exp Allergy. 1998; 28: 1264-1272.

[62] Blanca M, Leyva L, Torres MJ, Mayorga C, Cornejo-Garcia J, Antunez-Rodriguez C, Santamaria LF, Juarez C. Memory to the hapten in non-immediate cutaneous allergic reactions to betalactams resides in a lymphocyte subpopulation expressing both CD45RO and CLA markers. Blood Cells Mol Dis. 2003; 31: 75-79. S1079979603000615

[63] Koelle DM, Liu Z, McClurkan CM, Topp MS, Riddell SR, Pamer EG, Johnson AS, Wald A, Corey L. Expression of cutaneous lymphocyte-associated antigen by CD8(+) T cells specific for a skin-tropic virus. J Clin Invest. 2002 110: 537-548. 10.1172/JCI15537

[64] Ogg GS, Rod DP, Romero P, Chen JL, Cerundolo V. High frequency of skin-homing melanocyte-specific cytotoxic T lymphocytes in autoimmune vitilig. J Exp Med. 1998; 188: 1203-1208.

[65] Oh CJ, Das KM, Gottlieb AB. Treatment with anti-tumor necrosis factor alpha (TNF-alpha) monoclonal antibody dramatically decreases the clinical activity of psoriasis lesions. J Am Acad Dermatol. 2000; 42: 829-830. S0190962200907321

[66] Leonardi C, Matheson R, Zachariae C, Cameron G, Li L, Edson-Heredia E, Braun D, Banerjee S. Anti-interleukin-17 monoclonal antibody ixekizumab in chronic plaque psoriasis. N Engl J Med. 2012; 366: 1190-1199. 10.1056/NEJMoa1109997

[67] Papp KA, Leonardi C, Menter A, Ortonne JP, Krueger JG, Kricorian G, Aras G, Li J, Russell CB, Thompson EH, Baumgartner S. Brodalumab, an anti-interleukin-17-receptor antibody for psoriasis. N Engl J Med. 2012; 366: 1181-1189. 10.1056/NEJMoa1109017

[68] http://www.siliconinvestor.com/readmsgs.aspx?subjectid=24141&msgnum=97&batchsize=10&batchtype=Next

[69] https://business.highbeam.com/436989/article-1G1-110130198/fontolizumab-protein-design-discontinued-usa

[70] Bissonnette R, Papp K, Maari C, Yao Y, Robbie G, White WI, Le C, White B. A randomized, double-blind, placebo-controlled, phase I study of MEDI-545, an anti-interferon-alfa monoclonal antibody, in subjects with chronic psoriasis. J Am Acad Dermatol. 2010; 62: 427-436. S0190-9622(09)00686-0 [pii];10.1016/j.jaad.2009.05.042

[71] Antoniu SA. Discontinued drugs 2011: pulmonary, allergy, gastrointestinal and arthritis. Expert Opin Investig Drugs. 2012; 21: 1607-1618. 10.1517/13543784.2012.712112

Chapter 5

Psoriatic Animal Models Developed for the Study of the Disease

Sandra Rodríguez-Martínez, Juan C. Cancino-Diaz,
Isaí Martínez-Torrez, Sonia M. Pérez-Tapia and
Mario E. Cancino-Diaz

Additional information is available at the end of the chapter

http://dx.doi.org/10.5772/intechopen.68305

Abstract

Psoriasis is a skin disease mainly developed in humans, although it is also seen in monkeys and dogs. Animal models with psoriasis-like lesions have been a key factor for its understanding. Xenotransplants of human psoriatic skin in immunodeficient mice were the first approach for the association of immunologic problems with the development of psoriasis and have been also useful for the evaluation on new therapeutic agents. Imiquimod-induced murine psoriasis is nowadays one of the most used animal models to study this disease, perhaps because healthy wild-type mice are used, which means that it is an affordable model, easy to generate, and, more importantly, resembles the inflammatory, angiogenic and hyperproliferative characteristics of human psoriasis. Several transgenic (over-expressing VEGF, Tie2, TGFβ, STAT3, IL-36, PPARβ/γ) and knockout (lacking IκBα, JunB, IFNR-2, IL-36RA, CD18, IKK2) mice have been useful for the association of specific molecules for the development of psoriasis. Other approach has been the use of both transgenic/knockout mice and imiquimod treatment, where the importance of βTrCP, IκBζ, IL-35 and Tnip1 for the development of psoriasis was found. In this chapter, some of these animal models are discussed.

Keywords: psoriasis, animal models, skin immunology, angiogenesis, keratinocytes

1. Introduction

Psoriasis is a disease that has been accompanying the existence of humans. The ancient Greeks described an illness that seems to be psoriasis, but it could be confused with leprosy or Hansen's disease [1]. Because psoriasis develops naturally in humans but rarely in other species [2, 3], the study of this disease was possible only after progress was made on immunology and on genetic engineering knowledge. Although reports on animals with psoriatic lesions due spontaneous mutations exist, the phenotype does not completely resemble human psoriasis, as occur with the homozygous asebia (Scd1ab/Scd1ab) mutant mice, the Flaky skin mice (Ttcfsn/Ttcfsn) and the spontaneous chronic proliferative dermatitis mutation mice [4, 5]. Now, with the advances on genetic engineering, some transgenic animals and animals with targeted mutations (knockout and knock-in) have been developed to study psoriasis. In the case of knockout models, the targeted gene is inactivated and the phenotype is caused by the absence of the targeted gene product. In the case of knock-in model, the gene is modified through targeted point mutation, with the addition or deletion of a nucleotide, instead of complete disruption of the target gene expression, and the phenotype depends on the expression of modified gene products. Knockout and knock-in animals are also developed with the use of tissue specific promoters to eliminate or express the targeted gene, and even more, the expression or suppression of the gene could be controlled by specific promoter regulators, where antibiotics and hormones are frequently used [6].

Another strategy to study psoriasis and other dermatologic illnesses in vitro is the development of 2nd- or 3rd-dimensional cell co-cultures. These systems have the limitation that so far has not been possible to include all the cellular types that are part of the skin, but have been very useful to evaluate new drugs for treatment [7].

2. Immunological factors in psoriasis

2.1. Humanized animal models (xenotransplantation)

Xenotransplantation was the first approach generated as animal model for the study of psoriasis and for the evaluation of anti-psoriatic treatments that consists in the transplantation of human skin in the back of inmunodeficient mice. In 1994, the first murine psoriasis model done in mice with severe combined immunodeficiency (SCID) was described. These mice have the so-called scid mutation that affects the "protein kinase DNA activated catalytic polypeptide" (Prkdc/DNA-PKcs), causing a defect in the antigen receptor gene rearrangement of lymphocytes, and consequently a SCID of the T- and B-cell systems [8]. In these mice, the psoriatic phenotype is kept for 2 months, enough time for the analysis of the disease. Later, it was demonstrated that mice with non-psoriatic human skin transplants that received lymphocytes from the psoriatic skin developed psoriasis; these facts demonstrated the importance of the immunologic factor for the development of this disease [9]. Also, the so-called nude mice are used to study psoriasis; these mice have a mutation in the forkhead box transcription factor N1 that results in defective thymus development, and therefore in lack functional T cells, or nude mice that lack recombinase activating genes 1 (Rag1) and 2 (Rag2) involved in the development of T and B cells.

2.2. Imiquimod-induced murine psoriasis (IMQ-Mu-Pso)

This transient model of psoriasis-like disease was developed by Van der Fits et al. [10], using non-genetically modified healthy mice daily treated with topic imiquimod or resiquimod (TLR7-TLR8 ligand) for 6 days. This simple model shows wide characteristics described in the human psoriatic skin lesions, including: activation of pDC, Th17 cells producing IL-17, IL-22 and IL-23, activation of angiogenic process and hyperproliferacion of keratinocytes. IMQ-Mu-Pso model is generated due to an acute inflammation in the epidermis induced by imiquimod, hyperactivating the innate immunity and leading the adaptive immunity to produce great amounts of IL-17. IL-17, in turn, induces angiogenesis and proliferation of keratinocytes, as biological characteristics of psoriatic lesions. IMQ-Mu-Pso also demonstrated that undisrupted molecular and cellular mechanisms are able to break inflammation, as mice used for this model are healthy mice that show the highest production of inflammatory cytokines on the third day of treatment and show the highest development of psoriatic skin on the sixth day, but after this time, the mice are able to revert the inflammatory process as they are not genetically compromised. The short lasting presence of psoriatic lesions is an inconvenience of this model, although it has been widely used to elucidate the pathogenesis of psoriasis, and very interesting data have been published [10].

2.3. Intestinal microbiome affects the induction of psoriasis

The absence of 100% concordance between monozygotic twins suggests a crucial role of environmental factors for the development of psoriasis, as only 35–75% of monozygotic twins develop psoriasis; alcohol intake and smoking are considered non genetic factors that predispose individuals to develop psoriasis [11]. Intestinal microbiota has an important effect on the development and function of the immune system, for instance, a specific subset of microbiota has been shown to play roles in the development of Th17, meanwhile other subset favors the development of Treg cells [12]. Another study showed that microbiota from skin of psoriatic patients is different from healthy subjects; *Proteobacteria* were present at significantly higher levels in the psoriatic skin compared to limb skin used as control (52 vs. 32%, $p = 0.0113$), and in the same study, both *Staphylococci* and *Propionibacteria* were significantly lower in psoriasis versus control ($p = 0.051$, 0.046, respectively) [13]. In 2015, Zanvit et al. demonstrated that psoriasis is mediated by the early interaction between certain subset of bacterial microbiota and cells of immune system [14]. They treated 4-week-old mice with oral antibiotics (vancomycin and polymyxin B) showing a decrease in the severity of psoriasis compared to mice without antibiotics using the IMQ-Mu-Pso model. IL-17+ and IL-22+ T cells were significantly decreased in skin and gut in the antibiotic-treated mice; however, the Foxp3+ Treg cells were significantly increased in the skin of these mice. In contrast, when neonatal mice received the antibiotic treatment and the psoriasis was induced with imiquimod as 4-week old, they observed an increase in the severity of disease compared to mice without antibiotic treatment evidenced by the presence of immunological cells infiltration and by the increase of thickness in dermis; besides they did not find augment of IL-17+ cells, but significant increase of IL-22+ cells. The intestinal microbiota was also considerably different between mice treated with antibiotics as adults from those treated as neonates [14]. These results settle that among the factors that predispose to psoriasis is intestinal microbiota that depends on breast feed as neonates, type of food intake, but also on the use of antibiotics.

2.4. Disruption of NFκB and AP-1 to generate psoriasis in animal models

Innate immunity in skin is mediated by the activation of membrane receptors expressed on dendritic cells, Langerhans cells and macrophages activated by pathogens- or damage-molecular patterns (PAMP or DAMP). After ligand-receptor interaction, molecular signaling events occur into the cell leading to the activation of transcription factors, such as NFκB and AP-1 that translocate into the nucleus for the expression of cytokines and antimicrobial peptides [15]. The malfunctioning in the regulation of the activity of these transcription factors could lead to the development of psoriatic lesions, as we next describe.

In unstimulated cells, NFκB dimers are sequestered in the cytoplasm by a family of inhibitors called IκB (Inhibitor of κB), and the IκB proteins mask the nuclear localization signals (NLS) of NFκB proteins and keep them sequestered in an inactive state in the cytoplasm. Activation of NFκB is initiated by the signal-induced degradation of IκB proteins; this occurs primarily by the activation of a kinase called IκB kinase (IKK). When activated by PAMPs or DAMPs, IKK phosphorylates two serine residues located in IκBα's regulatory domain, and then IκBα is ubiquitinated and degraded by the proteasome. With the degradation of IκBα, NFκB dimer is freed to enter into the nucleus to initiate the expression of specific genes that have DNA-binding sites for NFκB at their promoter site. The transcription of the targeted genes initiates a physiological response, for example, inflammation, cell survival and cellular proliferation. In fact, NFκB turns on the expression of its own repressor, IκBα. The newly synthesized IκBα then inhibits NFκB activity controlling the function of NFκB in an oscillatory way [15].

In IMQ-Mu-Pso, the severity of psoriatic lesions has been associated with a reduced presence of IκBα due over-degradation and in consequence with an enhanced NFκB activation. IκBα knockout mice developed psoriasis and died within the 7th–10th day after birth. The histological analysis showed myelopoietic tissues enlarged and diffusely distributed, and also alterations in the liver with enhanced splenic extramedullary hematopoiesiswith increased presence of monocytes/macrophages was seen [16].

"β-transducin repeat-containing protein" (β-TrCP) serves as substrate recognition component of E3 ubiquitin ligase that control the stability of important regulators of signal transduction, including IκBα. Mice with down-regulation of βTrCP ameliorate IMQ-Mu-Pso skin lesions, as IκBα does not degrade, keeping NFκB into the cytoplasm. This interesting finding suggests that βTrCP could be a novel target for developing agents to treat psoriasis, since it is involved in the NFκB signaling to regulate inflammation [17].

IκBζ is another molecule that interacts with NFκB, but inside the nucleus. This molecule has been recently identified as a key regulator in the development of psoriasis [18]. IκBζ is increased in psoriatic skin compared to non-psoriatic skin from the same patient. Some studies suggest that IκBζ associates with NFκB p50 subunit and binds to specific IκBζ response elements located in the promoter region of targeted genes consisting of NFκB- and C/EBP (CCAAT/enhancer-binding protein)-binding sites and exerts its transcription-enhancing activity on secondary response genes primarily by chromatin remodeling [19]. IκBζ is expressed in human keratinocytes induced with IL-17 and is a direct transcriptional activator of TNFα/IL-17-inducible psoriasis-associated proteins such as IL-8, IL-17C, IL-17A22, IL-19, IL23, IL22, CCL20 and hBD220. Interestingly, in imiquimod-treated IκBζ-deficient mice, psoriatic skin is not observed, and the molecules induced by TNFα/IL-17 are significantly down-expressed [20].

The dysfunctional activity of other transcription factors, for instance, AP-1 and STAT3, also contributes to skin inflammation development [21]. Mice with deficient expression of JunB and c-Jun, and mice with over-expression of FOS, generate a phenotype resembling the histological characteristics of psoriasis, including the production pro-inflammatory cytokines. Besides, JunBexpression is reduced in epidermal keratinocytes of psoriatic patients in comparison with cells from healthy subjects [21]. Moreover, STAT3 transgenic mice and SOCS3 knockout mice (the negative regulator of STAT3) have constitutive activation of STAT3 and both develop murine IL-6-driven psoriasis [22, 23].

2.5. The role of cytokines in psoriasis

Other sort of psoriatic animal models includes those where cytokines and cells of immune system are involved. The importance of type I interferons in the psoriasis was demonstrated in "IFN regulatory factor-2" (IFNR-2)-deficient mice, a transcriptional repressor for IFN-$\alpha\beta$ signaling. These mice developed skin lesions similar to human psoriasis [24], in fact, type I interferons promote the activation of dermal dendritic cells (dDCs) [25].

Another cytokine with importance for the development of psoriasis is IL-36, an IL-1 family sub-member. The over-expression of IL-36α in transgenic murine (K14/IL-36) keratinocytes promotes acanthosis, hyperkeratosis, cells infiltration and increased expression of cytokines and chemokines [26]. The deficiency of IL-36RA (the natural antagonist of IL-36) in IL-36α (K14/IL-36, IL-36RA$^{-/-}$)-transgenic mice exacerbates the severity of psoriasis; histological analysis reveals intracorneal and intraepithelial pustules, parakeratotic and orthokeratotic hyperkeratosis, dilated superficial dermal blood vessels, and dermal inflammatory infiltrate. Additionally, mice deficient to IL-36 or in its receptor IL-36R are protected from IMQ-Mu-Pso [26]. In turn, IL-1β, TNFα, and IL-36 activate dDC and induce the production of IL-23, necessary for naive T cells to polarize to Th17, suggesting that IL-23 could be the link between the innate and adaptive immune response that occur in psoriasis [27]. In fact, it is possible to obtain psoriasiform skin in wild-type mice with nothing more but the inoculation of recombinant IL-23 or IL-17 [28]. In contrast, IL-35 has a potent immunosuppressive effect on HaCaT keratinocytes treated with TNF-α and IL-17 suppressing the expression of IL-6, CXCL8, and S100A7 [28]. In IMQ-Mu-Pso and K14-VEGF transgenic mice model, IL-35 reduced M1 macrophages (F4/80+CD80+), whereas anti-inflammatory M2 macrophages (F4/80+CD206+) were increased in the spleen and ear. IL-10–secreting CD4+, FoxP3+, CD25+ T cells were increased in those tissues, although IL-10–secreting CD25-T cells were also increased [29]. These results suggest that IL-35 treatment for psoriasis increases M2 macrophages as well as IL-10 production but suppresses Th17 cells development, consistent with the effect of IL-35 on Treg expansion, although not all IL-10 was secreted by Treg cells.

2.6. Cellular immunology in psoriasis

The insufficient regulation of specific cellular immune response is also involved in the development of psoriasis [30]. In normal conditions, Treg cells regulate the activity of auto-reactive Th1 and Th17 cells, but in psoriasis Treg cells might not be functional, as was evidenced in the CD18hypo mouse model [31]. Homozygous PL/J CD18 hypomorphic (CD18hypo)-mice developed spontaneously psoriasis-like skin in 12- to 14-week-old mice. CD18 is a molecule that together with CD11a constitutes an adhesion molecule of the β2 integrin family, important for the complete function of Treg cells. It has been suggested that CD18hypo mice induce psoriasis because CD18-low expressing Treg cells, or with a not fully active molecule, cannot regulate the activity of auto-reactive Th1 and Th17 cells, since these mice improve when Treg cells from normal mice are transferred [32]. In CD18hypo mice, psoriatic lesions meliorate when macrophages are eliminated by the use of clodronate liposomes in the skin [33]. These results show the importance of Treg cell and macrophages in the evolution of psoriasis.

2.7. Implantable synthetic cytokine-converter cells model

Schukur et al. [34] designed the so-called implantable synthetic cytokine converter cells system based on the observation that psoriatic patients have high concentrations of TNFα and IL-22, and on the fact that IL-4 and IL-10 cytokines have an important anti-psoriatic effect. Considering the previous, they generated by genetic engineering human cells to react to high concentrations of TNFα and IL-22; these cells would be implanted to psoriatic patients and activated by TNFα and IL-22 from a psoriatic flare, and as a result, they would produce therapeutic doses of IL-4 and IL-10 to control inflammation. To achieve the goal, HEK-293T cells were co-transfected with the plasmids pNFκB-hIL-22RA-pA, phCMV-hSTAT3-pA, pSTAT3-mIL-4-pA and pSTAT3-mIL-10-pA. The authors first confirmed that co-transfected cells produced important levels of IL-4 and IL-10 when stimulated with TNFα and IL-22 in vitro [34]. TNFα activated the production of IL-22 receptor, and in turn IL-22 activated STAT3 signaling to induce the production of IL-4 and IL-10, to generate an anti-inflammatory environment. When co-transfected HEK-293T cells were intraperitoneally implanted into mice with IMQ-Mu-Pso the cytokines associated with the pathogenesis of psoriasis, such as IL-17, IFNα and C-X-C motif chemokine 9 (CXCL9), decreased substantially and a considerable increase in the production of the anti-inflammatory cytokines IL-4 and IL-10 was observed on day 5. Only the skin of animals with implanted co-transfected cells containing the antipsoriatic cytokine converter showed reduced skin lesions, evidenced by the reduction of erythema, scaling, and thickening. This is an interesting approach to treat psoriasis, although the complexity relies on the requirement to co-transfect cells from every single patient to avoid transplant rejection. Meanwhile, this system was also evaluated in vitro using blood from psoriatic patients and from healthy individuals, and interestingly only in blood from psoriatic patients increased levels of anti-inflammatory cytokines were detected [34].

3. Angiogenic factor in psoriasis

The altered function of angiogenic molecules also produces psoriasis. "Vascular endothelial growth factor" (VEGF)-transgenic mice [35], "endothelial specific receptor tyrosine kinase" (K5-Tie2)-transgenic mice [36], and "transforming growth factor beta 1" (K5-TGFβ1)-transgenic mice [37] are psoriasis animal models that highlight the importance of angiogenesis in this pathology. VEGF is a crucial factor that mediates the angiogenesis of blood vessels and is highly expressed in the psoriatic skin lesions. VEGF induces microvascular alterations in the dermal papillae, which facilitate the development and persistence of the psoriatic lesions [35]. Moreover, the increased vasculature and permeability provide nutrition to the hyperproliferating keratinocytes and promote the migration of inflammatory cells. The 6-month- old

K14-VEGF mice develop psoriasis, but if these mice are treated with imiquimod at 8-week old, the skin thickens, chemokines CXCL-9/10, CCL-20 and CCR6 increase, cytokines IL-23, IL-17, TNFα, and (IFN)-γ rise, and the cells CD11c+ DCs, Th17, Th1, $\gamma\delta$-T increase. In wild-type mice IMQ-Mu-Pso skin lesions last until day 7 of treatment, but in K14-VEGF mice treated with imiquimod, all the parameters described above are stable until day 14 [38]. This combined model IMQ-K14-VEGF is more appropriate for long-term studies compared to IMQ-Mu-Pso model, which is only an acute chemical-stimulated model.

Tie2 is the angiopoietin receptor that together with VEGF is essential for proliferation, maturation and for the maintenance of blood vessels. Hyperproliferation of keratinocytes and abundance of immunological cells infiltration, including Th17 cells, are detected in psoriatic skin. The over-expression of VEGF is promoted by TGFβ but also can be regulated by HIF-1α, as it is over-expressed in the psoriatic skin [36].

4. The role of keratinocytes in psoriasis

4.1. PPAR β/δ

The "peroxisome proliferator-activated receptor" (PPAR β/δ) transgenic mice, and the human keratinocytes autocrine growth factor (amphiregulin) transgenic mice [39, 40] both resemble psoriasis because they participate in the proliferation and differentiation of keratinocytes [41]. PPAR β/δ receptor is induced by TNFα, contributes to STAT3 phosphorylation, blocks apoptosis in keratinocytes, induces angiogenesis, and is up-regulated in human psoriatic skin [42]. In fact, PPAR β/δ directly induces the differentiation of keratinocytes, and in the transgenic mouse model, a light augment of Th17 is observed [43].

4.2. NFκB inhibits proliferation in keratinocytes

Genome-wide association studies suggest a link between psoriasis and the NFκB pathway, and this proposal has been supported by mouse models. Evidence gathered from diverse studies has shown that NFκB has a growth inhibitory function in the skin. Mice with epidermis-specific deletion of IKK2 (which mediates canonical NFκB activation) develop severe inflammatory skin disease that is mediated by TNFα, suggesting the critical function of IKK2-mediated NFκB activity in epidermal keratinocytes to regulate mechanisms that maintain the immune homeostasis of the skin [44].

Grinberg-Bleyer, et al. [45] described a murine psoriasis model that lacks the expression of p65 and c-Rel in epidermal cells. After birth, these mice developed severe psoriasis; early lesions were well-demarcated, scattered and rigid, with scaly plaques without edematous or exudative reaction aspect. H&E staining revealed epidermal thickening, hyperkeratosis and focal parakeratosis, as well as mononuclear infiltrates in the epidermis, which are features of psoriatic lesions. In this model, psoriatic lesions were resolved 30 days after birth by Treg cells effect, but when these cells were eliminated by the use of anti-CD25 antibodies, the deficient mice showed a worsened pathology and the psoriatic lesions were reversed with anti-TNFα treatment [45]. Also RelA has a growth-inhibitory role in keratinocytes and prevents their differentiation [46]. Together, these results indicate that activation of canonical NFκB pathway in keratinocytes is required for their optimal differentiation and for the maintenance of immune homeostasis in the skin.

4.3. Prokineticin 2

Prokineticin2 (PK2), also named Bv8, is a small 8 KDa protein found in serum and dermis of psoriatic patients. PK2 participates in numerous important physiological processes including inflammation, neurogenesis, tissue development, angiogenesis, and even nociception [47, 48]. This peptide is mainly expressed in brain but can also be found in skin, bone marrow, lymphoid organs, granulocytes, dendritic cells and macrophages [49]. He et al. [50] found that bacterial products, including LPS and DNA, promoted in macrophages the production of PK2 and inflammatory factors, suggesting that infection is a primary inducer of PK2. The authors demonstrated that in macrophages PK2 induced high production of IL-1β, and in keratinocytes and fibroblast co-cultures PK2 induced IL-6, IL-8 and GM-SCF. In vivo PK2 promoted the differentiation of fibroblast and keratinocytes [51]. Besides, when PK2 was over-expressed in psoriasis-K14-VEGF transgenic mouse model, psoriatic lesions were gradually aggravated, as evaluated by increase of redness, swelling, weight, thickness, scaly epidermis, keratinocyte hyper-proliferation, and increase of IL-1β, TNFα, IFNγ, IL-12, IL-22, IL-23, IL-17 in the ear; moreover, increase of lymph node weight was also seen. On the contrary, in psoriatic-K14-VEGF transgenic mouse model with PK2 down-regulated, the psoriatic lesions were abrogated [50]. The results suggest that PK2 aggravates psoriasis by the promotion of keratinocytes and fibroblasts proliferation, inflammation, and angiogenesis.

4.4. Tnip1

The big dilemma about psoriasis is whether the root of the problem falls on keratinocytes or on immunological cells dysfunction. It has been well described that IL-23-producing myeloid cells and IL-17–producing T cells are abundant in psoriatic skin, and that IL-23 and IL-17 induce in keratinocytes and fibroblasts high production of chemokines, which in turn, recruit even more immunological cells creating a feedback loop that worsens the disease. In keratinocytes and immunological cells, "TNFAIP3-inter-acting protein 1" (Tnip1) down-regulates the chemokines production induced by IL-17 [50]. Ippagunta et al. [52], using the IMQ-Mu-Pso model under the Tnip-keratinocyte-specific-deletion mice (Tnip1flox/flox K14-Cre), found that keratinocytes contribute intrinsically to psoriasis because when keratinocytes lost Tnip1 function they could not control the production of chemokines induced by IL-17. Tnip1flox/floxK14-Cre mice developed severe psoriasis when low doses of imiquimod were used, even at concentrations on which WT mice do not develop psoriasis. Interestingly, when bone marrow cells from Tnip1-/- mice were transferred to WT mice and treated with low doses of imiquimod, they did not developed psoriasis, confirming that the lack of function of Tnip1 in keratinocytes and fibroblast, but not in hematopoietic lineage cells, generate psoriasis [52]. With these results, the authors provide evidence that specifically skin-resident keratinocytes contribute causally to psoriasis.

5. In vitro models for the study of psoriasis

As we previously mentioned, animal models have been very useful to dissect the molecular and cellular mechanisms for psoriasis development. These models have been also advantageous to evaluate new pharmaceuticals, nevertheless the physiology, anatomy and molecular differences between animal models and humans cause that only around 10% of new treatments assayed on phase I, be really useful in humans [53]. Although humanized models have also been developed, immunodeficient animals are most commonly used. Alternative methods have been developed to analyze the effect of new anti-psoriatic drugs; 2D, 2D+membrane, and 3D cell cultures have been designed [54]. 2D model consists of primary explants of keratinocytes or fibroblasts from psoriatic patients cultured over extracellular matrix proteins to evaluate cellular proliferation, cellular differentiation and cytokines production [55]. In the 2D+membrane model, two cell types are co-cultured separated by a synthetic membrane to evaluate the interconnection between two cell types in the pathology [56]. 3D cultures, also known as organotypic culture system (OCS), allow the growth of complex biological systems in vitro in a way that resembles part of their normal physiology and function. OCSs are powerful as experimental platforms in preclinical dermatological research, helping to validate mechanisms of diseases and to test the therapeutic potential of candidate drugs [57]. The new generation of 3D cultures connected to biosensors or chips allows real-time monitoring of biological parameters such as loss of water and electrophysiologic parameters [58].

6. Conclusion

The actual hypothesis about the cellular and molecular mechanisms that lead to the development of psoriatic lesions has been established by the use of animal models. The use of xenotransplants confirmed the important role of immunology in this disease. The studies done in genetically modified mice that overproduce (transgenic) or lack (knockout) certain proteins reveal specific protagonists of innate or adaptive immunity, angiogenesis or proliferation for the development of psoriasis.

In **Figure 1**, we represent a developing inflammation mechanism generated in the skin of healthy individuals denoted as a brown cogwheel system, where a trigger induces the innate and adaptive immune response, and in turn angiogenesis and keratinocytes proliferation are activated. Every cog represents one participant in inflammation: cell (DCs, macrophages, iLC IL-17+, Th1, Th17, keratinocytes, between others) or molecule (TLRs, NFκB, βTrCP, IκBζ, Stat3, TNFα, IFNα, IL-12, IL-36, IL-23, Th1, IL-6, Th17, IL-17, CCR6, VEGF, Tie2 TGFβ1, PPARαβ, PK2, between others). The red arrows indicate the movement of the cogwheels for the progression of inflammation. In healthy people, the inflammation is controlled by

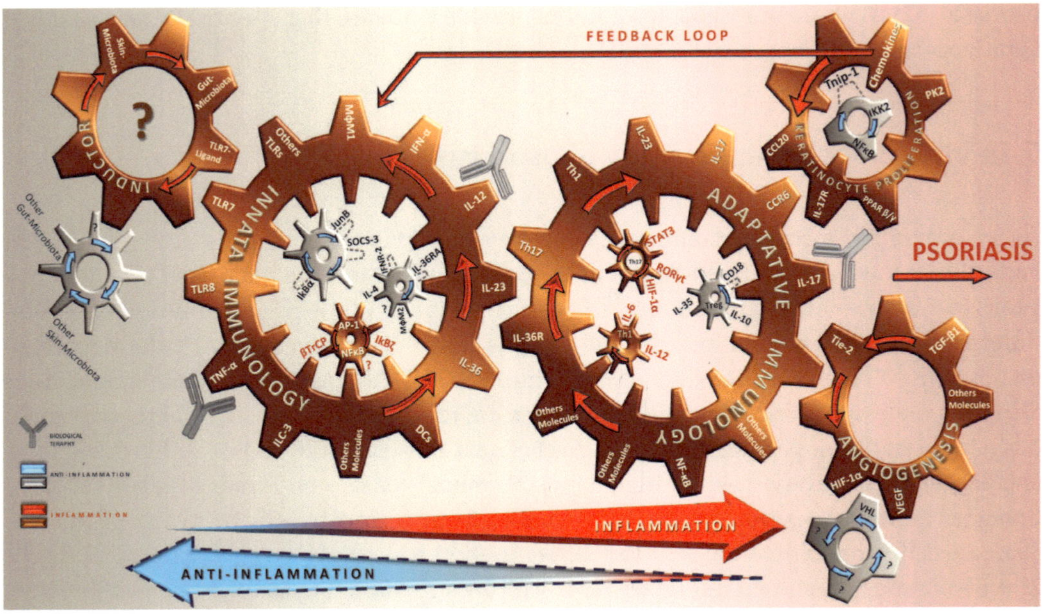

Figure 1. Inflammatory process. The developing inflammation mechanism generated in the skin is represented in this cogwheel system, where innate immune response, adaptive immune response, angiogenesis and cellular proliferation are represented in independent but interconnected cogwheels. Brown cogwheels represent inflammatory mechanisms moving in a pro-inflammatory sense (red arrows), where each cog represents one participant in inflammation (cell or molecule). Gray cogwheels represent the anti-inflammatory mechanism spinning the wheels in the opposite direction (blue arrows) to regulate inflammation. The "ghost" cogs (discontinuous lines) represent dysfunctional cells or molecules that disrupt effectiveness in the control of inflammation, favoring the development of psoriasis. Some antibodies interfere with the spinning of pro-inflammatory cogwheels, representing therapies with antibodies developed to control psoriasis. Question marks represent molecules to be discovered.

the activation of anti-inflammatory process after damage reparation. The cells (Treg and M2 macrophages) and molecules (IκBα, JunB, SOCS-3, IFNR-2, IL-36RA, IL-4, IL-10, IL-35, CD18, VHL, Tnip-1, between others) involved in the anti-inflammatory process are represented in the gray cogwheels. The blue arrows indicate the movement of the cogwheels for the progression of anti-inflammation. The "ghost" cogs (discontinuous lines) represent those dysfunctional molecules or cells that disrupt effectiveness in the control of inflammation, favoring the development of psoriasis.

Based on all the facts discussed in this chapter, we can conclude that psoriasis occurs in individuals with the anti-inflammatory regulation disrupted in immunological but also in non-immunological skin-resident cells.

Acknowledgements

This work was supported by a grant from the "SIP-IPN" (Num. SIP20161111). SRM, JCCD, SMPT and MECD belong to COFAA, EDI-IPN and SNI fellowships. IMT belongs to BEIFI and CONACyT fellowships.

Author details

Sandra Rodríguez-Martínez[1], Juan C. Cancino-Diaz[2], Isaí Martínez-Torrez[1], Sonia M. Pérez-Tapia[1,3] and Mario E. Cancino-Diaz[1]*

*Address all correspondence to: mecancinod@gmail.com

1 Immunology Department, Escuela Nacional de Ciencias Biológicas-IPN, Mexico City, Mexico

2 Microbiology Department, Escuela Nacional de Ciencias Biológicas-IPN, Mexico City, Mexico

3 UDIBI, Escuela Nacional de Ciencias Biológicas-IPN, Mexico City, Mexico

References

[1] Bechet PE. Psoriasis. A brief historical review.Archives of Dermatology and Syphilology. 1936;**33**:327-334

[2] Zanolli MD, Jayo MJ, Jayo JM, Blaine D, Hall J, Jorizzo JL. Evaluation of psoriatic plaques that spontaneously developed in a cynomolgus monkey (*Macacafascicularis*). Acta Dermato Venereologica – Supplementum (Stockh). 1989;**146**:58

[3] Regan SA, Marsell R, Ozmen I. First report of psoriatic-like dermatitis and arthritis in a 4-year-old female spayed pug mix. Case Reports in Veterinary Medicine. 2015;**2015**:1-4. DOI: 10.1155/2015/912509

[4] Gates AH, Karasek M. Hereditary absence of sebaceous glands in the mouse. Science. 1965;**148**:1471-1473. DOI: 10.1126/science.148.3676.1471

[5] Beamer WG, Pelsue SC, Shultz LD, Sundberg JP, Barker JE. The flaky skin (fsn) mutation in mice: map location and description of the anemia. Blood. 1995;**86**:3220-3226

[6] Chen J, Roop DR. Genetically engineered mouse models for skin research: Taking the next step. Journal of Dermatology Sciences. 2008;**52**:1-1. DOI: 10.1016/j.jdermsci.2008.03.012

[7] Bergers LI, Reijnders CM, van den Broek LJ, Spiekstra SW, de Gruijl TD, Weijers EM, Gibbs S. Immune-competent human skin disease models. Drug Discovery Today. 2016;**21**:1479-1488. DOI: 10.1016/j.drudis.2016.05.008

[8] Boehncke WH, Sterry W, Hainzl A, Scheffold W, Kaufmann R. Psoriasiform architecture of murine epidermis overlying human psoriatic dermis transplanted onto SCID mice. Archives of Dermatological Research. 1994;**286**:325-330

[9] Wrone-Smith T, Nickoloff BJ. Dermal injection of immunocytes induces psoriasis. Journal of Clinical Investigation.1996;**98**:1878-1887. DOI: 10.1172/JCI118989

[10] van der Fits L, Mourits S, Voerman JS, Kant M, Boon L, Laman JD, Cornelissen F, Mus AM, Florencia E, Prens EP, Lubberts E. Imiquimod-induced psoriasislike skin inflammation in mice is mediated via the IL-23/IL-17 axis. The Journal of Immunology. 2009;**182:**5836-5845. DOI: 10.4049/jimmunol.0802999; PMID: 19380832

[11] Duffy DL, Spelman LS, Martin NG. Psoriasis in Australian twins. Journal of the American Academy of Dermatology. 1993;**29**:428-434

[12] Ivanov II, Atarashi K, Manel N, Brodie EL, Shima T, Karaoz U, Wei D, Goldfarb KC, Santee CA, Lynch SV, Tanoue T, Imaoka A, Itoh K, Takeda K, Umesaki Y, Honda K, Littman DR. Induction of intestinal Th17 cells by segmented filamentous bacteria. Cell. 2009;**139**:485-498.DOI: 10.1016/j.cell.2009.09.033

[13] Fahlén A, Engstrand L, Baker BS, Powles A, Fry L. Comparison of bacterial microbiota in skin biopsies from normal and psoriatic skin. Archives of Dermatological Research. 2012;**304**:15-22. DOI: 10.1007/s00403-011-1189-x

[14] Zanvit P, Konkel JE, Jiao X, Kasagi S, Zhang D, Wu R, Chia C, Ajami NJ, Smith DP, Petrosino JF, Abbatiello B, Nakatsukasa H, Chen Q, Belkaid Y, Chen ZJ, Chen W. Antibiotics in neonatal life increase murine susceptibility to experimental psoriasis. Nature Communications. 2015;**6**:8424. DOI: 10.1038/ncomms9424

[15] Newton K, Dixit VM. Signaling in innate immunity and inflammation. Cold Spring Harbor Perspectives in Biology. 2012;**4:**a006049. DOI: 10.1101/cshperspect.a006049

[16] Klement JF, Rice NR, Car BD, Abbondanzo SJ, Powers GD, Bhatt PH, Chen CH, Rosen CA, Stewart CL. IκBα deficiency results in a sustained NF-κB response and severe widespread dermatitis in mice. Molecular and Cellular Biology. 1996;**16**:2341-2349

[17] Li R, Wang J, Wang X, Zhou J, Wang M, Ma H, Xiao S. Increased βTrCP are associated with imiquimod-induced psoriasis-like skin inflammation in mice via NF-κB signaling pathway. Gene. 2016;**592**:164-171. DOI:10.1016/j.gene.2016.07.066. PubMed PMID: 27476970

[18] Johansen C. IκBζ: A key protein in the pathogenesis of psoriasis. Cytokine. 2016;**78**:20-21. DOI:10.1016/j.cyto.2015.11.015

[19] Trinh DV, Zhu N, Farhang G,Kim BJ, Huxford T. The nuclear IκB protein IκBζ specifically binds NF-κB p50 homodimers and forms a ternary complex on κB DNA. Journal of Molecular Biology.2008;**379**:122-135. DOI: 10.1016/j.jmb.2008.03.060

[20] Johansen C, Mose M, Ommen P, Bertelsen T, Vinter H, Hailfinger S, Lorscheid S, Schulze-Osthoff K, Iversen L. IκBζ is a key driver in the development of psoriasis. Proceedingsof the National Academy of Sciences U S A. 2015;**112**:E5825-E5833. DOI: 10.1073/pnas.1509971112

[21] Zenz R, Eferl R, Kenner L, Florin L, Hummerich L, Mehic D, Scheuch H, Angel P, Tschachler E, Wagner EF. Psoriasis-like skin disease and arthritis caused by inducible epidermal deletion of Jun proteins. Nature. 2005;**437**:369-375. DOI: 10.1038/nature03963

[22] Sano S, Chan KS, Carbajal S, Clifford J, Peavey M, Kiguchi K, Itami S, Nickoloff BJ, DiGiovanni J. Stat3 links activated keratinocytes and immunocytes required for development of psoriasis in a novel transgenic mouse model. Nature Medicine. 2005;**11**:43-49. DOI: 10.1038/nm1162

[23] Uto-Konomi A, Miyauchi K, Ozaki N, Motomura Y, Suzuki Y, Yoshimura A, Suzuki S, Cua D, Kubo M. Dysregulation of suppressor of cytokine signaling 3 in keratinocytes causes skin inflammation mediated by interleukin-20 receptor-related cytokines. PLoS One. 2012;**7**:e40343. DOI: 10.1371/journal.pone.0040343

[24] Hida S, Ogasawara K, Sato K, Abe M, Takayanagi H, Yokochi T, Sato T, Hirose S, Shirai T, Taki S, Taniguchi T. CD8(+) T cell-mediated skin disease in mice lacking IRF-2, the transcriptional attenuator of interferon-alpha/beta signaling. Immunity. 2000;**13**:643-655. DOI:10.1016/S1074-7613(00)00064-9

[25] Nestle FO, Conrad C, Tun-Kyi A, Homey B, Gombert M, Boyman O, Burg G, Liu YJ, Gilliet M. Plasmacytoidpredendritic cells initiate psoriasis through interferon-alpha production. The Journal of Experimental Medicine. 2005;**202**:135-143

[26] Blumberg H, Dinh H, Trueblood ES, Pretorius J, Kugler D, Weng N, Kanaly ST, Towne JE, Willis CR, Kuechle MK, Sims JE, Peschon JJ. Opposing activities of two novel members of the IL-1 ligand family regulate skin inflammation. The Journal of Experimental Medicine. 2007;**204**:2603-2614. DOI: 10.1084/jem.20070157

[27] Towne E, Sims JE. IL-36 in psoriasis. Current Opinion in Pharmacology. 2012;**4**:486-490. DOI: 10.1016/j.coph.2012.02.009

[28] Lindroos J, Svensson L, Norsgaard H, Lovato P, Moller K, Hagedorn PH, Olsen GM, Labuda T. IL-23-mediated epidermal hyperplasia is dependent on IL-6. Journal of Investigative Dermatology. 2011;**131**:1110-1118. DOI: 10.1038/jid.2010.432

[29] Zhang J, Lin Y, Li C, Zhang X, Cheng L, Dai L, Wang Y, Wang F, Shi G, Li Y, Yang Q, Cui X, Liu Y, Wang H, Zhang S, Yang Y, Xiang R, Li J, Yu D, Wei Y, Deng H. IL-35 decelerates the inflammatory process by regulating inflammatory cytokine secretion and M1/M2 macrophage ratio in psoriasis. The Journal of Immunology. 2016;**197**:2131-2144. DOI: 10.4049/jimmunol.1600446

[30] Torales-Cardeña A, Martínez-Torres I, Rodríguez-Martínez S, Gómez-Chavez F, Cancino-Diaz JC, Vázquez-Sánchez EA, Cancino-Diaz- ME. Cross Talk between Proliferative, Angiogenic, and Cellular mechanisms orchestred by HIF-1α in psoriasis. Mediators of Inflammation. 2015;**2015**:1-11. DOI:10.1155/2015/607363

[31] Bullard DC, Scharffetter-Kochanek K, McArthur MJ, Chosay JG, McBride ME, Montgomery CA, Beaudet AL. A polygenic mouse model of psoriasiform skin diseas in CD18-deficient mice. Proceedings of the National Academy of Sciences U S A. 1996;**93**:2116-2121. DOI: 10.1073/pnas.93.5.2116

[32] Singh K, Gatzka M, Peters T, Borkner L, Hainzl A, Wang H, Sindrilaru A, Scharffetter-Kochanek K. Reduced CD18 levels drive regulatory T cell conversion into Th17

cells in the CD18hypo PL/J mouse model of psoriasis. The Journal of Immunology. 2013;**190**:2544-2553. DOI: 10.4049/jimmunol.1202399

[33] Wang H, Peters T, Kess D, Sindrilaru A, Oreshkova T, Van Rooijen N, Stratis A, Renkl AC, Sunderkötter C, Wlaschek M, Haase I, Scharffetter-Kochanek K. Activated macrophages are essential in a murine model for T cell-mediated chronic psoriasiform skin inflammation. Journal of Clinical Investigation. 2006;**116**:2105-2114. DOI: 10.1172/JCI27180

[34] Schukur L, Geering B, Charpin-El Hamri G, Fussenegger M. Implantable synthetic-cytokine converter cells with AND-gate logic treat experimental psoriasis. Science Translational Medicine. 2015;7**318**:318ra201. DOI: 10.1126/scitranslmed.aac4964

[35] Xia YP, Li B, Hylton D, Detmar M, Yancopoulos GD, Rudge JS. Transgenic delivery of VEGF to mouse skin leads to an inflammatory condition resembling human psoriasis. Blood. 2003;**102**:161-168. PMID: 12649136

[36] Wolfram JA, Diaconu D, Hatala DA, Rastegar J, Knutsen DA, Lowther A, Askew D, Gilliam AC, McCormick TS, Ward NL. Keratinocyte but not endothelial cell-specific overexpression of Tie2 leads to the development of psoriasis. American Journal of Pathology. 2009;**174:**1443-1458. DOI: 10.2353/ajpath.2009.080858

[37] Li AG, Wang D, Feng XH, Wang XJ. Latent TGFbeta1 overexpression in keratinocytes results in a severe psoriasis-like skin disorder. EMBO Journal. 2004;**23**:1770-1781. PubMed PMID: 15057277; PubMed Central PMCID: PMC394237

[38] Wang X, Sun J, Hu J. IMQ induced K14-VEGF mouse: A stable and long-term mouse model of psoriasis-like inflammation. PLoS One. 2015;**10**:e0145498. DOI: 10.1371/journal.pone.0145498. eCollection 2015

[39] Cook PW, Piepkorn M, Clegg CH, Plowman GD, DeMay JM, Brown JR, Pittelkow MR. Transgenic expression of the human amphiregulin gene induces a psoriasis-like phenotype. Journal of Clinical Investigation. 1997;**100**:2286-2294. PMID: 9410906

[40] Cook PW, Brown JR, Cornell KA, Pittelkow MR. Suprabasal expression of human amphiregulin in the epidermis of transgenic mice induces a severe, early-onset, psoriasis-like skin pathology: Expression of amphiregulin in the basal epidermis is also associated with synovitis. Experimental Dermatology. 2004;**13**:347-356. PubMedPMID: 15186320

[41] Romanowska M, Reilly L, Palmer CN, Gustafsson MC, Foerster J. Activation of PPAR beta/delta causes a psoriasis-like skin disease in vivo. PLoS One. 2010;**5**:e9701. DOI: 10.1371/journal.pone.0009701. PubMed PMID: 20300524

[42] Romanowska M, al Yacoub N, Seidel H, Donandt S, Gerken H, Phillip S, Haritonova N, Artuc M, Schweiger S, Sterry W, Foerster J. PPARdelta enhances keratinocyte proliferation in psoriasis and induces heparin-binding EGF-like growth factor. Journal of Investigative Dermatology. 2008;**128**:110-124. PubMed PMID: 17637826.

[43] Tan NS, Michalik L, Noy N, Yasmin R, Pacot C, Heim M, Flühmann B, Desvergne B, Wahli W. Critical roles of PPAR beta/delta in keratinocyte response to inflammation. Genes & Development.2001;**15**:3263-3277. PubMed PMID: 11751632

[44] Pasparakis M, Courtois G, Hafner M, Schmidt-Supprian M, Nenci A, Toksoy A, Krampert M, Goebeler M, Gillitzer R, Israel A, Krieg T, Rajewsky K, Haase I. TNF-mediated inflammatory skin disease in mice with epidermis-specific deletion of IKK2. Nature. 2002;**417**:861-866. PubMed PMID: 12075355

[45] Grinberg-Bleyer Y, Dainichi T, Oh H, Heise N, Klein U, Schmid RM, Hayden MS, Ghosh S. Cutting edge: NF-κB p65 and c-Rel control epidermal development and immune homeostasis in the skin. The Journal of Immunology. 2015;**194**:2472-2476. DOI: 10.4049/jimmunol.1402608

[46] Zhang JY, Green CL, Tao S, Khavari PA. NF-κB RelA opposes epidermal proliferation driven by TNFR1 and JNK. Genes & Development. 2004;**18**:17-22

[47] Monnier J, Samson M. Prokineticins in angiogenesis and cancer. Cancer Letters. 2010;**296**:144-149. DOI: 10.1016/j.canlet.2010.06.011

[48] Shojaei F, Singh M, Thompson JD, Ferrara N. Role of Bv8 in neutrophil-dependent angiogenesis in a transgenic model of cancer progression. Proceedings of the National Academy of Sciences U S A. 2008;**105**:2640-2645. DOI:10.1073/pnas.0712185105

[49] Martucci C, Franchi S, Giannini E, Tian H, Melchiorri P, Negri L, Sacerdote P. Bv8, the amphibian homologue of the mammalian prokineticins, induces a proin-flammatory phenotype of mouse macrophages. British Journal of Pharmacology. 2006;**147**:225-234. DOI: 10.1038/sj.bjp.0706467

[50] He X, Shen C, Lu Q, Li J, Wei Y, He L, Bai R, Zheng J, Luan N, Zhang Z, Rong M, Lai R. Prokineticin 2 Plays a Pivotal Role in Psoriasis. EBioMedicine. 2016;**13**:248-261. DOI: 10.1016/j.ebiom.2016.10.022

[51] Callahan JA, Hammer GE, Agelides A, Duong BH, Oshima S, North J, Advincula R, Shifrin N, Truong HA, Paw J, Barrera J, DeFranco A, Rosenblum MD, Malynn BA, Ma A. Cutting edge: ABIN-1 protects against psoriasis by restricting MyD88 signals in dendritic cells. The Journal of Immunology. 2013;**191**:535-539. DOI:10.4049/jimmunol.1203335

[52] Ippagunta SK, Gangwar R, Finkelstein D, Vogel P, Pelletier S, Gingras S, Redecke V, Häcker H. Keratinocytes contribute intrinsically to psoriasis upon loss of Tnip1 function. Proceedings of the National Academy of Sciences U S A. 2016;**113**:E6162-E6171. PubMed PMID: 27671649

[53] Hay M, Thomas DW, Craighead JL, Economides C, Rosenthal J. Clinical development success rates for investigational drugs. Nature Biotechnology. 2014;**32**:40-51. DOI: 10.1038/nbt.2786

[54] Krueger GG, Jorgensen CM. Experimental models for psoriasis. Journal of Investigative Dermatology. 1990;**95**:56S-58S. DOI: 10.1111/1523-1747.ep12505791

[55] Van Ruissen F, de Jongh GJ, Zeeuwen PL, Van Erp PE, Madsen P, Schalkwijk J. Induction of normal and psoriatic phenotypes in submerged keratinocyte cultures. Journal of Cellular Physiology. 1996;**168**:442-452. DOI: 10.1002/(SICI)1097-4652(199608)168:2<442::AID-JCP23>3.0.CO;2-3

[56] Auriemma M, Brzoska T, Klenner L, Kupas V, Goerge T, Voskort M, Zhao Z, Sparwasser T, Luger TA, Loser K. α-MSH-stimulated tolerogenic dendritic cells induce functional regulatory T cells and ameliorate ongoing skin inflammation. Journal of Investigative Dermatology. 2012;**132**:1814-1824. DOI: 10.1038/jid.2012.59

[57] Van den Bogaard EH, Tjabringa GS, Joosten I, Vonk-Bergers M, van Rijssen E, Tijssen HJ, Erkens M, Schalkwijk J, Koenen HJ. Crosstalk between keratinocytes and T cells in a 3D microenvironment: A model to study inflammatory skin diseases. Journal of Investigative Dermatology. 2014;**134**:719-727. DOI: 10.1038/jid.2013.417

[58] Wufuer M, Lee G, Hur W, JeonB, KimB, ChoiT,LeeS. Skin-on-a-chip model simulating inflammation, edema and drug-based treatment. Scientific Reports. 2016;**6**:37471. DOI:10.1038/srep37471

Chapter 6

Immune System Links Psoriasis-Mediated Inflammation to Cardiovascular Diseases via Traditional and Non-Traditional Cardiovascular Risk Factors

Rodolfo A. Kölliker Frers, Matilde Otero-Losada, Eduardo Kersberg, Vanesa Cosentino and Francisco Capani

Additional information is available at the end of the chapter

http://dx.doi.org/10.5772/intechopen.68559

Abstract

Background. Cutaneous psoriasis and psoriatic arthritis increase the risk of cardiovascular diseases though the reasons are not clear. Here we discuss the role of the immune system in atherosclerosis and of the proinflammatory status in psoriasis and psoriatic arthritis diseases.

Methods. We performed a Pubmed query covering publications within the last ten years including epidemiological studies, cross-sectional case-control studies, and reviews. Articles were selected according critical associations using arthritis, immune-mediated inflammatory diseases, and psoriasis as key fields. These were crossed and combined with atherogenesis, endothelial dysfunction, intima-media thickness, subclinical atherosclerosis, plaque, thrombosis, thrombus, fibrinolysis, coagulation, and reactive oxygen species, all closely related to cardiovascular diseases. Both types of disease selected terms were separately combined with cardiovascular risk factors both non-traditional (innate and adaptive pro- and anti-inflammatory immune molecules and cells), and traditional (metabolic conditions and related molecules).

Results and conclusions. Immune-activated crossroads came out as the main contributors to proatherogenic inflammation in psoriasis and psoriatic arthritis disease. Traditional and non-traditional cardiovascular risk factors′ interactions result from an active cross-talk between proatherogenic mediators derived from metabolic, vascular and autoimmune joint and skin inflammation in target tissues. Consistently, psoriasis and psoriatic arthritis diseases offer an invaluable scenario to deepen our knowledge on atherosclerotic cardiovascular disease.

Keywords: psoriasis, psoriatic arthritis, inflammation, immune system, cardiovascular risk factors

1. Introduction

Traditional cardiovascular risk factors like smoking, diabetes mellitus, hypertension, and hypercholesterolemia can barely account for the high prevalence of cardiovascular disease.

At the beginning of the last century, Nikolai N. Anichkov demonstrated that cholesterol per se was able to produce atheromatous lesions in the vascular wall [1]. He also described the presence of inflammatory cells in the lesions, but these findings were dismissed for many decades. In 1995, Hansson and others established that atherosclerosis exhibited many features of a chronic inflammatory process, giving rise to the immune-mediated hypothesis behind atherogenesis [2]. At the time, however, preventive medicine was not a priority. Nowadays, such discoveries can be highly valuable in immune-mediated inflammatory disorders (IMID) in general, and in psoriasis (Ps) and psoriatic arthritis (PsA) in particular. It is known that adaptive and innate immunity participate in every step of atherogenesis. In fact, both traditional and non-traditional cardiovascular risk (CVR) factors increase in the course of these diseases [3]. This provides a comprehensive basis to explain the immune-mediated nature of atherogenesis beyond autoimmune condition while outlining the different crossroads of inflammation.

2. Psoriasis and psoriatic arthritis

Psoriasis (Ps) and psoriatic arthritis (PsA) belong to the family of IMID, affecting predominantly skin and joints. The prevalence of Ps varies between 2 and 3% worldwide with a similar distribution according to sex [4]. Epidemiological studies show peak incidence between the second and third decades in life [5]. It has been estimated that 7–42% of Ps patients develop inflammatory arthropathy, usually manifesting as a mono or asymmetrical oligo-arthritis [6]. Substantial body of evidence suggests that PsA patients are at higher risk of developing atherosclerotic cardiovascular disease (CVD) [7–9] and mortality [10, 11]. To date, the pathogenesis of Ps and PsA remains unknown. Autoantigens have not been identified and the specificity of infiltrating lymphocytes is still unknown [2]. Genetically predisposed background and several suspected environmental triggering factors (e.g., infections, drugs, physical, and emotional stress) have been implicated in the initial stages of these diseases [9]. PsA is considered a seronegative (rheumatoid factor negative) arthritis. In Ps and PsA, the inflammatory features/reactions in skin and joints are very similar regarding composition of inflammatory infiltrates and vascular changes as explained in **Figure 1** [12]. Moreover, the cellular infiltrate is predominantly perivascular and due to mononuclear cells [13].

The contribution of B lymphocytes to Ps and PsA pathogenesis is poorly understood. However, none of the forms of Ps or PsA have been associated with serum auto-antibodies [14]. In contrast, T lymphocytes are the most abundant in both skin and the synovial fluid of joints, with

http://dx.doi.org/10.5772/intechopen.68559

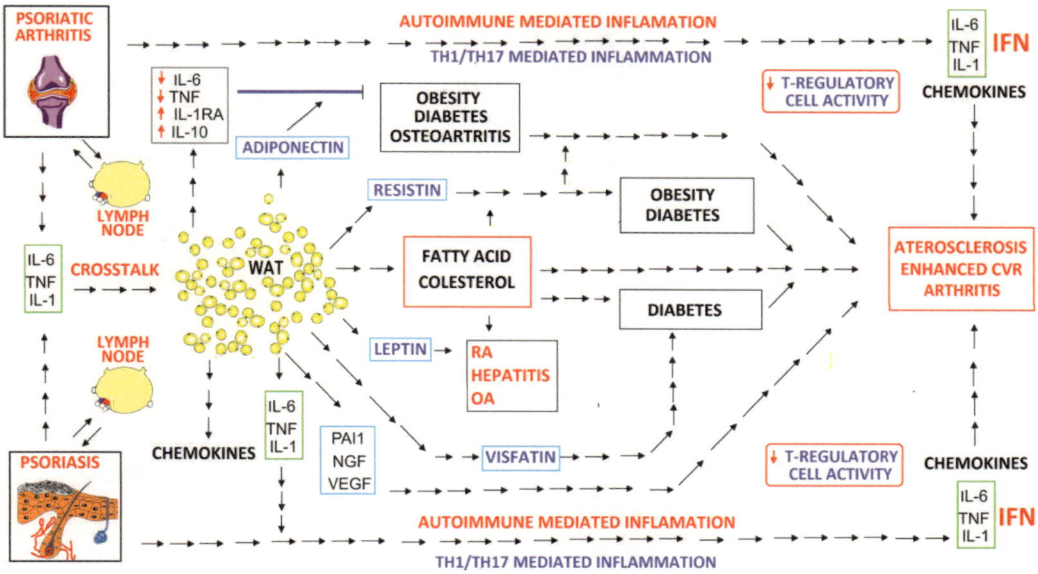

Figure 1. Schematic representation of the immune system-derived crosstalk between IMID and metabolic tissue, with events that worsen cardiovascular risk profile. Chronic inflammation of the skin and joints have many common immunopathological features, including genetic predisposition, composition of inflammatory infiltrates, vascular changes, early immune events, and proangiogenicity. Antigen is presented to naive CD4 T cells during immune synapse in the lymph node. Emerging lymphocytes migrate preferentially to skin and joints, where the above-mentioned infiltrating T lymphocytes (CD4 and CD8) interact with local APC (Langerhans cells, myeloid-DC, and plasmacytoid-DC) to produce chronic inflammatory conditions. Local re-activated T cells secrete chemokines and cytokines that amplify the inflammatory environment, resulting in the formation of psoriatic plaque, induction of cartilage degradation, and perhaps formation of atherosclerotic plaque. Since the suppressive activity of regulatory T cells is decreased in both tissue and blood, chronic production of proinflammatory cytokines (IFN-γ and TNF-α) crucially contributes to perpetuate the disease. In addition, deregulated adipose tissue (WAT) that secretes cytokines and chemokynes enhances systemic inflammatory burden leading to metabolic diseases (diabetes, metabolic syndrome, and dislipemia).

predominance of Tc1 (subpopulation of CD8+ cytotoxic T cells that secrete interferon (IFN) and IL-4), T-helper 1 lymphocyte subpopulation (Th1) and Th17 (IL-17+ T-helper cells) which interact with dendritic cells, macrophages, and target tissue cells [15]. Positive chemotaxis is observed between these cells and MCP-1 as found in synovial fluid [16] and skin biopsies obtained from Ps and PsA patients [17]. The role of lymphocytes in Ps and PsA pathogenesis is discussed later.

3. Atherosclerosis

Atherosclerosis is a complex inflammatory disease characterized by disturbances in the metabolic and immune system homeostasis that lead to pathogenic chronic progressive vascular damage and production of atherosclerosis plaque containing macrophages, lymphocytes, and other immune cells.

Classical knowledge distinguishes between inflammatory and non-inflammatory diseases. However, this distinction is no longer appropriate following the identification of inflammatory mechanisms associated with the traditionally called "non-inflammatory diseases."

Although atherogenesis belonged to this group for several decades, now it is confirmed that the immune system acts on the endothelial wall and triggers an inflammatory cascade, leading to a progressive low-grade inflammatory process of the arterial vascular wall in response to accumulation and oxidation of lipoproteins. Yet, further considerations pinpoint a prominent and severely pathogenic role of the immune system in these diseases [18].

Studies in hypercholesterolemia-induced immune activation in mouse models of atherosclerosis highlight the critical balance between Th1 cells [19] and Treg [20]. Inflammation in the intima layer appears to be related with protective and pathogenic immune responses against modified self-antigens in the atherosclerotic plaque [21].

The paradigm of atherosclerosis as an inflammatory disease is widely accepted. Interestingly, systemic inflammatory rheumatic diseases might share several immune-mediated inflammatory pathways with atherosclerosis. In fact, molecules and cells from innate and adaptive immune system (described below) mediate chronic inflammatory pathways activation derived from both diseases interacting in a positive feedback pathogenic circuit.

Increasing evidence suggests that even in clinically heterogeneous diseases, both of them could share common immunological pathways that might damage the cardiovascular (CV) system (**Table 1**). The contribution of chronic inflammation to CVR has mainly been investigated in rheumatoid arthritis (RA), the prototypical inflammatory disorder [22–24]. Consistently,

Author, year	**Number of patients and study profile**	**Findings**
Han et al., 2006 [33]	3066 PsA patients vs. clinically asimptomatic controls matched by age, sex, and geographic region.	Higher prevalence for CHF, PVD, IHD atherosclerosis, type II diabetes, HL, and HTN in PsA patients than controls.
Sattar et al., 2007 [34]	127 patients with active Ps/PsA after at least first failure with DMARDS treatment, PsA- with 6 months duration or more with active arthritis in 3 or 4 swollen joints. Double-blind placebo (n = 42) controlled study performed with two doses of Onercept for 12 weeks.	Result compared against baseline before and after the end of treatment with Onercept. Results indicate higher CRP, that positively correlate with reduced Lp (a); higher ICAM-1; reduced IL6; reduced Homocysteine; same levels Apo-I, higher Apo-B, and higher TG.
Gonzalez-Juanatey et al., 2007 [35]	59 PsA patients vs. 59 control patients without clinically evident CVD adjusted for age and ethnia.	Carotid artery IMT correlated with age, time of PsA diagnosis, disease duration, total cholesterol, and LDL.
Eder et al., 2008 [36]	40 PsA patients compared with 40 controls matched by age, sex, and CVR factors.	Multivariate analysis indicates that PsA status, age, and TG levels were associated with IMT and carotid plaque.
Tam et al., 2008 [37]	102 PsA patients from Southern China.	Increased prevalence of DM and HTN was found in PsA group compared with age- and sex and BMI-matched controls.
Kimhi et al., 2007 [38]	Carotid artery IMT from 47 patients with PsA were compared with 43 healthy controls matched for age and sex.	The average IMT (mean/standard deviation) in PsA patients was significantly higher compared to CP even after adjustment for age, GR, BMI, HTN, and HL.

Author, year	Number of patients and study profile	Findings
Gladman et al., 2009 [39]	648 patients with Ps and PsA.	Enhanced CV risk. Severity of skin involvement is an independent CVR factor.
Shang et al., 2011 [40]	94 PsA patients without clinical evidence of CVD and 63 healthy subjects.	PsA patients without established CVD and in the absence of TRF have a high prevalence of subclinical ED via imaging studies.
Eder et al., 2013 [29]	Cross-sectional study comparing 125 PsA with 114 Ps patients.	PsA patients suffer from more severe subclinical atherosclerosis compared with Ps patients.This difference is independent of CVR factors.
Ogdie et al., 2014 [27]	Longitudinal cohort study comparing 8706 PsA, 41,752 RA, 138,424 Ps and 82,258 controls.	Patients with RA and Ps have increased mortality compared with the GP but patients with PsA do not.
Svedbom et al., 2015 [41]	The study compared the risk of death in 39,074 patients with mild and severe psoriasis vs. 154,775 sex-, age-matched referents.	Cardiovascular disease was the main driver of excess mortality patients with mild and severe psoriasis.
Cea-Calvo et al., 2016 [42]	PSO-RISK was a cross-sectional, multicenter, single-visit study of 368 patients (≥18) with Ps on systemic therapy.	CVR factors were detected in 27.5% (n = 101) of patients with previously unknown cardiovascular risk factors.
Tejón et al., 2016 [43]	The study compared age- and sex-matched case-control study PsA patients who developed CV events during the study (2010–2014) vs. control group CV events.	Traditional CV risk factors as well non-inflammatory CV risk factors of the disease were the main predictors of CV complications in this PsA population.

AC: Alcohol consumption; BMI: Body mass index; CAD: Coronary artery disease; CCF: Controlled for confounding factors; CHF: Congestive heart failure; CP: Control population; CVD: Cardiovascular disease; DM: Diabetes mellitus; DMARDS: Disease-modifying antirheumatic drugs; ED: Endothelial dysfunction; GR: Gender: GP: General population; HDL: High-density lipoprotein; HL: Hyperlipidemia; HTN: Hypertension; ICAM-1: Intercellular adhesion molecule 1; IHD: Ischemic heart disease; IL6: Interleukin 6; LDL: Low-density lipoprotein; Lp (a): Lipoprotein A; MI: Myocardial infarction; OB: Obesity; PVD: Peripheral vascular disease; TC: Total cholesterol; TG: Triglycerides; TRF: Traditional risk factors; VLDL: Very low-density lipoprotein.

Table 1. Representative summary of epidemiological studies (prospective and retrospective) linking Ps to associated Cardiovascular Risk and Comorbidities (RCM), published between 2006 and 2016.

chronic activation of immune-mediated pathways is believed to accelerate or trigger critical atherosclerosis events in Ps and PsA.

A multidisciplinary expert committee was designated a few years ago in accordance with European League against Rheumatism (EULAR) suggests apart from the management of conventional risk factors, an aggressive inflammation suppressive therapy to further reduce [3] death in PsA patients [25]. Chronic inflammatory state seems to be the potential driving force behind the accelerated atherogenesis [26]. In this regard, few papers have been published related to CVR factors (**Table 1**) [7, 8, 27]. Some representative prospective and retrospective epidemiological surveys, published between 2006 and 2015 (**Table 1**), indicate that Ps and PsA patients exhibit higher prevalence of myocardial infarction (MI), ischemic heart disease, hypertension, diabetes, and dyslipidemia compared with normal controls. Although multiple CVR factors are associated with Ps, key components of the metabolic syndrome are more strongly connected with more severe Cutaneous psoriasis (PsC) [28]. Recent studies [29] suggest an increased inflammatory burden in PsA compared with Ps (**Table 1**). In contrast, the risk of developing a CV event (MI, ischemic stroke, and transient ischemic attack) was not elevated in early Ps patients in a matched follow-up study, case-control analysis [30, 31].

4. Inflammatory and classical cardiovascular risk factors

4.1. Inflammatory risk factors

Since a substantial amount of data accumulates in the past of this issue, we provide a brief insight into the most common inflammation-related and non-inflammatory factors involved in accelerated atherogenesis in Ps and PsA. As previously mentioned, Ps and atherosclerosis have a similar immune innate and adaptive pathogenic hallmark and an active crosstalk between "traditional" or "non-traditional" (**Figure 1**) [32].

4.1.1. Innate immunity

Toll-like receptor 2 (TLR-2) and toll-like receptor 4 (TLR-4) trigger receptor-mediated events, including cytokine-mediated inflammation, are involved in atherosclerosis [44], Ps, and other pathologies [34]. TLR expression is positively correlated with plasma tumor necrosis factor-alpha (TNF-α) levels [45]. Cytokine-triggered TLRs activation is known to modulate major pathological processes, including inflammation, angiogenesis, tissue remodeling, and fibrosis. Although joints are the most obvious inflammation sites in PsA, proinflammatory cytokines, most likely TNF-α and interleukin 6 (IL-6), are released in blood circulation and act on distant organs (immune system, adipose tissue, liver, hematopoietic tissue, skeletal muscle, glands, and endothelium). These effects are linked to systemic inflammation and lead to a proatherogenic profile. Cytokines orchestrate endothelial adhesiveness, matrix metalloproteinases (MMPs) activation, reactive oxygen species (ROS) production, C-reactive protein (CRP), fibrinogen, and plasminogen activator inhibitor-1 (PAI-1) release [46].

Indeed, atherogenic lipid alterations, oxidative stress abnormalities, vascular injury repair failure, arterial stiffness, insulin resistance induction, endothelial dysfunction, hypercoagulable state, homocysteine elevation, and pathogenic T cell up-regulation could all be attributed in part to the proinflammatory actions of cytokines. Common inflammatory mechanisms in Ps and atherosclerosis may be related to other factors by the high number of overlapping molecules, including cytokines [interleukins (IFN-α, IL-2, IL-6, IL-10, IL-13, IL-15, IL-17, IL-18, IL-20, and IL-23)], interferon alpha (IFN-α), Oncostatin M, (TNF-α), chemokines [Fractalkine, growth-regulated oncogene (GRO) alpha], CCL-3(MIP-1α), CCL-4 (MIP-1α), CCL-11 (Eotaxin), IL-8, MCP-1, monokine induced by interferon gamma (MIG/CXCL9), adipokines

(Resistin, Leptin, and PAI-1), adhesion molecules (ICAM/LFA-1(leukocyte function-associated antigen-1), CD154 (OX40L)/CD134 (OX40), epidermal growth factor (EGF), vascular endothelial growth factor (VEGF), fibroblast growth factors (FGF), and GCSF, co-stimulatory molecules (CD80, CD28, and CD40/CD40L), lymphocyte profile Th1/Th17 up-regulation, Treg down-regulation, CTL effect or activity, NK cells, natural killer T (NKT) cells, myeloid dendritic cells, plasmacytoid dendritic cells, monocytes/macrophages, mast cells and neutrophils, complement activation [47], TLR-mediated inflammation (TLR-2, TLR-4, and TLR-9) [27–29], and other important factors, such as CRP, endothelin-1, inducible nitric oxide synthase (iNOS), heat shock protein (HSP60, HSP65, and HSP70), matrix metalloproteinases (MMP-2 and MMP-9), and oxidized low-density lipoprotein (LDL) [45, 48, 49]. Some molecules listed before and other PsA-related serum cytokine patterns have been demonstrated by multiplex cytokine array systems in Norwegian PsA patients [50, 51]. Few of these cytokines previously mentioned [52, 53] and their pathogenic contribution at different stages in the pathobiology of atherothrombosis and PsA are not clear yet [36].

NK cells increase the susceptibility to PsA [51] and the inflammatory infiltrate in psoriatic skin lesions. Although more studies must be done, emerging evidence supports a role for NK cells in Ps. Inverse correlation exists between NK cell population and body mass index (BMI). Therefore, adipose immune cell phenotype and function may provide greater insight into cardio-metabolic pathophysiology in psoriasis [54, 55].

NKT cells are a heterogeneous subset of T cell lineage lymphocytes that bear NK cell molecules and T cell receptors, which recognize microbial glycolipids and their own endogenous mammalian lipids presented by the MHC I-like molecule (CD1d) and have been implicated in the pathogenesis of various autoimmune diseases including Ps. Due to the numerous functions of NKT cells that link innate and adaptive immunity, their role in Ps is complex and still elusive. ApoE and LDL receptors have been involved in antigen uptake for presentation to NKT cells [56] NKT cells may represent a potential new therapy for atherosclerosis [57].

Our knowledge of biologically active serum molecules and cells involved in the pathogenesis of both PsA and atherosclerosis is still not clear enough. Taken together, cytokines seem to play a pivotal role as the major link between PsA and atherosclerosis. Compiled data show that untreated PsA inflammation could produce damage to the CV system even before it affects the joints [50]. Current evidence suggests that the pathway of inflammation in atherosclerosis culminates in altered concentrations of various markers in peripheral blood, including oxidative stress molecules [58–60] and markers of vascular inflammation like CRP [59], IL-6, ICAM-1, and MCP-1 [61].

4.1.1.1. Tumor necrosis factor-α

The pleiotropic cytokine TNF-α is among the most potent mediators of inflammation. Circulating T lymphocytes and monocyte-derived macrophages isolated from PsA patients produce increased amounts of TNF-α in comparison with macrophages isolated from healthy controls [8]. Furthermore, levels of TNF-α in PsA patients are elevated in the synovial tissue and skin lesions and correlate with disease activity. TNF-α is a key regulator of vascular homoeostasis [34], leading to proatherogenic effects, lipid abnormalities, including high LDL cholesterol and low HDL cholesterol [62], hypercoagulable state via induction of cell surface expression of tissue factor (TF) on the endothelial wall and suppress anticoagulant activity via the thrombomodulin-activated protein C system [63]. The majority of epidermal CTL and Th1 effector lymphocyte populations and molecules are elevated in Ps vulgaris lesions and in circulating blood in psoriatic patients [64]. TNF-α also induces endothelial dysfunction including low nitric oxide availability and up-regulation of endothelial adhesion molecules such as vascular cell adhesion molecule 1 (VCAM-1) [65, 66], a critical early step in atherogenesis. On the other hand, TNF-α blockade leads to a significant decrease in the levels of lipoprotein a (Lpa) homocysteine and an increase in apolipoprotein A-I (Apo A-I), triglyceride, and Apo-B concentration [62]. Long-term use of TNF-α blocking agents interferes with TNF-α function reducing the high incidence of cardiovascular events and associated vascular complications in CV diseases [67]. Taken together, the above-mentioned studies confirm a critical role for TNF-α in altering a number of well-studied putative vascular, thrombotic, and metabolic risk parameters (lipids and lipoproteins).

4.1.1.2. Interleukin 6

As an inflammatory cytokine, IL-6 regulates chemokine-directed leukocyte trafficking and directs transition from innate to adaptive immunity through the regulation of leukocyte activation, differentiation, and proliferation [68]. During acute and chronic inflammatory response, macrophages release TNF-α in the presence of a great variety of stimuli, including atherogenic and poorly characterized arthritogenic factors. TNF-α action on macrophages triggers the release of more TNF-α and IL1-β, which stimulate endothelial cells to produce IL-6 and IL-8. IL-6 and their signaling events contribute to hepatic release of acute-phase reactants including CRP levels, atherosclerotic plaque development and destabilization [69, 70]. IL-6 may also contribute to atherosclerosis and arterial thrombosis by activating the production of tissue factor, fibrinogen and factor VIII; increasing endothelial cell adhesiveness and stimulating platelet production and aggregation [71]. In addition, IL-6 is produced by smooth muscle cells (SMC) of many blood vessels and by adipocytes and, together with CRP and TNF-α, is involved in metabolic syndrome pathophysiology, insulin resistance [72] and coronary artery disease and the risk of MI [73–76], and cardiovascular mortality [77]. In addition, IL-6 locally produced in the endothelium and in SMC is an important autocrine and paracrine regulator of SMC proliferation and migration. IL-6 decreases cardiac contractility via a nitric oxide (NO)-dependent pathway activating STAT3-dependent anti-inflammatory signal transduction [78].

Numerous studies show a strong association between IL-6 and joint immune-mediated diseases. In the joint, macrophages and mast cells trigger a proinflammatory cascade in the presence of unknown stimuli, releasing great amounts of TNF-α, which induce the expression of IL-1 and IL-6. Mice deficient in mast cells are comparatively resistant in experimentally induced arthritis. In addition, it is a major promoter of bone resorption in pathological conditions [79]. In particular, IL-6 has a pivotal role in synovitis, bone erosion, and in the systemic features of inflammation [80].

http://dx.doi.org/10.5772/intechopen.68559

In Ps, most available evidence indicates that the pathogenic action of IL-6 is important. In fact, IL-6 co-localizes with CD45+ perivascular cells within lesional tissue and reverses the suppressive function of human T-regulatory cells [81].

The successful treatment of certain autoimmune conditions with the humanized antibody anti-IL-6 receptor (IL-6R) (Tocilizumb) has emphasized the clinical importance of cytokines that signal through the β-receptor subunit glycoprotein 130 [82].

IL-6 may, in both cardiovascular and joint-diseases involving Th1/Th17 mechanisms, alter the balance between the effector and regulatory arms of the immune system and drive a proinflammatory phenotype reinforcing innate and adaptive immune-mediated positive feedback [83], potentiating the immune effector mechanism. In both arterial disease and Ps/PsA, IL-6 seems to be a critical mediator of long-term chronic inflammation and to have deleterious effect in the arterial wall and in the joint.

4.1.1.3. Endothelin-1

The family of endothelins (ET) includes three 21-aminoacid isoforms endothelin-1 (ET-1), endothelin-2 (ET-2), and endothelin-3 (ET-3), which have endogenous pressor activity and are secreted by different tissues and cells. In addition, ET-1 is a vasoactive peptide that induces vasoconstriction, inflammation, and fibrosis and has mitogenic potential for SMC [84]. In the skin, ET-1 participates in keratinocyte proliferation, neoangiogenesis, and chemotaxis. Its levels are elevated in psoriatic lesions and serum of patients with Ps [85]. Synovial tissue and serum of patients with PsA all show strongly enhanced ET-1 receptor expression [86].

4.1.1.4. C-reactive protein

A considerable amount of evidence implicates C-reactive protein (CRP) as a predictive marker for future CV events and mortality in different settings, particularly under metabolic syndrome conditions in the general population [87, 88]; CRP has also been implicated as a direct partaker [7, 89, 90]. In addition, CRP stimulates the production of plaque destabilizing MMPs and MCP-1, a decrease in the activity of endothelial nitric oxide synthase (eNOS) and impairment in endothelium dependent vasodilation [91]. In vitro, studies provide evidence for direct proatherogenic effects of CRP, including increased endothelial dysfunction [92]. Baseline CRP levels were elevated in patients with Ps with and without psoriatic arthritis and Etanercept, a biologic TNF antagonist, treatment may reduce CRP levels in both groups [93].

4.1.1.5. Adipokines

Interestingly, in metabolic disorders associated with Ps/PsA, inflamed adipose tissue may enhance inflammatory proatherogenic status via adipokine production (leptin, adiponectin, and resistin) and cytokine (TNF-α and IL-6) secretion. Adipose tissue influences both natural and adaptive immunities and links inflammation, metabolic dysfunction, and cardiovascular disease [94].

4.1.1.6. Matrix metalloproteinases (MMPs)

MMPs are endoproteases with collagenase and/or gelatinase activity which exert deleterious effects on the endothelium integrity and collagen fibers, promoting atherosclerotic plaque destabilization and accelerating the process of atherothrombosis [95]. MMP-1 serum levels and gene expression are elevated in PsA [96].

4.1.2. Adaptive immunity

As previously mentioned, Ps/PsA and atherosclerosis share certain common underlying pathogenic inflammatory mechanisms. Specifically, both are associated with Th1 and CTL (cytotoxic T lymphocyte) effector cell-mediated events in vivo [68], and are elevated in circulating blood [63]. In contrast, the T-regulatory activity is reduced.

4.1.2.1. Cellular immune response

Myeloid dendritic cells can stimulate both memory and naive T cells, and are the most potent of all the antigen-presenting cells in normal and various pathophysiological conditions [97]. In turn, activated T cells undergo firm adhesion and transendothelial migration to inflammatory focus. Extravasation is orchestrated by the combined action of cellular adhesion receptors and chemotactic factors in a wide variety of cardiovascular and autoimmune disorders that involve inflammation.

The development and maintenance of psoriatic plaque are dependent on the participation of infiltrating T lymphocytes (CD4 and CD8) and local antigen-presenting cells (APCs) (Langerhans cells, myeloid, and plasmacytoid-DC). DCs are increased in psoriatic lesions and are critically involved in the induction of Th1 and Th17 cell proliferation, which, in turn, release IFN-γ and IL-17, respectively. Activated mDCs produce IL-23 [98, 99] and TNF-α. IL-23 stimulates the secretion of IL-22 by Th17 cells, which may be involved in epidermal hyperplasia [5]. The effects of IL-17A-producing T-helper 17 (Th17) cells include suppressive effects of T-regulatory (Treg) subsets, which have also been implicated in both pathologies. The association of IL-17A with Ps and PsA has been extensively described [98, 99] and a growing body of evidence suggests that IL-17A might also be involved in atherosclerosis [100]. IL-17 seems to have a modulatory role in atherosclerosis, but studies available show contrasting results, which could be attributed to different approaches and models. Coronary syndrome correlates with increased IL-17 levels [101]. In addition, TNF-α and IL-17 synergistically up-regulate further cytokine transcription in both diseases, Ps and atherogenesis [102]. These observations make IL-17A an interesting therapeutic target to modulate both PsA/Ps disease activity and atherosclerosis/cardiovascular risk. Obesity may play an important role by amplifying the inflammation of arthritis through the Th1/Th17 response [103]. Limited evidence from Ps patients indicates that induction therapy with infliximab, with moderate to severe plaque Ps, led to decrease in clinical disease scores and circulating levels of Th17, Th1 cells, and associated TNF-α release [104].

T cell activation is under control from T-regulatory immune cell (Treg) activity via IL-10 and TGF-β [105–107]. Reduced numbers and/or activity of Treg cells may produce hyperactivity of Th1/Th17 subsets in both pathologies [21, 108, 109]. Ps and coronary artery disease patients show impaired inhibitory function of Treg [110, 111]. Serum and epidermal levels [105, 106] of TGF-β in Ps patients are associated with Ps disease severity [112, 113] and are diminished in low Ps [5]. In atherosclerosis, high serum levels of TGF-β and IL-10 may inhibit plaque formation [114, 115] and plaque stabilization exerting protective effect due its inhibition of T cells [116].

4.1.2.2. Humoral immune response

Humoral response seems to protect rather than harm the host. Several lines of evidence support the hypothesis that humoral immunity protects patients against atherosclerosis. First, the injection of immunoglobulin preparations inhibits atherosclerosis. Second, spleen removal (a B-cell rich lymphoid organ) seems to deteriorate vascular disease condition. Third, oxidized LDL plus adjuvant immunization promote atheroprotection [2]. Evidence so far indicates that atheroprotection is due to a T cell dependent B-cell-mediated mechanism, probably involving antibody dependent clearance of LDL and humoral dependent regulation of pathogenic T cell [17]. This atheroprotective response must be confirmed in humans.

4.1.3. Genes related to the innate and adaptive immune system associated with psoriasis and atherogenesis

At least 10 chromosomal locus associated with psoriasis have been identified as PSORS (PSORS, psoriasis susceptibility) [117]. Additionally, certain human leucocyte antigen (HLAs) are more common in psoriatic arthritis. HLA alleles that are specific for psoriatic arthritis are HLA-B27 and possibly HLA-B7, HLA-B38, and HLA-B39.

There is a strong association of psoriasis with the HLA-Cw6 allele, which increases 10–20 times the risk of psoriasis and is present in 90% of the patients with early onset psoriasis and in 50% of those with late onset psoriasis [118].

Some molecules of the innate immune system have an important influence on the pathophysiology of psoriasis, such as TLR2 and TLR4 play a key role in the pathogenesis of autoimmune diseases, including rheumatoid arthritis, systemic lupus erythematosus, systemic sclerosis, Sjogren's syndrome, psoriasis, multiple sclerosis, and autoimmune diabetes [119].

Additionally, the expression of TLR2 and TLR4 correlates with the degree and severity of coronary disease [120, 121] oxidized phospholipids stimulate the TLR signaling pathway to induce inflammatory cytokine secretion by macrophages and endothelial cells [122].

Anti-CD14 and anti-TLR antibodies significantly inhibit the binding of fluorescein-labeled LDL to monocytes and interfering with cytokine release [123]. TNF-binding proteins are encoded by genes unrelated to PSORS, conferring susceptibility to psoriasis. Tumor necrosis factor, alpha-induced protein 3 (TNFAIP3) and tumor necrosis factor interacting protein 1 (TNIP1) are related to the inflammatory signal NF-κB, which regulates the release of TNF-α [124, 125].

TNFAIP3 promotes the survival of T-CD4 lymphocytes [126]. Certain cytokine genes have been implicated with psoriasis, including IL-12, IL-23, IL-4/IL-13 [127] conferring an increased risk of psoriatic arthritis [128].

These genes strengthened the assertion that psoriasis is an immune disorder, as these genes are linked to both the innate and adaptive immune response [129–131]. In summary, defects in these genes could amplify an inflammatory response by interfering with normal negative feedback of the NF-kB signal and therefore would link to psoriasis with other IMID and coronary pathology.

4.2. Non-inflammatory risk factors

Ps, PsA, and atherosclerosis share disturbances in different metabolic pathways involving insulin-dependent diabetes mellitus (IDDM), dyslipidemia, hypertension, obesity, and mostly metabolic syndrome, which may be related to an increase in the prevalence of CVD to their capability of inducing inflammation on the endothelial lining to initiate the process of atherosclerosis. So far, no pathophysiological mechanism for this association has been identified [63].

4.2.1. Hypertension

Several studies have found an increase in the prevalence of hypertension in Ps patients, although the definition of hypertension is very heterogeneous among these studies [117–121, 132]. Other authors have not observed a significant association between Ps and hypertension [122].

4.2.2. Diabetes mellitus

IDDM is responsible for metabolic alterations, accompanied by chronic inflammation and endothelium dysfunction. Observational studies show that the risk of IDDM is higher in patients with Ps compared with a healthy control group. This risk increases with the duration and severity of Ps and it is not related to a high body mass index (BMI) alone [133]. In a case-control study from Israel, the risk of diabetes was significantly higher in individuals with Ps [124]. Similarly, PsA patients have a higher prevalence of IDDM, even after adjusting for the BMI [125]. TNF-α antagonist therapy in patients with Ps seems to improve insulin sensitivity in limited preliminary data [126]. Finally, a few isolated cases of Ps patients with diabetes develop unpredictable hyperglycemia after starting treatment with TNF-α inhibitors [127].

4.2.3. Obesity

Recent studies have shown that obesity may precede the onset of Ps as a risk factor [120], whereas a higher BMI is associated with more severe skin disease activity [3]. The influence of obesity on psoriatic diseases is the result of complex interactions of inflammatory and metabolic factors. The proinflammatory cytokines stimulate adipocytes to synthesize neuropeptides and more cytokines, which are critical in the pathogenesis of the psoriatic and CVD [69].

4.2.4. *Smoking*

Heavy and long-term smoking [128] have been associated with increased Ps risk in both men and women [129], particularly pustular Ps [116, 117, 120]. Smoking increases oxidative damage, promotes inflammatory changes, and enhances Ps-associated gene expression [121] and CVR [50, 122].

4.2.5. *Dyslipidemia*

Ps patients have a higher prevalence of dyslipidemia and triglycerides and lower prevalence of HDL levels. However, associations with total cholesterol and LDL have not been found statistically significant in a multivariate analysis study [116–118].

4.2.6. *Metabolic syndrome*

The metabolic syndrome consists of a constellation of clinical features involving abdominal obesity (waist circumference from >94 cm in men and >80 cm in women), and two or more of the following clinical situations:

HDL ≤ 40 mg/dl in men and 50 mg/dl in women, TG > 150 mg/dl, fasting blood glucose > 100 mg/dl, blood pressure > 130/85 mm Hg or treatment for hypertension. The metabolic syndrome is characterized by increases in the immunological activity of Th1, which suggests it may be associated with Ps because of shared inflammatory pathways.

Gisondi et al. [134] reported that, among Ps patients without systemic medication, 40-year-old and older people have a higher prevalence of metabolic syndrome [124].

Recently, Raychaudhuri et al. observed an increased prevalence of metabolic syndrome in patients with PsA; DM type 2 [58] and increased risk for CVD and mortality [125–129]. Ps with metabolic syndrome [130] associates with high serum uric acid levels that correlate with an increased risk of carotid intima-media thickness (IMT) or with the presence of carotid plaques [131].

5. Common angiogenic factors for Ps and atherosclerosis

Angiogenesis appears to be pathological in some chronic inflammatory diseases, like Ps and RA. It is possible for reactive homeostatic or pathological angiogenesis to play an important role in atherosclerosis. Serum levels of proangiogenic cytokines (TGF-β, TNF-α, IL-8, and IL-17), growth factors, including VEGF, and hypoxia-induced factor-1 have been shown to be significantly elevated in Ps patients compared to healthy controls [132, 133].

6. Oxidative mechanisms common to atherosclerosis and Ps

Cellular deregulation and damage [51] could be the result of overproduction or insufficient removal of ROS. In the skin, ROS can be generated either endogenous or exogenously.

Endogenously, ROS are produced through the electron transport chain and enzymes, such as cyclooxygenases (COX) [33], lipoxygenases [38], NADPH oxidases [135], and myeloperoxidases [39]. Exogenous sources that trigger ROS production include UV radiation and heavy metals [51]. In Ps, antioxidant defense mechanisms seem to be impaired, including superoxide dismutases (SODs), glutathione peroxidases, glutathione reductase, catalase, thioredoxin/thioredoxin reductase system, and metallothioneins. Augmented ROS production in the skin leads to downstream molecular events that promote atherosclerosis [51, 136, 137].

The antioxidant activity of vitamin D is well known/widely characterized. The knowledge of non-classical functions emerges from studies that indicate a close association between a low vitamin D status and increased risk of IMID and CVD [138]. It is also known that vitamin D insufficiency induces metabolic, procoagulant, and inflammatory perturbations. Recent studies indicate that it also increases the risk of MI by promoting established CVR factor-mediated mechanisms that predispose to atherothrombosis [139].

Immunomodulatory role of vitamin D in human health implicates appropriate signaling for both innate and adaptive immune responses (T and B lymphocyte function) [140–142] that amplify inflammation in Ps [143] and promote the development of different types of Treg cells [144].

7. Some lessons from CVD and rheumatic-associated therapies

Whether antirheumatic therapies increase or decrease CV risk is controversial. Glucocorticoids (GCs) are known to cause hypercholesterolemia, hypertriglyceridemia, weight gain, hypertension, and glucose intolerance, all factors promoting CVD. However, GCs are not ever conflicting. In RA patients with a known history of CVD, steroid therapy surprisingly attenuated the risk of CV death [145]. The mechanism of this apparent discrepancy with GC exposure is still unknown, but it seems to be related with dose, duration, and intensity of the exposure.

Although coronary artery disease and acute myocardial infarction are inflammatory disorders, the only drugs with anti-inflammatory effect so far widely used in ischemic heart disease are aspirin and statins (e.g., atorvastatin and simvastatin).

The contribution of coxibs and most nonsteroidal anti-inflammatory drugs (NSAIDs) to lowering CVR is not well established and the evidence available so far is controversial. Multiple studies provide evidence that methotrexate is protective against CV events and CV mortality, although the protective benefit is under discussion [146]. Immunomodulatory or immunosuppressive therapies, such as cyclosporine and colchicine, may have benefits in coronary artery disease [147]. Other studies have found that glucocorticoids plus cytotoxic immunosuppressive agents (azathioprine, cyclosporine, and leflunomide) are associated with an increased amount of CV events when compared with methotrexate alone [148].

The new targeted biological therapies, such as the suppression of systemic inflammation by anti-TNF therapies, seem to be associated with concomitant reduction in the risk of CV events

http://dx.doi.org/10.5772/intechopen.68559

[149], although the effect of TNF-α antagonists in lowering proatherogenic status needs further investigation. In addition, cardiovascular therapy drugs could change the proinflammatory status of PsA patients under treatment with 3-hydroxy-3-methylglutaryl coenzyme A reductase inhibitors (statins), angiotensin converting-enzyme (ACE) inhibitors, and/or angiotensin II receptor antagonists (AT-II blockers). Hence, their prescription should be managed cautiously, especially for patients with a documented CV disease or in the presence of CVR factors.

Other drugs with potential benefits may include the thiazolidinedione (TZD) family, which produces positive effects on both CVR factors and Ps [14]. Targeted therapeutic interventions along with an effective control of the inflammation may have more beneficial CV effects than direct CV toxicity. There is a need for more studies addressing the role of current biological therapies on patients with a CV risk profile [3].

8. The central role of the immune system

Atherosclerosis is a complex disease but, as specific knowledge increases, the immune system can be clearly recognized to be involved in all steps of vascular pathology. Both classical and non-classical CVR factors are closely interconnected in the production of chronic inflammation through loss of immune homeostasis; indeed, either molecules or cells involved in atherogenesis present altered regulatory and/or effector immune functions, attenuating and promoting atherogenesis.

Some authors have proposed an autoimmune origin in atherosclerosis [82, 83]. Immune system homeostasis alterations against the patient's own antigens and the increasing prevalence of atherosclerosis in immune-mediated diseases, such as diabetes, periodontal disease, systemic sclerosis, antiphospholipid syndrome, RA, SLE, ankylosing spondylitis (AS), and PsA strongly reinforce the involvement of autoimmune mediators and the key role of inflammation in atherosclerosis [150]. This autoimmune response to oxidized LDL is a driving force for cell activation in the human atherosclerotic plaque [151]. The fact that low and high grade chronic inflammatory disorders present an accelerated progression of atherosclerosis constitutes indirect but critical evidence that strengthens the above-mentioned immune-mediated inflammation. The Ps/PsA proatherosclerotic profile seems to be related to chronic inflammation through classical and non-classical factors. Important insights reviewed in this article indicate that most, if not all inflammatory factors, are the result of immune activation and cytokine-driven inflammation.

For example, Th1, CTL, and Th17 effector cells are the dominant types in the pathogenesis of the psoriatic and cardiovascular diseases and are the most abundant T lymphocytes in skin, joints, and human atherosclerotic plaque [63]. In addition, reduced levels of circulating anti-inflammatory mediators and Treg may increase CV risk in both diseases [146, 152] inducing up-regulation of adhesion molecules [153] and promoting a more procoagulant [154] and vasoconstrictor phenotype [155]. Although anti-atherogenic humoral response could be verified, its anti-atherogenic action must be confirmed [2].

Indirect evidence indicating that immune-mediated inflammation is a key regulator in the crossroad of pathogenesis between Ps/PsA and atherogenesis derives from the role of certain therapies. Some drugs used in the treatment of CV disease, such as statins and ACE inhibitors, have anti-inflammatory activity. In addition, systemic treatments for Ps that decrease inflammation also reduce CV risk [156]. TLRs are the best candidates to explain what triggers and sustains the natural and adaptive immune response, maintaining proinflammatory cytokine gene expression in chronic inflammation, worsening atherosclerosis [145] in general population and in Ps patients.

Finally, the role of obesity, metabolic syndrome (possible via hypertriglyceridemia and associated abdominal adiposity in Ps/PsA patients), and probably DM, in this scenario of severe Ps and accelerated CVR. Adipose tissue is not just an "endocrine organ." Now, we know adipocytes express TLRs, which are involved in the innate immune response reacting to exogenous and endogenous stimuli by releasing inflammatory cytokines, adipokines, and other key mediators of Ps and atherogenesis. In addition, a consistent association was described between increasing obesity and lower serum 25-hydroxy vitamin D (25D) concentrations [147, 157].

In summary, chronic immune-mediated inflammation plays a key role in the pathogenesis of atherosclerosis in Ps, acting independently and/or synergistically with the conventional risk factors.

Framingham risk score (FRS), which only takes into account traditional CV risk factors for estimating the 10-year risk of CV events like metabolic syndrome and diabetes, may underestimate CVR related to underlying inflammatory factors associated with this disease, also known as non-traditional risk factors. Improvement by inflammatory suppression argues strongly for immune-mediated inflammation as the central risk factor for CVD in PsA. However, many of the studies investigating mechanisms of PsA associated with atherogenesis are not definitive or conclusive enough. Larger, more systematic, and controlled studies are needed to confirm many of the findings previously reviewed.

9. Conclusions

Most evidence reviewed in this chapter strongly supports the hypothesis that the inflammatory immune-mediated pathogenesis is probably the mayor force beyond the atherogenesis, from its initiation to plaque formation, rupture, and associated thrombotic complications. Taken together, evidence so far strongly suggests immune-mediated inflammation is the central actor in atherogenesis beyond all risk factors, regardless of whether they are "traditional" or "non-traditional." Although certain crossroads between immune-mediated inflammation pathways are activated in general population under cardiovascular risk conditions, it seems to be potentiated in psoriasis patients and other IMID. This is in agreement with accumulated evidence so far that indicates an enhanced CVR associated with Ps via both traditional and non-traditional factors immune-modulation.

Evidence so far suggests that patients with PsA and aggressive clinical presentation of Ps should be treated more aggressively for CVR prevention and modification. Therefore, selective long-term anti-atherosclerotic immunomodulation-oriented therapy might improve atherogenesis in both general population and Ps patients.

The existence of proatherogenic immunological pathways in CID that could damage the CV system reveals potential targets for more efficient therapies. This much more selective therapy requires long-term studies until it is available and accurate enough (**Figure 2**).

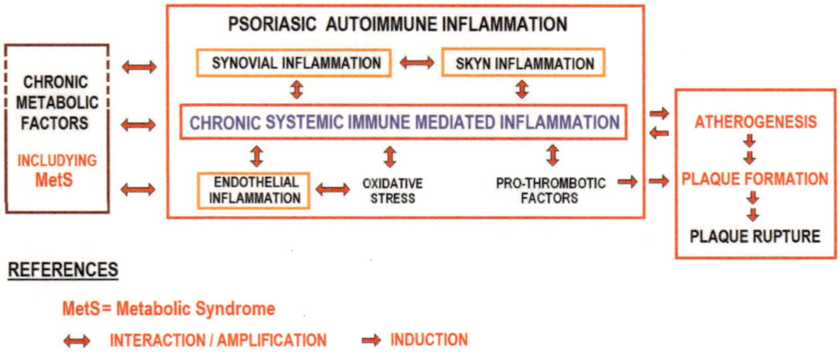

Figure 2. Interactions between autoreactive, metabolic, and endothelial inflammation. Adipose tissue releases numerous inflammatory cytokines (TNF, IL6, resistin, leptin, and vistatin) that contribute to elevate systemic inflammatory burden. The inflammatory load is also increased by the contribution of inflammatory cytokines derived from the affected tissues derived autoimmune diseases. The total inflammatory load is increased only in these patients. These molecules perpetuate and potentiate the inflammatory process, exerting a relevant proatherogenic effect. Increased uncontrolled inflammation also leads to increased oxidative stress and prothrombotic risk. Then, burden psoriatic disease is likely to be aggravated by the concurrence of augmented inflammatory burden along with disregulated activity.

Abbreviations

CV	Cardiovascular
CVD	Cardiovascular disease
CVR	Cardiovascular risk
CID	Chronic inflammatory disease
CRP	C-reactive protein
CLA	Cutaneous lymphocyte-associated antigen
EGF	Epidermal growth factor
eNOS	Endothelial nitric oxide synthase
ET	Endothelins
FGF	Fibroblast growth factors
GCs	Glucocorticoids
GCSF	Granulocyte colony-stimulating factor
GMCSF	Granulocyte macrophage colony-stimulating factor
CXCL-1 GRO-a	Growth-regulated oncogene-a

HSP	Heat shock protein
HDL	High-density lipoprotein
HIF-1	Hypoxia-induced factor-1
ICAM	Intercellular adhesion molecule
IL	Interleukin
iNOS	Inducible nitric oxide synthase
IFN-γ	Interferon gamma
IP-10	Interferon-inducible protein 10
ICAM1	Intercellular cell-adhesion molecule 1
IMT	Intima-media thickness
LDL	Low-density lipoprotein
LFA	Lymphocyte function-associated antigen-1
MMPs	Matrix metalloproteinases
MAPK	Mitogen-activated protein kinases
MCP-1	Monocyte chemoattractant protein 1

Conflict of interest statement

The authors have no competing interests or financial, political, personal, religious, ideological, academic, intellectual, commercial, or any other issues to declare in relation to this manuscript.

Author details

Rodolfo A. Kölliker Frers[1,2]‡, Matilde Otero-Losada[3]‡, Eduardo Kersberg[2], Vanesa Cosentino[2] and Francisco Capani[1,4*]

*Address all correspondence to: franciscocapani@hotmail.com

1 Laboratory of Cytoarchitecture and Neuronal Plasticity, Institute of Cardiological Research, University of Buenos Aires, Natl. Res. Council. ININCA.UBA.CONICET., Buenos Aires, Argentina

2 Rheumatology Department, J. M. Ramos Mejia Hospital, Buenos Aires, Argentina

3 Laboratory of HPLC, Institute of Cardiological Research, University of Buenos Aires, Natl. Res. Council. ININCA.UBA.CONICET., Buenos Aires, Argentina

4 Department of Biology, University John F. Kennedy, Buenos Aires, Argentina

‡ Rodolfo A. Kölliker Frers RA and Matilde Otero-Losada share authorship based on their participation in this work.

References

[1] Anitschkow N, Chalatow S. Über experimentelle Cholesterinsteatose and ihre Bedeutung fur die Entstehung einiger pathologischer Prozesse. Zentralbl Allg Path Path Anat (Zentralblatt für allgemeine Pathologie und pathologische Anatomie) 1913; 24:1-9.

[2] Hansson GK. Atherosclerosis—an immune disease: The Anitschkov Lecture 2007. Atherosclerosis. 2009;**202**:2-10

[3] Peters MJ, Symmons DP, McCarey D, Dijkmans BA, Nicola P, Kvien TK, et al. EULAR. Evidence-based recommendations for cardiovascular risk management in patients with rheumatoid arthritis and other forms of inflammatory arthritis. Annals of the Rheumatic Diseases. 2010;**69**:325-331

[4] Parisi R, Symmons DP, Griffiths CE, Ashcroft DM. Global epidemiology of psoriasis: A systematic review of incidence and prevalence. Journal of Investigative Dermatology. 2013;**133**:377-385

[5] Nickoloff BJ, Nestle FO. Recent insights into the immunopathogenesis of psoriasis provide new therapeutic opportunities. Journal of Clinical Investigation. 2004;**113**:1664-1675

[6] Gladman DD. Psoriatic arthritis. Dermatology and Therapy. 2009;**22**:40-55

[7] Bisoendial RJ, Stroes ES, Tak PP. Where the immune response meets the vessel. Wall. The Netherlands Journal of Medicine. 2009;**67**:328-333

[8] Gladman DD, Farewell VT, Wong K, Husted J.Mortality studies in psoriatic arthritis: Results from a single outpatient center. II. Prognostic indicators for death. Arthritis and Rheumatism. 1998;**41**:1103-1110

[9] Nickoloff BJ. The cytokine network in psoriasis. Archives of Dermatology. 1991;**127**:871-884

[10] Ludwig RJ, Herzog C, Rostock A, Ochsendorf FR, Zollner TM, Thaci D, et al. Psoriasis: A possible risk factor for development of coronary artery calcification. British Journal of Dermatology. 2007;**156**:271-276

[11] Gelfand JM, Neimann AL, Shin DB,Wang X, Margolis DJ, Troxel AB. Risk of myocardial infarction in patients with psoriasis. The Journal of the American Medical Association. 2006;**296**:1735-1741

[12] Racz E, Prens EP. Molecular pathophysiology of psoriasis and molecular targets of antipsoriatic therapy. Expert Reviews in Molecular Medicine. 2009;**11**:e38

[13] Vollmer S, Menssen A, Prinz JC. Dominant lesional T cell receptor rearrangements persist in relapsing psoriasis but are absent from nonlesional skin: Evidence for a stable antigen-specific pathogenic T cell response in psoriasis vulgaris. Journal of Investigative Dermatology. 2001;**117**:1296-1301

[14] Kölliker Frers RA, Bisoendial RJ, Montoya SF, Kerzkerg E, Castilla R, Tak PP, et al. Psoriasis and cardiovascular risk: Immune-mediated crosstalk between metabolic, vascular and autoimmune inflammation. IJC Metabolic & Endocrine. 2015;**6**:43-54

[15] Pot C, Apetoh L, Awasthi A, Kuchroo VK. Molecular pathways in the induction of interleukin-27-driven regulatory type 1 cells. Journal of Interferon and Cytokine Research. 2010;**30**:381-388

[16] Ross EL, D'Cruz D, Morrow WJ. Localized monocyte chemotactic protein-1 production correlates with T cell infiltration of synovium in patients with psoriatic arthritis. Journal of Rheumatology. 2000;**27**:2432-2443

[17] Deleuran M, Buhl L, Ellingsen T, Harada A, Larsen CG, Matsushima K, et al. Localization of monocyte chemotactic and activating factor (MCAF/MCP-1) in psoriasis. Journal of Dermatological Science. 1996;**13**:228-236

[18] Milei J, Parodi JC, Alonso GF, Barone A, Grana D, Matturri L. Carotid rupture and intraplaque hemorrhage: Immunophenotype and role of cells involved. American Heart Journal. 1998;**136**:1096-1105

[19] Nilsson J, Wigren M, Shah PK. Vaccines against atherosclerosis. Expert Review of Vaccines. 2013;**12**:311-321

[20] Klingenberg R, Gerdes N, Badeau RM, Gistera A, Strodthoff D, Ketelhuth DF, et al. Depletion of FOXP3+ regulatory T cells promotes hypercholesterolemia and atherosclerosis. Journal of Clinical Investigation. 2013;**123**:1323-1334

[21] Cheng X, Yu X, Ding YJ, Fu QQ, Xie JJ, Tang TT, et al. The Th17/Treg imbalance in patients with acute coronary syndrome. Clinical Immunology. 2008;**127**:89-97

[22] Beinsberger J, Heemskerk JW, Cosemans JM. Chronic arthritis and cardiovascular disease: Altered blood parameters give rise to a prothrombotic propensity. Seminars in Arthritis and Rheumatism. 2014; 44:345-352

[23] Scarno A, Perrotta FM, Cardini F, Carboni A, Annibali G, Lubrano E, et al. Beyond the joint: Subclinical atherosclerosis in rheumatoid arthritis. World Journal of Orthopedics. 2014;**5**:328-335

[24] García-Gómez C, Bianchi M, de la Fuente D, Badimon L, Padró T, Corbella E, et al. Inflammation, lipid metabolism and cardiovascular risk in rheumatoid arthritis: a qualitative relationship? World Journal of Orthopedics. 2014;**5**:304-311

[25] Gladman DD, Antoni C, Mease P, Clegg DO, Nash P. Psoriatic arthritis: Epidemiology, clinical features, course, and outcome. Annals of the Rheumatic Diseases. 2005;**64**(Suppl. 2):ii14

[26] Angel K, Provan SA, Gulseth HL, Mowinckel P, Kvien TK, Atar D. Tumor necrosis factor-alpha antagonists improve aortic stiffness in patients with inflammatory arthropathies: A controlled study. Hypertension. 2010;**55**:333-338

[27] Ogdie A, Haynes K, Troxel AB, Love TJ, Hennessy S, Choi H, et al. Risk of mortality in patients with psoriatic arthritis, rheumatoid arthritis and psoriasis: a longitudinal cohort study. Annals of the Rheumatic Diseases. 2014;**73**:149-153

[28] Neimann AL, Shin DB, Wang X, Margolis DJ, Troxel AB, Gelfand JM. Prevalence of cardiovascular risk factors in patients with psoriasis. Journal of the American Academy of Dermatology. 2006;**55**:829-835

[29] Eder L, Jayakar J, Shanmugarajah S, Thavaneswaran A, Pereira D, Chandran V, et al. The burden of carotid artery plaques is higher in patients with psoriatic arthritis compared with those with psoriasis alone. Annals of the Rheumatic Diseases. 2013;**72**: 715-720

[30] Brauchli YB, Jick SS, Miret M, Meier CR. Psoriasis and risk of incident myocardial infarction, stroke or transient ischaemic attack: An inception cohort study with a nested case-control analysis. British Journal of Dermatology. 2009;**160**:1048-1056

[31] Prodanovich S, Kirsner RS, Kravetz JD, Ma F, Martinez L, Federman DG. Association of psoriasis with coronary artery, cerebrovascular, and peripheral vascular diseases and mortality. Archives of Dermatology. 2009;**145**:700-703

[32] Ritchlin C. Psoriatic disease—from skin to bone. Nature Clinical Practice Rheumatology. 2007;**3**:698-706

[33] Han C, Robinson Jr DW, Hackett MV, Paramore LC, Fraeman KH, Bala MV. Cardiovascular disease and risk factors in patients with rheumatoid arthritis, psoriatic arthritis, and ankylosing spondylitis. Journal of Rheumatology. 2006;**33**:2167-2172

[34] Sattar N, Crompton P, Cherry L, Kane D, Lowe G, McInnes IB. Effects of tumor necrosis factor blockade on cardiovascular risk factors in psoriatic arthritis: A double blind, placebo-controlled study. Arthritis and Rheumatism. 2007;**56**:831-839

[35] Gonzalez-Juanatey C, et al. Endothelial dysfunction in psoriasis arthritis patients without clinically evidente cardiovascular disease or classic atheroesclerosis risk factors. Arthrtis and Rheumatism (Arthritis Care and Research). 2007;**55**:287

[36] Eder L, et al. Subclinical Atheroesclerosis in psoriatic arthritis: a case control study. Journal of Rheumatology. 2008;**35**:877-882

[37] Tam LS, Shang Q, Li EK, Tomlinson B, Chu TT, Li M, et al. Subclinical carotid atherosclerosis in patients with psoriatic arthritis. Arthritis and Rheumatism. 2008;**59**:1322-1331

[38] Kimhi O, Caspi D, Bornstein NM, Maharshak N, Gur A, Arbel Y, et al. Prevalence and risk factors of atherosclerosis in patients with psoriatic arthritis. Seminars in Arthritis and Rheumatism. 2007;**36**:203-209

[39] Gladman DD, Ang M, Su L, Tom BD, Schentag CT, Farewell VT. Cardiovascular morbidity in psoriatic arthritis. Annals of the Rheumatic Diseases. 2009;**68**:1131-1135

[40] Shang Q, Tam LS, Yip GW, Sanderson JE, Zhang Q, Li EK, Yu CM. High prevalence of subclinical left ventricular dysfunction in patients with psoriatic arthritis. Journal of Rheumatology. 2011;**38**:1363-1370

[41] Svedbom A, Dalén J, Mamolo C, Cappelleri JC, Mallbris L, Petersson IF and Ståhle M. Increased Cause-specific mortality in patients with mild and severe psoriasis: A Population-based Swedish Register Study. Acta Dermato-Venereologica. 2015;**95**:809-815

[42] Cea-Calvo L, Vanaclocha F, Belinchón I, Rincón O, Juliá B and Puig L. Underdiagnosis of cardiovascular risk factors in outpatients with psoriasis followed at hospital dermatology offices: The PSO-RISK Study. Acta Dermato-Venereologica. 2016;**96**:972-973

[43] Tejón P, Morante PI, Cabezas I, Sarasqueta C, Coto P, Queiro R. A polyarticular onset and diabetes could be the main predictors of cardiovascular events in psoriatic arthritis. Clinical and Experimental Rheumatology. 2016;**34**:276-281

[44] Pryshchep O, Ma-Krupa W, Younge BR, Goronzy JJ, Weyand CM. Vessel-specific toll-like receptor profiles in human medium and large arteries. Circulation. 2008;**118**:1276-1284

[45] Alexandroff AB, Pauriah M, Camp RD, Lang CC, Struthers AD, Armstrong DJ. More than skin deep: Atherosclerosis as a systemic manifestation of psoriasis. British Journal of Dermatology. 2009;**161**:1-7

[46] Kashiwagi M, Imanishi T, Ozaki Y, Satogami K, MasunoT,Wada T, et al. Differential expression of toll-like receptor 4 and human monocyte subsets in acute myocardial infarction. Atherosclerosis. 2012;**221**:249-253

[47] Palikhe A, Sinisalo J, Seppanen M, Haario H, Meri S, Valtonen V, et al. Serum complement C3/C4 ratio, a novel marker for recurrent cardiovascular events. American Journal of Cardiology. 2007;**99**:890-895

[48] Griffiths CE, Barker JN. Pathogenesis and clinical features of psoriasis. Lancet. 2007;**370**: 263-271

[49] Kumar N, Armstrong DJ. Cardiovascular disease—the silent killer in rheumatoid arthritis. Clinical Medicine Journal. 2008;**8**:384-387

[50] Szodoray P, Alex P, Chappell-Woodward CM, Madland TM, Knowlton N, Dozmorov I, et al. Circulating cytokines in Norwegian patients with psoriatic arthritis determined by a multiplex cytokine array system. Rheumatology (Oxford). 2007;**46**:417-425

[51] Chandran V, Bull SB, Pellett FJ, Ayearst R, Pollock RA, Gladman DD. Killer-cell immunoglobulin-like receptor gene polymorphisms and susceptibility to psoriatic arthritis. Rheumatology (Oxford). 2014;**53**:233-239

[52] Ballara S, Taylor PC, ReuschP, Marme D, Feldmann M, Maini RN, et al. Raised serum vascular endothelial growth factor levels are associated with destructive change in inflammatory arthritis. Arthritis and Rheumatism. 2001;**44**:2055-2064

[53] Winterfield LS, Menter A, Gordon K, Gottlieb A. Psoriasis treatment: Current and emerging directed therapies. Annals of the Rheumatic Diseases. 2005;**64**(Suppl. 2):ii87–ii90 [discussion ii1-2]

[54] Rose S, Stansky E, Dagur PK, SamselL, Weiner E, Jahanshad A, et al. Characterization of immune cells in psoriatic adipose tissue. Journal of Translational Medicine. 2014;**12**:258

[55] Xia M, Guerra N, Sukhova GK, Yang K, Miller CK, Shi GP, Raulet DH, Xiong N. Immune activation resulting from NKG2D/ligand interaction promotesatherosclerosis. Circulation. 2011;**124**:2933-2943

[56] van den Elzen P, Garg S, Leon L, Brigl M, Leadbetter EA, Gumperz JE, et al. Apolipoprotein-mediated pathways of lipid antigen presentation. Nature. 2005;**437**:906-910

[57] Tupin E, Nicoletti A, Elhage R, Rudling M, Ljunggren HG, Hansson GK, et al. CD1ddependent activation of NKT cells aggravates atherosclerosis. Journal of Experimental Medicine. 2004;**199**:417-422

[58] Armstrong AW, Voyles SV, Armstrong EJ, Fuller EN, Rutledge JC. Angiogenesis and oxidative stress: Common mechanisms linking psoriasis with atherosclerosis. Journal of Dermatological Science. 2011;**63**:1-9

[59] Libby P. Inflammation in atherosclerosis. Nature. 2002;**420**:868-874

[60] Tsimikas S, Willerson JT, Ridker PM. C-reactive protein and other emerging blood biomarkers to optimize risk stratification of vulnerable patients. Journal of the American College of Cardiology. 2006;**47**:C19-C31

[61] Pearson TA, Mensah GA, Alexander RW, Anderson JL, Cannon 3rd RO, Criqui M, et al. Markers of inflammation and cardiovascular disease: application to clinical and public health practice: A statement for healthcare professionals from the Centers for Disease Control and Prevention and the American Heart Association. Circulation. 2003;**107**:499-511

[62] FonTacer K, Kuzman D, Seliskar M, Pompon D, Rozman D. TNF-alpha interferes with lipid homeostasis and activates acute and proatherogenic processes. Physiological Genomics. 2007;**31**:216-227

[63] Raychaudhuri SP. Comorbidities of psoriatic arthritis 440 metabolic syndrome and prevention: A report from the GRAPPA 2010 annual meeting. Journal of Rheumatology. 2012;**39**:437-440

[64] Danning CL, Illei GG, Hitchon C, Greer MR, Boumpas DT, McInnes IB. Macrophage-derived cytokine and nuclear factor kappaB p65 expression in synovial membrane and skin of patients with psoriatic arthritis. Arthritis and Rheumatism. 2000;**43**:1244-1256

[65] Mestas J, Ley K. Monocyte-endothelial cell interactions in the development of atherosclerosis. Trends in Cardiovascular Medicine. 2008;**18**:228-232

[66] Fenyo IM, Gafencu AV. The involvement of themonocytes/macrophages in chronic inflammation associated with atherosclerosis. Immunobiology. 2013;**218**:1376-1384

[67] Zhang H, Park Y, Wu J, Chen X, Lee S, Yang J, et al. Role of TNF-alpha in vascular dysfunction. Clinical Science (Journal). 2009;**116**:219-230

[68] Uyemura K, Demer LL, Castle SC, Jullien D, Berliner JA, Gately MK, et al. Crossregulatory roles of interleukin (IL)-12 and IL-10 in atherosclerosis. Journal of Clinical Investigation. 1996;**97**:2130-2038

[69] Schuett H, Luchtefeld M, Grothusen C, Grote K, Schieffer B. How much is too much? Interleukin-6 and its signalling in atherosclerosis. Thrombosis and Haemostasis. 2009;**102**:215-222

[70] Kibler JL, Tursich M, Ma M, Malcolm L, Greenbarg R. Metabolic, autonomic and immune markers for cardiovascular disease in posttraumatic stress disorder. World Journal of Cardiology. 2014;**6**:455-461

[71] Ingegnoli F, Fantini F, Favalli EG, Soldi A, Griffini S, Galbiati V, et al. Inflammatory and prothrombotic biomarkers in patients with rheumatoid arthritis: Effects of tumor necrosis factor-alpha blockade. Journal of Autoimmunity. 2008;**31**:175-179

[72] Matsuzawa Y. Adipocytokines and metabolic syndrome. Seminars in vascular Medicine. 2005;**5**:34-39

[73] Yin YW, Hu AM, Sun QQ, Liu HL, Wang Q, Zeng YH, et al. Association between interleukin-6 gene -174 G/C polymorphism and the risk of coronary heart disease: A meta-analysis of 20 studies including 9619 cases and 10,919 controls. Gene. 2012;**503**:25-30

[74] Rauramaa R, Vaisanen SB, Luong LA, Schmidt-Trucksass A, Penttila IM, Bouchard C, et al. Stromelysin-1 and interleukin-6 gene promoter polymorphisms are determinants of asymptomatic carotid artery atherosclerosis. Arteriosclerosis, Thrombosis, and Vascular Biology. 2000;**20**:2657-2662

[75] Rundek T, Elkind MS, Pittman J, Boden-Albala B, Martin S, Humphries SE, et al. Carotid intima-media thickness is associated with allelic variants of stromelysin-1, interleukin-6, and hepatic lipase genes: The Northern Manhattan Prospective Cohort Study. Stroke. 2002;**33**:1420-1423

[76] Hingorani AD, Casas JP. The interleukin-6 receptor as a target for prevention of coronary heart disease: A Mendelian randomisation analysis. Lancet. 2012;**379**:1214-1224

[77] Tedgui A, Mallat Z. Cytokines in atherosclerosis: Pathogenic and regulatory pathways. Physiological Reviews. 2006;**86**:515-581

[78] Sikorski K, Czerwoniec A, Bujnicki JM, Wesoly J, Bluyssen HA. STAT1 as a novel therapeutical target in pro-atherogenic signal integration of IFN-γ, TLR4 and IL-6 in vascular disease. Cytokine and Growth Factor Review. 2011;**22**:211-219

[79] Schubert N, Dudeck J, Liu P, Karutz A, Speier S, Maurer M, Tuckermann J, Dudeck A. Mast cell promotion of T cell-driven antigen-induced arthritis despite being dispensable for antibody-induced arthritis in which T cells are bypassed. Arthritis and Rheumatology. 2015;**67**:903-913

[80] Lee DM, Friend DS, Gurish MF, Benoist C, Mathis D, Brenner MB. Mast cells: A cellular link between autoantibodies and inflammatory arthritis. Science. 2002;**297**(5587):1689-1692

[81] Goodman WA, Levine AD, Massari JV, Sugiyama H, McCormick TS, Cooper KD. IL-6 signaling in psoriasis prevents immune suppression by regulatory T cells. Journal of Immunology. 2009;**183**:3170-1376

[82] Jones SA, Scheller J, Rose-John S. Therapeutic strategies for the clinical blockade of IL-6/gp130 signaling. Journal of Clinical Investigation. 2011;**121**:3375-3383

[83] Veldhoen M, Hocking RJ, Atkins CJ, Locksley RM, Stockinger B. TGFβ in the context of an inflammatory cytokine milieu supports de novo differentiation of IL-17-producing T cells. Immunity. 2006;**24**:179-189

[84] Hamed SA, Hamed EA, Ezz Eldin AM, Mahmoud NM. Vascular risk factors, endothelial function, and carotid thickness in patients with migraine: relationship to atherosclerosis. Journal of Stroke and Cerebrovascular Diseases. 2010;**19**:92-103

[85] Bonifati C, Ameglio F. Cytokines in psoriasis. International Journal of Dermatology. 1999; **38**:241-251

[86] Maurer M,Wedemeyer J, Metz M, Piliponsky AM, Weller K, Chatterjea D, et al. Mast cells promote homeostasis by limiting endothelin-1-induced toxicity. Nature. 2004; **432**:512-516

[87] Ridker PM, Cook N. Clinical usefulness of very high and very low levels of C-reactive protein across the full range of Framingham Risk Scores. Circulation. 2004;**109**:19551959

[88] Wick G, Knoflach M, Xu Q. Autoimmune and inflammatory mechanisms in atherosclerosis. Annual Review of Immunology. 2004;**22**:361-403

[89] Jialal I, Devaraj S, Venugopal SK. C-reactive protein: Risk marker or mediator in atherothrombosis? Hypertension. 2004;**44**:6-11

[90] Bisoendial R, Birjmohun R, Keller T, van Leuven S, Levels H, Levi M, et al. In vivo effects of C-reactive protein (CRP)-infusion into humans. Circulation Research. 2005;**97**:e115-e116

[91] Qamirani E, Ren Y, Kuo L, Hein TW. C-reactive protein inhibits endothelium dependent NO-mediated dilation in coronary arterioles by activating p38 kinase and NAD (P) H oxidase. Arteriosclerosis, Thrombosis, and Vascular Biology. 2005;**25**:995-1001

[92] Venugopal SK, Devaraj S, Yuhanna I, Shaul P, Jialal I. Demonstration that C-reactive protein decreases eNOS expression and bioactivity in human aortic endothelial cells. Circulation. 2002;**106**:1439-1441.

[93] Strober B, Teller C, Yamauchi P, Miller JL, Hooper M, Yang YC, et al. Effects of etanercept on C-reactive protein levels in psoriasis and psoriatic arthritis. British Journal of Dermatology. 2008;**159**:322-330

[94] Kaur S, Zilmer K, Leping V, Zilmer M. The levels of adiponectin and leptin and their relation to other markers of cardiovascular risk in patients with psoriasis. Journal of the European Academy of Dermatology and Venereology. 2011;**25**:1328-1333

[95] Cowan KN, Jones PL, Rabinovitch M. Elastase and matrix metalloproteinase inhibitors induce regression, and tenascin-C antisense prevents progression, of vascular disease. Journal of Clinical Investigation. 2000;**105**:21-34

[96] Shi Y, Patel S, Niculescu R, Chung W, Desrochers P, Zalewski A. Role of matrix metalloproteinases and their tissue inhibitors in the regulation of coronary cell migration. Arteriosclerosis, Thrombosis, and Vascular Biology. 1999;**19**:1150-1155

[97] McKenna K, Beignon A-S, Bhardwaj N. Plasmacytoid dendritic cells: Linking innate and adaptive immunity. Journal of Virology. 2005;**79**:17-27

[98] Aggarwal S, Ghilardi N, Xie MH, de Sauvage FJ, Gurney AL. Interleukin-23 promotes a distinct CD4 T cell activation state characterized by the production of interleukin-17. Journal of Biological Chemistry. 2003;**278**:1910-1094

[99] Kirkham BW, Kavanaugh A, Reich K. IL-17A: A unique pathway in immune mediated diseases: Psoriasis, psoriatic arthritis, and rheumatoid arthritis. Immunology. 2014;**141**: 133-142

[100] Madhur MS, Funt SA, Li L, Vinh A, Chen W, Lob HE, et al. Role of interleukin 17 in inflammation, atherosclerosis, and vascular function in apolipoprotein e-deficient mice. Arteriosclerosis, Thrombosis, and Vascular Biology. 2011;**31**:1565-1572

[101] Hashmi S, Zeng QT. Role of interleukin-17 and interleukin-17-induced cytokines interleukin-6 and interleukin-8 in unstable coronary artery disease. Coronary Artery Disease. 2006;**17**:699-706

[102] Chabaud M, Miossec P. The combination of tumor necrosis factor alpha blockade with interleukin-1 and interleukin-17 blockade is more effective for controlling synovial inflammation and bone resorption in an ex vivo model. Arthritis and Rheumatism. 2001;**44**:1293-1303

[103] Jhun JY, Yoon BY, Park MK, Oh HJ, Byun JK, Lee SY, et al. Obesity aggravates the joint inflammation in a collagen-induced arthritis model through deviation to Th17 differentiation. Experimental and Molecular Medicine. 2012;**44**:424-431

[104] Kagami S, Rizzo HL, Lee JJ, Koguchi Y, Blauvelt A. Circulating Th17, Th22, and Th1 cells are increased in psoriasis. Journal of Investigative Dermatology. 2010;**130**:1373-1383

[105] George J. Mechanisms of disease: The evolving role of regulatory T cells in atherosclerosis. Nature Clinical Practice Cardiovascular Medicine. 2008;**5**:531-540

[106] Sakaguchi S, Yamaguchi T, Nomura T, Ono M. Regulatory T cells and immune tolerance. Cell. 2008;**133**:775-787

[107] Tang Q, Bluestone JA. The Foxp3+ regulatory T cell: A jack of all trades, master of regulation. Nature Immunology. 2008;**9**:239-244

[108] de Boer OJ, van der Meer JJ, Teeling P, van der Loos CM, van der Wal AC. Low numbers of FOXP3 positive regulatory T cells are present in all developmental stages of human atherosclerotic lesions. PLoS One. 2007;**2**:e779

[109] Chen L, Shen Z, Wang G, Fan P, Liu Y. Dynamic frequency of CD4+CD25+Foxp3+ Treg cells in psoriasis vulgaris. Journal of Dermatological Science. 2008;**51**:200-203

[110] Armstrong AW, Voyles SV, Armstrong EJ, Fuller EN, Rutledge JC. A tale of two plaques: Convergent mechanisms of T-cell-mediated inflammation in psoriasis and atherosclerosis. Experimental Dermatology. 2011;**20**:544-549.

[111] Kagen MH, McCormick TS, Cooper KD. Regulatory T cells in psoriasis. Ernst Schering Research Foundation Workshop Journal. 2006;**56**:193-209

[112] Flisiak I, Chodynicka B, Porebski P, Flisiak R. Association between psoriasis severity and transforming growth factor beta(1) and beta(2) in plasma and scales from psoriatic lesions. Cytokine. 2002;**19**:121-125

[113] Flisiak I, Zaniewski P, Chodynicka B. Plasma TGF-beta1, TIMP-1, MMP-1 and IL-18 as a combined biomarker of psoriasis activity. Biomarkers. 2008;**13**:549-556

[114] Mallat Z, Besnard S, Duriez M, Deleuze V, Emmanuel F, Bureau MF, et al. Protective role of interleukin-10 in atherosclerosis. Circulation Research. 1999;**85**:e17-e24

[115] Mallat Z, Gojova A, Marchiol-Fournigault C, Esposito B, Kamate C, Merval R, et al. Inhibition of transforming growth factor-beta signaling accelerates atherosclerosis and induces an unstable plaque phenotype in mice. Circulation Research. 2001;**89**:930-934

[116] Tuluc F, Lai JP, Kilpatrick LE, Evans DL, Douglas SD. Neurokinin 1 receptor isoforms and the control of innate immunity. Trends in Immunology. 2009;**30**:271-276

[117] Bowes J, Barton A. The genetics of psoriatic arthritis: lessons from genome-wide association studies. Discovery Medicine. 2010;**10**:177-183

[118] Chandra A, Lahiri A, Senapati S, et al. Increased Risk of Psoriasis due to combined effect of HLA-Cw6 and LCE3 risk alleles in Indian population. Scientific Reports. 2016;**6**:24059

[119] Liu Y, Yin H, Zhao M, Lu Q. TLR2 and TLR4 in autoimmune diseases: a comprehensive review. Clinical Reviews in Allergy and Immunology. 2014;**47**:136-147

[120] Liu P, Yu YR, Spencer JA, Johnson AE, Vallanat CT, Fong AM, Patterson C, Patel DD. CX3CR1 deficiency impairs dendritic cell accumulation in arterial intima and reduces atherosclerotic burden. Arteriosclerosis Thrombosis and Vascular Biology. 2008;**28**:243-250

[121] Mizoguchi E, Orihara K, Hamasaki S, Ishida S, Kataoka T, Ogawa M, Saihara K, OkuiH, Fukudome T, Shinsato T, Shirasawa T, Ichiki H, Kubozono T, Ninomiya Y, OtsujiY, Tei C. Pathophysiology and Natural History Association between toll-like receptors and the extent and severity of coronary artery disease in patients with stable angina. Coronary Artery Disease. 2007;18:31-38

[122] Miller Yury I. Toll-like receptors and atherosclerosis: Oxidized LDL as an endogenous toll-like receptor ligand. Future Cardiology. 2005;**1**:785-792

[123] Van Furth AM, Verhard-Seijmonsbergen EM, Langermans JAM, van Dissel JT, van Furth R. Anti-CD14 monoclonal antibodies inhibit the production of tumor necrosis factor alpha and interleukin-10 by human monocytes stimulated with killed and live haemophilus influenzae or *Streptococcus pneumoniae* organisms. In: Moore RN, editor. Infection and Immunity. 1999; 67: 3714-3718 (American Society for Microbiology, Washington DC)

[124] Rahman P, Elder JT. Genetic epidemiology of psoriasis and psoriatic Arthritis. Annals of the Rheumatic Diseases. 2005;**64**:1137-1139

[125] Elder JT. Genome-wide association scan yields new insights into the immunopathogenesis of psoriasis. Genes and Immunity. 2009;**10**:201-209

[126] Matsuzawa Y, Oshima S, Takahara M, Maeyashiki C, Nemoto Y, Kobayashi M, Nibe Y, Nozaki K, Nagaishi T, Okamoto R, Tsuchiya K, Nakamura T, Ma A, Watanabe M. TNFAIP3 promotes survival of CD4 T cells by restricting MTOR and promoting autophagy. Autophagy. 2015;**11**:1052-1062

[127] Nestle FO, Kaplan DH, Barker J. Mechanisms of disease: Psoriasis. The New England Journal of Medicine. 2009;**361**:496-509

[128] Duffin KC, Krueger GG. Genetic variations in cytokines and cytokine receptors associated with psoriasis found by genome wide association. Journal of Investigative Dermatology. 2009;**129**:827-833

[129] Oudot T, Lesueur F, Guedj M, De Cid R, et al. An association study of 22 candidate genes in psoriasis families reveals shared genetic factors with other autoimmune and skin disorders. Journal of Investigative Dermatology. 2009;**129**:2637-2645

[130] Valdimarsson H. The genetic basis of psoriasis. Clinical Dermatology. 2007;**25**:563-567

[131] Ammar M, Souissi-Bouchlaka C, Gati A, Zaraa I, Bouhaha R, Kouidhi S, Ben Ammar-Gaied A, Doss N, Mokni M, Marrakchi R. Psoriasis: Physiopathology and immunogenetics. Pathologie Biologie (Paris). 2014;**62**:10-23

[132] Ahmed N, Prior JA, Chen Y, Hayward R, Mallen CD, Hider SL. Prevalence of cardiovascular-related comorbidity in ankylosing spondylitis, psoriatic arthritis and psoriasis in primary care: A matched retrospective cohort study. Clinical Rheumatology. 2016;**35**:3069-3073

[133] Eder L, Chandran V, Cook R, Gladman DD. The risk of developing diabetes mellitus in patients with psoriatic arthritis: A cohort study. Journal of Rheumatology. 2017;**44**:286-291

[134] Gisondi P, Cotena C, Tessari G, Girolomoni G. Anti-tumour necrosis factor-alpha therapy increases body weight in patients with chronic plaque psoriasis: A retrospective cohort study. Journal of the European Academy of Dermatology and Venereology. 2008;**22**:341-344

[135] Tam LS, Tomlinson B, Chu TT, Li M, Leung YY, Kwok LW, et al. Cardiovascular risk profile of patients with psoriatic arthritis compared to controls—the role of inflammation. Rheumatology (Oxford). 2008;**47**:718-723

[136] Cassano N, Carbonara M, Panaro M, Vestita M, Vena GA. Role of serum uric acid in conditioning the association of psoriasis with metabolic syndrome. European Journal of Dermatology. 2011;**21**:808-809

[137] Gonzalez-Gay MA, Gonzalez-Juanatey C, Vazquez-Rodriguez TR, Gomez-Acebo I, Miranda-Filloy JA, Paz-Carreira J, et al. Asymptomatic hyperuricemia and serum uric acid concentration correlate with subclinical atherosclerosis in psoriatic arthritis patients without clinically evident cardiovascular disease. Seminars in Arthritis and Rheumatism. 2009;**39**:157-162

[138] Takahashi H, Tsuji H, Hashimoto Y, Ishida-Yamamoto A, Iizuka H. Serum cytokines and growth factor levels in Japanese patients with psoriasis. Clinical and Experimental Dermatology. 2010;**35**:645-649

[139] Heidenreich R, Röcken M, Ghoreschi K. Angiogenesis drives psoriasis pathogenesis. International Journal of Experimental Pathology. 2009;**90**:232-248

[140] Nofal A, Al-Makhzangy I, Attwa E, Nassar A, Abdalmoati A. Vascular endothelial growth factor in psoriasis: An indicator of disease severity and control. Journal of the European Academy of Dermatology and Venereology. 2009;**23**:803-806

[141] Celletti FL, Waugh JM, Amabile PG, Brendolan A, Hilfiker PR, Dake MD. Vascular endothelial growth factor enhances atherosclerotic plaque progression. Nature Medicine. 2001;**7**:425-429

[142] Stannard AK, Khurana R, Evans IM, Sofra V, Holmes DI, Zachary I. Vascular endothelial growth factor synergistically enhances induction of E-selectin by tumor necrosis factor-alpha. Arteriosclerosis, Thrombosis, and Vascular Biology. 2007;**27**:494-502

[143] Kuehl Jr FA, Egan RW. Prostaglandins, arachidonic acid, and inflammation. Science. 1980;**210**:978-984

[144] Kuhn H, Thiele BJ. The diversity of the lipoxygenase family. Many sequence data but little information on biological significance. FEBS Letters. 1999;**449**:7-11

[145] Icen M, Nicola PJ, Maradit-Kremers H, Crowson CS, Therneau TM, Matteson EL, et al. Systemic lupus erythematosus features in rheumatoid arthritis and their effect on overall mortality. Journal of Rheumatology. 2009;**36**:50-57

[146] Stemme S, Faber B, Holm J, Wiklund O, Witztum JL, Hansson GK. T lymphocytes from human atherosclerotic plaques recognize oxidized low density lipoprotein. Proceedings of the National Academy of Sciences of the United States. 1995;**92**:3893-3897

[147] Moreira DM, da Silva RL, Vieira JL, Fattah T, Lueneberg ME, Gottschall CA. Role of vascular inflammation in coronary artery disease: potential of anti-inflammatory drugs in the prevention of atherothrombosis. Inflammation and anti-inflammatory drugs in coronary artery disease. American Journal of Cardiovascular Drugs. 2015;**15**:1-11

[148] Listing J, Strangfeld A, Kekow J, Schneider M, Kapelle A, Wassenberg S, et al. Does tumor necrosis factor alpha inhibition promote or prevent heart failure in patients with rheumatoid arthritis? Arthritis and Rheumatology. 2008;**58**:667-677

[149] Avouac J, Allanore Y. Cardiovascular risk in rheumatoid arthritis: Effects of anti-TNF drugs. Expert Opinion on Pharmacotherapy. 2008;**9**:1121-1128

[150] Suissa S, Bernatsky S, Hudson M. Antirheumatic drug use and the risk of acute myocardial infarction. Arthritis and Rheumatology. 2006;**55**:531-536

[151] Skaaby T, Husemoen LL, Martinussen T, Thyssen JP, Melgaard M, Thuesen BH, et al. Vitamin D status, filaggrin genotype, and cardiovascular risk factors: A Mendelian randomization approach. PLoS One 2013;**8**:e57647

[152] Deleskog A, Piksasova O, Silveira A, Samnegard A, Tornvall P, Eriksson P, et al. Serum 25-hydroxyvitamin D concentration, established and emerging cardiovascular risk factors and risk of myocardial infarction before the age of 60 years. Atherosclerosis. 2012;**223**:223-229

[153] Mahon BD, Wittke A, Weaver V, Cantorna MT. The targets of vitamin D depend on the differentiation and activation status of CD4 positive T cells. Journal of Cellular Biochemistry. 2003;**89**:922-932

[154] Hewison M. Vitamin D and innate and adaptive immunity. Vitamins and Hormones. 2011;**86**:23-62

[155] Hegyi Z, Zwicker S, Bureik D, Peric M, Koglin S, Batycka-Baran A, et al. Vitamin D analog calcipotriol suppresses the Th17 cytokine-induced proinflammatory S100 "alarmins" psoriasin (S100A7) and koebnerisin (S100A15) in psoriasis. Journal of Investigative Dermatology. 2012;**132**:1416-1424

[156] van der Aar AM, Sibiryak DS, Bakdash G, van Capel TM, van der Kleij HP, Opstelten DJ, et al. Vitamin D3 targets epidermal and dermal dendritic cells for induction of distinct regulatory T cells. Journal of Allergy and Clinical Immunology. 2011;**127**:1532-1540

[157] Babior BM. NADPH oxidase: an update. Blood. 1999;**93**:1464-1476

Section 2

Psoriasis Monitoring

Chapter 7

Clinical and Epidemiological Factors Predicting the Severity of Psoriasis

Anca Chiriac, Cristian Podoleanu and Doina Azoicai

Additional information is available at the end of the chapter

http://dx.doi.org/10.5772/intechopen.68728

Abstract

Introduction: Psoriasis, a systemic disease with a chronic course, is associated with a high degree of comorbidities and decreased quality of life.

Aims: The aims of the study were to analyze epidemiological data of a large cohort of patients diagnosed with psoriasis over 8 years and to assess factors related to psoriasis severity and impact on quality of life.

Research methods: A transversal study was performed on 1236 persons diagnosed with psoriasis in an OutPatient Dermatology Center between January 1, 2004 and December 31, 2011.

Clinical examination was done and medical records were complied including: type of psoriasis, number of body locations at the onset and at the moment of examination, severity index, family history of psoriasis, comorbidities, past and current treatments, demographic characteristics, residence, level of education, working status and income, smoking, and alcohol intake. Linear regression was used for multivariable analysis.

Key results of the chapter: Comorbidities were present in 36.1% of patients with mild form of psoriasis, 44.05% with moderate forms, and in 19.64% of severe psoriasis.

Onset and clinical examination age, education level, residence, job, gender, and smoking were significant factors associated with severity of psoriasis.

Keywords: psoriasis, epidemiological data, comorbidities, risk factors, severity index

1. Introduction

One of the most common T-cell-mediated diseases, psoriasis, is widely spread, potentially affecting 125 million people, or nearly 3% of the world's population [1–3]. Reports show that psoriasis affects as much as 2% of the UK population [4]. A significant number of UK psoriatic patients have a Dermatology Life Quality Index (DLQI) of >10, indicating that the disease strongly affects their lives [4]. Social factors such as stigmatization, psychological factors such as depression, and physical factors such as pruritus, pain, and other comorbidities have a great impact on the patient's life [5, 6].

Psoriasis involves high costs in the health-care system, represented by diagnosis, psychological counseling, investigations, treatments, and further research, which cannot be entirely quantified. A systematic review including 22 studies, published in *JAMA Dermatology 2015*, takes a comprehensive look at the cost of psoriasis in the USA by analyzing the expenses reported between 2008 and 2013, associated with the disease. In 2013, the US cost of psoriasis was estimated around $112 billion. Researchers have described four categories of expenses associated with psoriasis. Direct costs represented by doctor's appointments, investigations, and therapies, have the highest expenses, estimated to be $8000 annually per person. The cost of dealing with comorbidities such as heart disease and depression, extends the costs with almost $5000 per person annually. Indirect costs are considered absences from work or lost productivity on the job, caused by psoriasis, and estimated to be upwards of $4000 annually per person. The decreased quality of life with reduced selfconfidence and substantial stigmatization cannot be quantified or calculated in terms of cost—impalpable costs. US psoriatic patients would pay a lifetime cost of $11,498 for treatment, relief of physical symptoms, emotional health, and reintegration into society. The direct psoriasis costs ranged from $51.7 to $63.2 billion, the indirect costs ranged from $23.9 to $35.4 billion, and medical comorbidities were estimated to be $36.4 billion in 2013 [7]. On the strength of such high costs and the burden of seeking the right therapy, it is of great importance to assess psoriatic patients with comorbidities associated with severe disease and decreased quality of life.

Recent studies show that psoriatic patients have relatively higher risks of heart disease, stroke, hypertension, and diabetes. Furthermore, due to social isolation, patients are more prone to develop depression and anxiety compared to the general population [4–6, 8]. A national study in Taiwan performed on 51,800 patients diagnosed with psoriasis revealed a high prevalence ratio (relative risk (RR); [95% confidence interval (CI)]) for rheumatoid arthritis (3.02; [2.68, 3.41]), alopecia areata (4.71; [2.98, 7.45]), vitiligo (5.94; [3.79, 9.31]), pemphigus (41.81; [12.41, 140.90]), pemphigoid (14.75; [5.00, 43.50]), heart disease (1.32; [1.26, 1.37]), hypertension (1.51; [1.47, 1.56]), hyperglyceridemia (1.61; [1.54, 1.68]), diabetes (1.64; [1.58, 1.70]), hepatitis B viral infection (1.73; [1.47, 2.04]), hepatitis C viral infection (2.02; [1.67, 2.44]), systemic lupus erythematosus (6.16; [4.70, 8.09]), sleep disorder (3.89; [2.26, 6.71]), asthma (1.29; [1.18, 1.40]), allergic rhinitis (1.25; [1.18, 1.33]), chronic airways obstruction (1.47; [1.34, 1.61]), lip, oral cavity, and pharynx cancer (1.49; [1.22, 1.80]), digestive organs and peritoneum cancer (1.57; [1.41, 1.74]), and depression (1.50; [1.39, 1.61]) [8].

Psoriasis, a systemic disease with a chronic course, is associated with a high degree of comorbidities and decreased quality of life.

Psoriasis can vary tremendously in its severity. A number of studies investigated the factors that affect severity [9, 10]. They reported significant associations between psoriasis severity and comorbid diseases [10], male gender, younger age [11, 12], localization of the lesions [13], the presence of family history of psoriasis [14], smoking, and alcohol consumption [15]. The factors that affect severity are still not well characterized.

2. An overview of the transversal study

2.1. Aims and objectives of the study: methods and materials

The aim of this study was to evaluate clinical and epidemiological characteristics of the psoriatic population for establishing prevention strategies and optimal clinical management.

The objectives of this transversal study were to analyze epidemiological data of a large cohort of patients diagnosed with psoriasis over a period of 8 years and to assess factors related to psoriasis severity and impact on their quality of life (validated by Psoriasis Area and Severity Index (PASI) index and DLQI).

All the investigations were conducted in an outpatient clinic specialized for psoriasis and investigative dermatology, in the north-eastern region of Romania, over a period of 8 years. **Study** was performed on **1236 persons** diagnosed with psoriasis **between January 1, 2004 and December 31, 2011**.

Participants were examined for psoriasis by the same two dermatologists, under similar conditions. All patients had a complete physical examination and their medical history was recorded.

Psoriasis was diagnosed by dermatological examination and was confirmed by punch skin biopsy, when needed. Skin biopsies were performed at a representative psoriatic plaque of each patient.

In other articles [16, 17], psoriasis is classified as mild, moderate, and severe, based on clinical evaluation tools such as the extent of the affected skin surface. In this study, in order to quantify the severity of the disease, PASI was used; patients were categorized into mild (PASI: 0.0–4.0), moderate (4.1–9.9), and severe (10 or higher) psoriasis.

Patient data and medical history were collected from the Specialized Psoriasis Clinic, over a period of 8 years. Written informed consent was obtained from all patients.

The data collected by our dermatologists included the following:

1. **demographic characteristics**: gender, date of birth, age of the patients at the moment of examination, level of education, occupation (jobs distribution, respectively, socioeconomic status), residence;

2. **psoriasis—clinical-related data:** family history of psoriasis, age distribution at the onset of psoriasis, distribution of psoriatic lesions at the moment of diagnosis and at the moment of clinical inspection, number of areas involved, symptoms such as pruritus;
3. **comorbidities** such as thyroid abnormalities, cardiovascular disease (CVD), hypertension, other concomitant skin disorders, and others;
4. **severity of lesions in relation to evolution characteristics:** smoking history, alcohol consumption, past and current therapies with topical steroids.

2.1.1. Statistical analysis

All statistical analyses were conducted using Statistical Analysis System software.

Patient data were presented as proportions, standard deviations, means, and ranges. Linear regression was used for multivariable analysis of factors affecting psoriasis severity. Specified variables were included in the analysis of index severity. Spearman's rank coefficient of correlation was used as a nonparametric measure of dependence. Pearson's chi-squared test to quantify differences was used. All statistical tests had a confidence interval of 95% and the significance level was set at $p < 0.05$.

2.2. Results and discussion

2.2.1. Demographic data

2.2.1.1. Gender distribution

Out of the 1236 patients diagnosed with psoriasis, 669 were men (54.13%) and 567 (45.87%) were women, showing a ***predominance of male*** *over female gender* **(1.18/1)**.

2.2.1.2. Age distribution at the moment of examination

The highest incidence of the disease was noticed for the *age group 30–50 years old* (43.12%); **the minimal incidence** was *over 70 years* (5.83%) and *under 20 years* (5.5%). Statistically 50% of cases were over 40 years and 25% under 33 years.

The median value for age was 44.94 ± 15.84 standard deviation (SD), with a great variability from 6 to 91 years old. Psoriasis can occur at any age; patients should seek medical advice regardless of age.

2.2.1.3. Distribution of cases reported to residence

As shown in **Table 1**, urban patients prevail. People living in villages have low incidence of psoriasis, reflecting a real reduced number of cases or a smaller addressability to medical care (**Figure 1**).

Residence	Nr. cases	%
Urban	1036	83.82
Rural	200	16.18
Total	1236	

Table 1. Results of the study: number of patients reported to residence.

2.2.1.4. Level of education

The level of education correlates with the prevalence of psoriasis (**Table 2**). This can be explained by stress, underlying the western modern lifestyle.

2.2.1.5. Occupational characteristics at the moment of medical examination: jobs distribution, respectively, socioeconomic status

Present data confirm the high prevalence of psoriasis in working people, especially in stressful activities: engineers, students, professors, managers, drivers, salesmen, and medical staff. Physical activity, alcohol consumption, smoking, pollution from the working place, repeated trauma, and irritants are linked to psoriasis on workers.

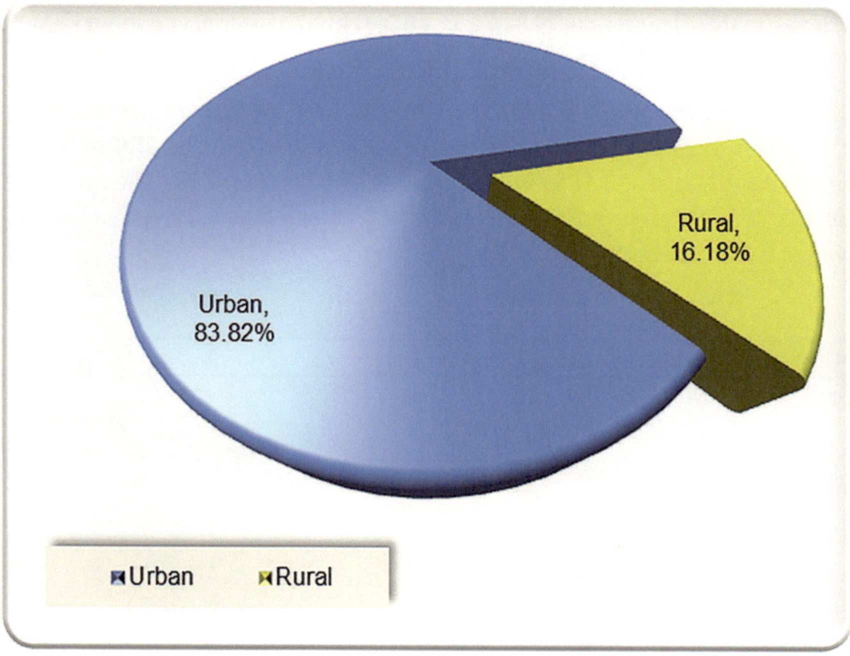

Figure 1. Results of the study: distribution of cases reported to residence.

Retired persons encounter a frequent diagnosis of psoriasis after a long evolution of the disease (psoriasis march), even though they allocate time and money in search of medical help. This can be explained by the fact that chronic infections, comorbidities, and drug administration could be a potential trigger for psoriasis flares.

2.2.2. *Diagnosis of psoriasis and clinical data*

2.2.2.1. *Family history of psoriasis*

Out of the 1236 patients, a positive family history of psoriasis was found in 380 patients (59.37%); of these, 174 (27.18%) had at least one parent with psoriasis, with a λR of 13.59, while 106 patients (16.56%) had at least one second-degree relative with psoriasis, and 34 patients (5.31%) had one-third-degree relative with psoriasis (**Figure 2**). No parent-of-origin effect in transmission of psoriasis from affected parent to offspring was observed, and there were no significant differences in the clinical profiles of the disease between patients grouped by transmission pattern of psoriasis.

2.2.2.2. *Age of the patients at the onset of psoriasis*

Results of the study showed the following: 7.77% of patients did not recall the age at which the first lesions appeared, 46.04% had the first diagnosis of psoriasis somewhere between 10 and 30 years old, and the fewest cases were detected over the age of 50 (11.17%).

The median age at the diagnosis is 29.34 ± 15.24 SD, with the youngest patient being 6 months (neonatal psoriasis) and oldest 76 years.

Statistically 50% of cases were less than 27 years old at the moment of first medical seek and 25% over 39 years old when they accepted psoriasis as a diagnosis (**Table 3**). Within this group, there were 104 cases (8.41%) with the onset of psoriasis under the age of 10 and 263 (21.28%) of cases had the first certified diagnosis of psoriasis before 19 years old. The majority of cases were adult psoriasis 869 (70.31%).

Level of education	**Nr. cases**	**%**
Middle school	54	4.37
College	148	11.97
Vocational school	48	3.88
High school	345	27.91
Postsecondary school	47	3.80
Students	182	14.72
University graduates	412	33.33
Total	1236	

Table 2. Results of the study: level of education among patients diagnosed with psoriasis.

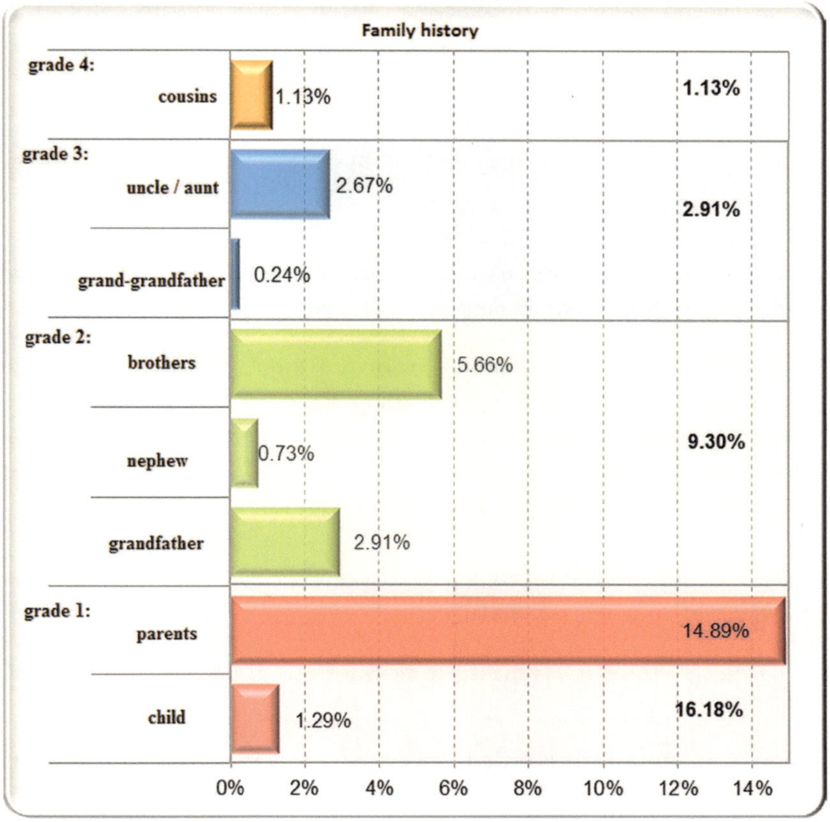

Figure 2. Results of the study: family history reported.

Onset age (years)	Nr. cases	%
Age ≤10	104	8.41
10 < age ≤19	263	21.28
Over 20	869	70.31

Table 3. Results of the study: age of the patients at the onset of psoriasis.

Psoriasis has been reported as a chronic disease that begins in one-third of the patients during the first two decades of life [18]. Several prevalence studies have published their results showing that one-third of psoriatic patients develop the disease during childhood [19]. A fast increase in the incidence rate of psoriasis until the age of 30–35 years was recently reported [20].

Childhood onset of psoriasis was not proven to be a risk factor for higher frequencies of cardiovascular and metabolic comorbidities during adulthood in a recent French study [21]. Moreover, the age of onset of psoriasis had no impact on the severity of the disease in another retrospective study conducted in Greece [22]. No evidence was found that under 18 years may influence the disease severity in later life [23].

Similar data have been obtained by present analysis: 70.31% of patients enrolled in the study were diagnosed after the age of 20, only 104 cases (8.41%) had the onset before the age of 10; 263 (21.28%) of cases were diagnosed between 10 and 19 years old.

Psoriasis in children should not be considered as underreported because parents seek for medical care for their children at the first signs of skin injury. Children with psoriatic arthritis (PsA) were not included in the study.

2.2.2.3. The distribution of psoriatic lesions at the moment of diagnosis (Single lesion or multiple distributions of cutaneous manifestations declared by patients)

The majority of cases **(91.18%)** had ***a unique lesion*** of psoriasis *when they were first diagnosed*, multiple locations being much rarer (8.82%). Among the unique first clinical signs, most of the patients (28.07%) reported **scalp** being involved, followed by **elbows** (11.89%), **palms** (7.93%), **feet** (7.12%), and **trunk** (5.18%). A significant number of persons involved in the study were not able to remember the first location of psoriasis (10.36%).

2.2.2.4. The distribution of psoriatic lesions at the moment of clinical inspection (Single lesion or multiple distributions of cutaneous manifestations)

The majority of patients **(82.85%)** *had* **multiple skin lesions** *at the moment of clinical inspection* (**Table 4**).

The distribution of psoriasis was recorded. Active lesions were noted on the scalp, face, trunk, anogenital area, arms, legs, hands, feet, or nails, that is, in 10 different locations (**Figure 3**):

	Nr. cases	%
Nail psoriasis	165	13.35
Psoriatic arthritis	309	25.00
Koebner phenomena	173	14.00
Scalp psoriasis	681	55.10
Gutate psoriasis	146	11.81
Superior limbs	788	63.75
Inferior limbs	736	59.55
Trunk	462	37.38
Face	55	4.45
Palmo-plantar	205	16.59
Others	265	21.44
Total	1236	

Table 4. Results of the study: distribution of multiple skin lesions at the moment of clinical inspection.

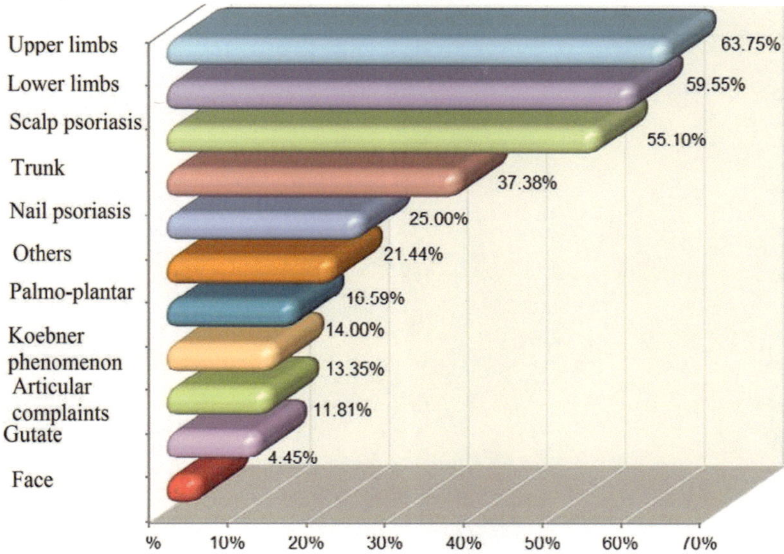

Figure 3. Distribution of multiple skin lesions at the moment of clinical inspection.

2.2.2.5. Number of areas involved at the moment of clinical inspection (By single or multiple cutaneous lesions)

Out of the 1236 patients enrolled in the study, an *approximately equal distribution* was observed among patients with **solitary lesion or two, three, or four body areas involved** (**Table 5**). More generalized forms were very rare (**Figure 4**).

2.2.2.6. Evolution of psoriatic lesions from diagnosis to present clinical inspection

Few patients (1.21%) with ***multiple onset lesions*** later **turned to have** *unique lesions*, while 7.61% of them **preserved** the initial multiple lesions; 15.94% of patients with *onset single lesions* remained with a unique cutaneous psoriasis stigma (the same of different location) (**Table 6**).

The vast majority of cases (75.24%) with declared unique psoriatic lesion at the onset of the disease **developed** *multiple skin manifestations* over short or long periods of time.

The statistical report shows **no marked relationship** between the lesions location at the time of the first diagnosis of psoriasis and at the moment of onset evaluation ($r = 0.1406$, $\chi^2 = 1.018$, $p = 0.312$, 95% CI).

The comparison between unique onset lesion and multiple lesions at the moment of clinical examination is presented in (**Table 7**).

2.2.2.7. Symptoms: pruritus and psoriasis

Previous dermatology dogma suggested that atopic dermatitis is itchy and psoriasis is not!

Location	Nr. cases	%
Unique lesion	212	17.15
Multiple lesions	1024	82.85
Two body areas	266	21.55
Three body areas	244	19.74
Four body areas	240	19.41
Five body areas	155	12.54
Six body areas	76	6.15
Seven body areas	30	2.43
Eight body areas	12	0.97
10 body areas	1	0.08
Total	1236	

Table 5. Number of areas involved.

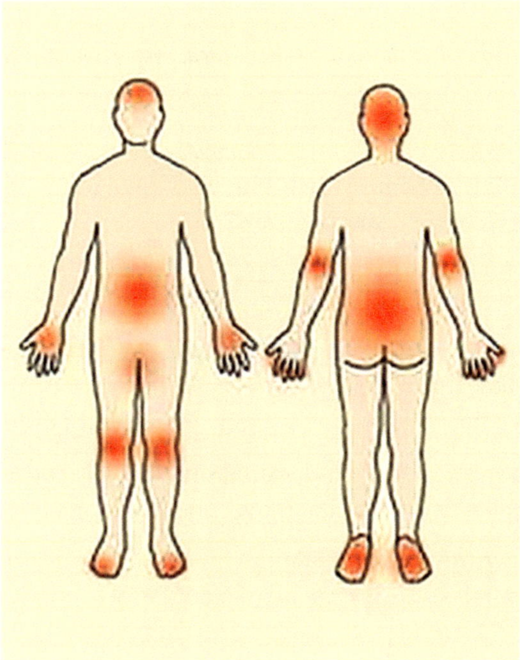

Figure 4. Body areas frequently involved.

The aim of the present study was to assess the incidence of pruritus in patients diagnosed with psoriasis (**Figure 5**); data were collected based on patients' responses and pruritus was certified by declaration.

Onset *unique lesion*	**Nr. cases**	**%**	**Associations of *multiple lesions* at the onset of evaluation**	**Nr. cases**	**%**
Unknown	128	10.36	Scalp, auxiliary	1	0.08
Scalp	347	28.07	Scalp, presternal	2	0.16
Elbows	147	11.89	Scalp, elbows	9	0.73
Palms	98	7.93	Scalp, elbows, knees	1	0.08
Feet	88	7.12	Scalp, face	3	0.24
Trunk	64	5.18	Scalp, knees	2	0.16
Hands	51	4.13	Scalp, intraauricular	3	0.24
Knees	34	2.75	Scalp, feet	1	0.08
Goutate	23	1.86	Scalp, buttocks	1	0.08
Abdomen	18	1.46	Scalp, trunk	5	0.40
Fingers	16	1.29	Trunk, axillary	1	0.08
Plantar	16	1.29	Trunk, face	1	0.08
Face	12	0.97	Trunk, palms	1	0.08
Thighs	11	0.89	Trunk, fingers	1	0.08
Retroauricular	11	0.89	Trunk, knees	1	0.08
Perimaleolar	10	0.81	Elbows, palms	5	0.40
Erythrodermic	9	0.73	Elbows, knees	42	3.40
Periumbilical	9	0.73	Elbows, palms	2	0.16
Occipital	6	0.49	Elbows, feet	4	0.32
Cervical	8	0.64	Elbows, plantar	1	0.08
Palpebral	4	0.32	Palms, fingers	1	0.08
Retrooccipital	4	0.32	Palms, pretibial	1	0.08
Genital	3	0.24	Palms, dorsal aspect of the hands	1	0.08
Buttocks	3	0.24	Palms, occipital	1	0.08
Preauricular	2	0.16	Palmo-plantar	6	0.49
Lumbo-sacral	2	0.16	Knees, plantar	1	0.08
Temporal	2	0.16	Knees, pretibial	2	0.16
Frontal	1	0.08	Knees, dorsal aspects of the hands	1	0.08
			Knees, buttocks	1	0.08
			Dorsal aspects of the hands, feet	4	0.32

Onset *unique lesion*	Nr. cases	%	Associations of *multiple lesions* at the onset of evaluation	Nr. cases	%
			Dorsal aspects of the hands, face	1	0.08
			Plantar, abdomen	1	0.08
			Cervical, retroauricular	1	0.08
Total	1127		Total	109	

Table 6. Number of areas involved.

Onset location	Location at the moment of examination		Total
	Unique location	Multiple locations	
ONSET: unique location	197	930	1127
	15.94%	75.24%	
ONSET: multiple location	15	94	109
	1.21%	7.61%	
Total	212	1024	1236

Table 7. The number of psoriatic lesions found in time of diagnosis as compared with the number found at clinical inspection.

Pruritus was admitted by 293 persons **(23.7%)** and *denied* by 943 **(76.3%)**. The presence and intensity of pruritus were independent of age, gender, marital status, family history of psoriasis, job, level of education, type of psoriasis, alcohol, smoking, duration of the disease, number of lesions, and severity index.

Pruritus may be unrecognized and underestimated by the patients and/or medical staff.

2.2.3. Comorbidities

2.2.3.1. Comorbidities: overview

Comorbidities present at the moment of diagnosis and/or in the medical history of patients (**Figure 6**, **Table 8**).

Out of the 1236 patients enrolled in the study, 59.22% (732 psoriatic patients) had no comorbidities at the moment of diagnosis or in their medical history (**Table 8**).

2.2.3.2. Comorbidities: psoriasis and psoriatic arthritis

Psoriatic arthritis is a chronic, inflammatory, seronegative form of arthritis occurring in subjects with psoriasis. PsA usually occurs over the age of 40 and it affects both sexes equally [24, 25].

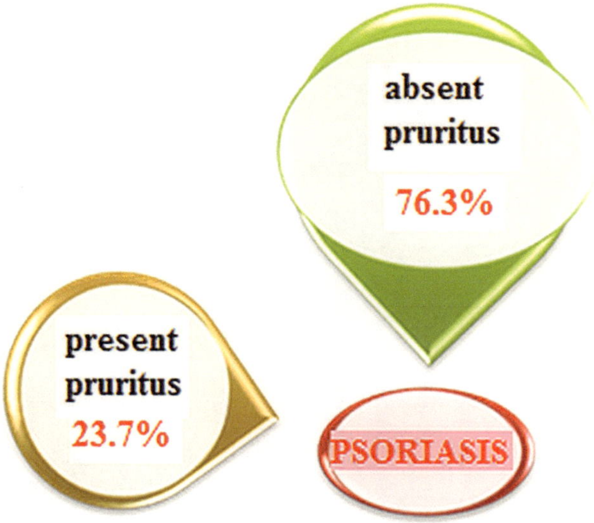

Figure 5. Results of the study: pruritus and psoriasis.

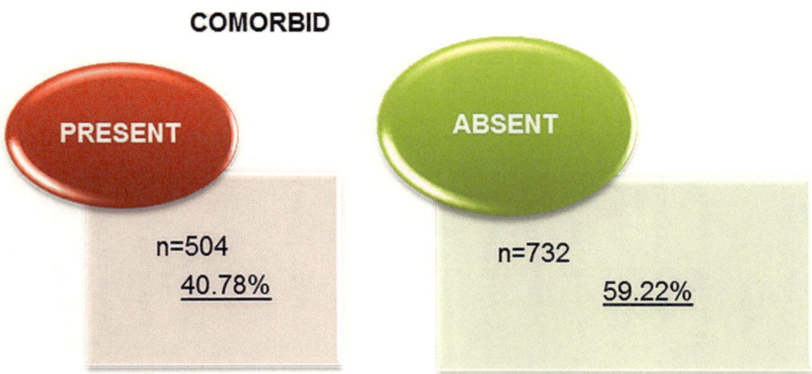

Figure 6. The number of patients with present/absent comorbidities at the moment of diagnosis and/or in their medical history.

The incidence and prevalence of PsA among patients with psoriasis varies between different studies based on the variety of criteria and methods used to study PsA such as patient history, questionnaires, Moll and Wright or Caspar and Grappa classification criteria [26]. Prey et al. published a review where prevalence ranged from 2.04 to 26% and 5.94 to 25% when evaluating PsA using only rheumatologic diagnostic criteria [26].

Likewise, geographical variations in PsA were notified: Europe and North America present higher PsA prevalence ranging between 20.6 and 30% compared with Asia where PsA is significantly lower (8.7%) as seen in a large study of 1149 patients, in Argentina the prevalence rate was found to be 17%, whereas in Brazil 35% [27–31].

Comorbidities	*N*	%	Comorbidities	*N*	%	Comorbidities	*N*	%
Absent	732	59.22	Chronic urticaria	2	0.16	Allergic rhinitis	1	0.08
Arterial hypertension	124	9.92	Lyell syndrome	1	0.08	Sinusitis	2	0.16
Cardiac dysrhythmia	18	1.44	Quincke edema	1	0.08	Hay fever	1	0.08
Ischemic heart disease	20	1.16	Acne	1	0.08	Gilbert syndrome	1	0.08
DZ II	47	3.79	Amygdalectomy	10	0.80	Chronic pancreatitis	3	0.24
DZ insulin-dependent	3	0.24	Adenoidectomy	13	1.04	Hiatal hernia	1	0.08
Dysmetabolic syndrome	18	1.44	Colecystectomy	16	1.28	Umbilical hernia	2	0.16
Morbid obesity	16	1.28	Splenectomy	1	0.08	Chronic cholecystitis	8	0.65
Chronic hepatitis B	10	0.08	Hysterectomy	1	0.08	Biliary lithiasis	4	0.32
Chronic hepatitis C	7	0.56	Ovarectomy	6	0.49	Renal lithiasis	9	0.73
Toxic chronic hepatitis	28	2.24	Inguinal hernia	5	0.40	Chronic pyelonephritis	2	0.16
Liver cirrhosis	2	0.16	Megacolon surgery	1	0.08	Enuresis	1	0.08
Hepatic steatosis	3	0.24	Ischemic stroke	5	0.40	Chronic glomerulonephritis	1	0.08
Hepatitis B virus carrier	1	0.08	Infantile paralysis	1	0.08	Chronic urinary tract infection	1	0.08
Hepatic cyst hydatid	1	0.08	Status epilepticus	1	0.08	Testicular ectopia	1	0.08
Tuberculosis	12	0.96	Meningitis	1	0.08	Hydrocele	5	0.40
Peptic ulcer	36	2.91	Parkinson disease	1	0.08	Azoospermia	1	0.08
Gastritis	8	0.64	Spastic tetraparesis	1	0.08	Phimosis	2	0.16
Gastric hemorrhage	2	0.16	Cervical cancer	2	0.16	Endometriosis	1	0.08
Disc herniation	21	1.68	Hodgkin disease	1	0.08	Fibroma uterus	14	1.12
Gout	3	0.24	Breast cancer	1	0.08	Ovarian cysts	8	0.64
Rheumatoid arthritis	4	0.32	Cancer colorectal	1	0.08	Fibrocystic breast disease	6	0.49

http://dx.doi.org/10.5772/intechopen.68728

Comorbidities	*N*	%	Comorbidities	*N*	%	Comorbidities	*N*	%
Ankylosing spondylitis	4	0.32	Thyroid cancer	1	0.08	Pituitary adenoma	1	0.08
Rheumatic fever	1	0.08	Gastric cancer	1	0.08	Chronic hypocalcemia	5	0.40
Osteitis	1	0.08	Chronic venous insufficiency	15	1.2	Asthma	11	0.88
Psoriatic arthritis	2	0.16	Peripheral arteriopathy	1	0.08	Chronic bronchitis	6	0.49
Knee meniscus graft	1	0.08	Crohn's disease	1	0.08	Spontaneous pneumothorax	1	0.08
Osteomyelitis	2	0.16	Erythematous-pultaceous angina	3	0.24	Pleural effusion	1	0.08
Cervical spondylotic	2	0.16	B streptococcal pharyngitis	3	0.24	Multiple sclerosis	1	0.08
Autoimmune thyroiditis	1	0.08	Anti-streptolyzin o	2	0.16	Duchenne muscular dystrophy	1	0.08
Thyroidectomy Hypothyroidism	8 9	0.64 0.73	Psychiatric disorders	10	0.80	Myasthenia gravis	1	0.08
Thyroid goiter	3	0.24	keratoconjunctivitis	1	0.08	Vestibular disorder	1	0.08
Vitiligo	10	0.80	Blepharitis Retinopathy	1 1	0.08 0.08	Secondary amenorrhea	1	0.08
Alopecia areata	2	0.16	Hypermetropia	1	0.08	Gastric prolapse	1	0.08
Dermatomyositis	3	0.24	Glaucoma	1	0.08	Chronic mastoiditis	1	0.08
Rosacea	3	0.24	Cataract	2	0.16	Polyposis coli	2	0.16
Keratosis pilaris	2	0.16	Anemia	3	0.24	Spina bifida	1	0.08
Celiac disease	1	0.08	Idiopathic thrombocytopenia	1	0.08			

Table 8. General comorbidities among psoriatic patients involved in the study.

In our study, the estimated PsA prevalence based on rheumatologic evaluation (Moll and Wright criteria) was **0.16%** among 1236 patients with psoriasis (**Table 9**), **NOT** in accord with several European revisions.

An extensive study in Germany on 1511 patients revealed a total PsA prevalence of 20.5% [31]. In Greece, a retrospective analysis on 278 patients with psoriasis revealed that PsA prevalence was 30%. This subgroup of patients with PsA showed significantly higher rates of comorbidities including CVD, hypertension, diabetes mellitus type 2, and hypercholesterolemia compared to non-PsA patients [24]. Other studies show PsA prevalence ranging between 0.17 and 0.35% in the general Greek population [32, 33]. Other two publications report remarkably lower rates of PsA prevalence among patients with psoriasis, 7.23% in Croatia, respectively, 9.3% in Serbia [26].

2.2.3.3. Comorbidities: coexistence of psoriasis with other skin diseases at the moment of diagnosis

Out of the 1236 patients enrolled in the study, only 26 psoriatic patients had other skin diseases at the moment of diagnosis (**Table 10**), including 10 with vitiligo, 3 with dermatomyositis, 3 with Rosacea, and 2 with Alopecia areata.

2.2.3.4. Comorbidities: coexistence of psoriasis with cardiovascular diseases at the moment of diagnosis

Psoriasis has been associated with high cardiovascular morbidity and mortality. Recent studies suggest that psoriasis, particularly if severe, has a 58% increased risk of major adverse cardiovascular events such as arrhythmia, myocardial infarction, or stroke, and has a 57% increased risk of cardiovascular death, beyond the risk of death associated with traditional cardiovascular risk factors [34–36].

Of the 1236 patients enrolled in the study, 162 psoriatic patients had cardiovascular diseases at the moment of diagnosis (**Table 11**), great majority accusing arterial hypertension.

Coexistence of rheumatologic diseases	Nr. cases	%
Disc herniation	21	1.68
Gout	3	0.24
Rheumatoid arthritis	4	0.32
Ankylosing spondylitis	4	0.32
Rheumatic fever	1	0.08
Osteitis	1	0.08
Psoriatic arthritis	2	0.16
Knee meniscus graft	1	0.08
Osteomyelitis	2	0.16
Cervical spondylotic	2	0.16
Total	68/1236	

Table 9. Coexistence of psoriasis with other rheumatologic diseases.

2.2.3.5. *Comorbidities: prevalence of thyroid abnormalities among psoriatic patients*

Of the 1236 patients diagnosed with psoriasis, only 22 were spotted with thyroid abnormalities (**Table 12**).

Coexistence of other skin diseases	Number of cases	%
Vitiligo	10	0.80
Alopecia areata	2	0.16
Dermatomyositis	3	0.24
Rosacea	3	0.24
Keratosis pilaris	2	0.16
Dermatitis herpetiformis	1	0.08
Chronic urticaria	2	0.16
Lyell syndrome	1	0.08
Quincke edema	1	0.08
Acne	1	0.08
Total	26/1236	

Table 10. Coexistence of psoriasis with other skin diseases.

Cardiovascular diseases	Nr. cases	%
Arterial hypertension	124	9.92
Cardiac dysrhythmia	18	1.44
Ischemic heart disease	20	1.16
Total	162/1236	

Table 11. Cardiovascular diseases among psoriatic patients involved in the study.

Thyroid abnormalities	Nr. cases	%
Autoimmune thyroiditis	1	0.08
Thyroidectomy	8	0.64
Hypothyroidism	9	0.73
Thyroid goiter	3	0.24
Thyroid cancer	1	0.08
Total	22/1236	1.77

Table 12. Coexistence of thyroid abnormalities at patients diagnosed with psoriasis.

2.2.3.6. Comorbidities: psoriasis and tuberculosis

In this transversal study, the incidence of tuberculosis was quantified from the medical history and at the moment of the clinical examination for patients diagnosed with psoriasis. Of the 1236 patients diagnosed with psoriasis, over a period of 8 years (2004–2011) comorbidities were present in **40.78%** of cases, and **12** of them **(0.97%)** had **a history of tuberculosis**: 5 were men (41.67%), 8 cases of pulmonary tuberculosis (66.67%), 2 pleural effusions (16.67%), 1 genital tuberculosis (8.34%), and 1 case of kerato-conjunctivitis (8.34%). Of the 12 patients with psoriasis and past tuberculosis, 1 had arterial hypertension and chronic nephritis, 1 obesity, 1 erythema nodosum, and 1 with gastric carcinoma (**Figure 7**).

Psoriasis could represent an independent risk factor for tuberculosis, because a high prevalence was reported in recent studies: 18.0%—Bordignon et al. [37]. In another study, latent tuberculosis infection was more reported in psoriasis (50%) than inflammatory bowel disease patients (24.2%), prior to the onset of any anti-tumor necrosis factor (TNF)-α treatment [38].

2.2.4. Evolution characteristics

2.2.4.1. Severity of lesions in relation to risk factors

The number of psoriatic lesions is in direct relation with the risk factors, including residence, gender, index severity, presence of comorbidities, alcohol intake, smoking, work status, and family history of psoriasis (**Table 13**).

2.2.4.2. Severity of lesions in relation to risk factors: smoking and psoriasis

Most of the patients enrolled in the study were **nonsmokers**, *by declaration* (**Figure 8**) but **there is a significant correlation between the smoking and the severity of the disease** ($r = 0.254$, $\chi^2 = 10.49$, $p = 0.00527$, 95% CI).

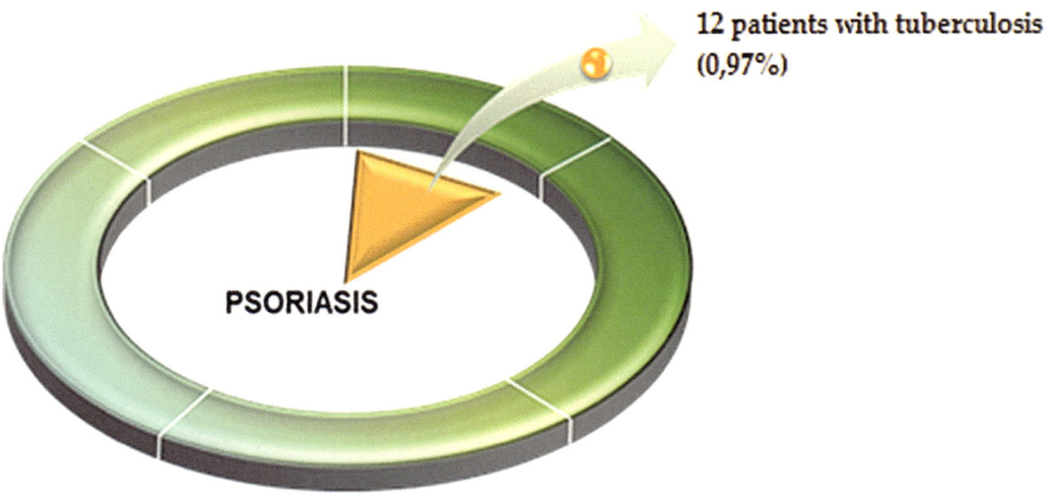

Figure 7. Tuberculosis among psoriatic patients involved in the study.

	Location			
	Unique lesion		Multiple lesions	
	Nr. patients	%	**Nr. patients**	%
Urban residence	192	18.53	844	81.47
Rural residence	20	10	180	90
Male gender	103	15.40	566	84.60
Female gender	109	19.22	458	84.60
Mild psoriasis	132	24.63	404	75.37
Moderate psoriasis	65	13	435	87.00
Severe psoriasis	15	7.5	185	92.50
Comorbidities absent	135	18.44	597	81.56
Comorbidities present	77	15.28	427	84.72
Alcohol consumer	45	10.98	365	89.02
Nonalcohol consumer	167	20.22	659	79.78
Nonsmoker	171	19.06	726	80.94
Smoker	41	12.09	298	87.91
Pupil/student	45	3.64	137	11.08
Worker	130	10.52	622	50.32
Retired	20	1.62	129	10.44
Social assisted	1	0.08	27	2.18
Jobless	16	1.29	109	8.82
Family history absent	150	17.22	721	82.78
First-degree relatives diagnosed with psoriasis	38	19.00	162	81.00
Second-degree relatives diagnosed with psoriasis	15	13.04	100	86.96
Third-degree relatives diagnosed with psoriasis	7	19.44	29	80.56
Fourth-degree relatives diagnosed with psoriasis	2	14.29	12	85.71

Table 13. Number of lesions in relation to risk factors (residence, gender, index severity, presence of comorbidities, alcohol intake, smoking, work status, and family history of psoriasis).

2.2.4.3. *Severity of lesions in relation to risk factors: alcohol intake (by declaration) and psoriasis*

Of 1236 patients with psoriasis, alcohol consumption was declared by 410 persons, representing 33.17% of all (**Table 14**).

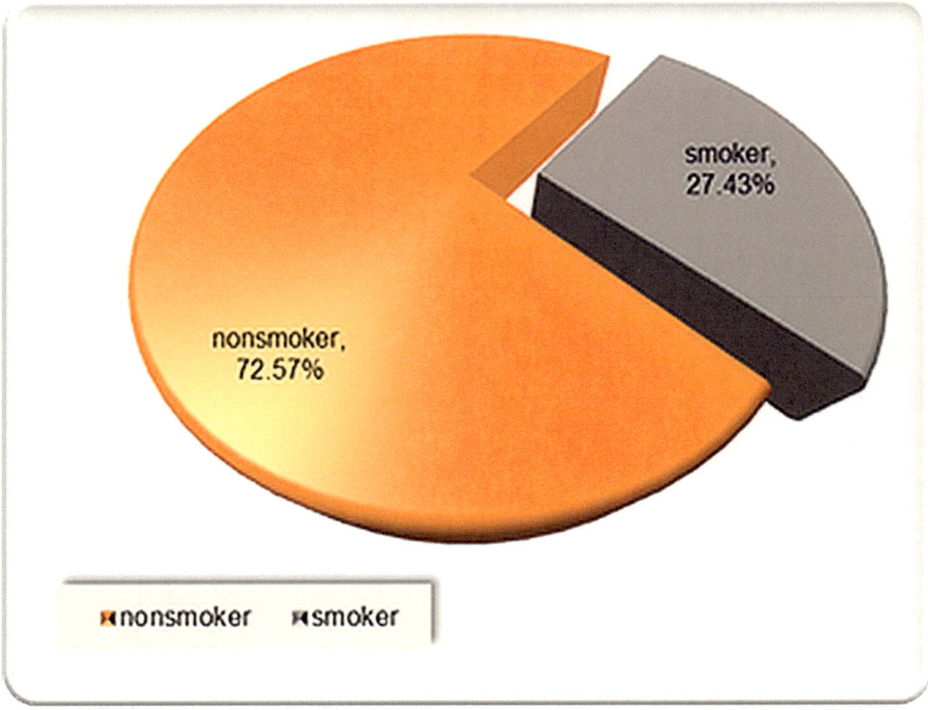

Figure 8. Results of the study: smokers and nonsmokers involved in the study.

Alcohol consumption	Nr. cases	%
Positive	410	33.17
Negative	826	66.83
Total	1236	

Table 14. Results of the study: number of patients in relation with alcohol consumption.

2.2.4.4. Severity of lesions in relation to PASI

The number of psoriasis lesions correlates with (**Table 15**):

- age at the moment of clinical examination ($F = 8.902$, $p = 0.0029$);
- residence in rural area ($\chi^2 = 8.589$, $p = 0.00338$, 95% CI);
- alcohol intake ($\chi^2 = 16.47$, $p = 0.00005$, 95% CI);
- smoking ($\chi^2 = 8.408$, $p = 0.00373$, 95% CI);
- occupation: workers/pupils/students ($\chi^2 = 14.11$, $p = 0.0069$, 95% CI).

2.2.4.5. Severity of lesions in relation with topical steroids

Topical steroids: most of the patients were several years treated with steroids topically before presenting to the clinical appointment (**Table 16**).

2.3. Correlations with the severity of psoriasis (Risk factors)

Severity index of the disease at the moment of clinical examination (**Table 17**) are as follows:

Within psoriasis patients, 43.37% were diagnosed with mild form of the disease, 40.45% with moderate, and only 16.18% with severe type.

2.3.1. Correlations between demographic data and the severity index of psoriasis

2.3.1.1. Gender distribution versus severity index

There is a strong correlation between gender and severity of the disease ($r = 0.378$, $p = 0.00023$, $\chi^2 = 16.706$, $p = 0.00024$, 95% CI) (**Table 18**). Among severe cases, 19.8% were men and only 11.82% women, in comparison with mild cases where 47.62% were women (**Figure 9**).

Parameter/factor	PASI index-correlation	Number of psoriatic lesions-correlation
Onset age	Yes	No
Age at the moment of clinical examination	Yes	Yes
Gender (male)	Yes	No
Residence in rural area	Yes	Yes
History family of psoriasis	Yes	No
Presence of comorbidities	Yes	No
Alcohol and smoking	Yes	Yes
Work status-education	Retired persons/jobless	Workers/pupils-students

Table 15. Results of the study: severity of lesions in relation to PASI.

Topical steroids	Nr. cases	%
Yes	1073	86.81
No	110	8.90
Unknown	53	4.29
Total	1236	

Table 16. Results of the study: number of patients treated with topical steroids.

Type of psoriasis	Nr. cases	%
Severe (PASI > 10)	200	16.18
Moderate (PASI: 3/5–10)	500	40.45
Mild	536	43.37
Total	1236	

Table 17. Results of the study: severity index of the disease.

Psoriasis severity	Gender of the patient		Total
	Male	Female	
Mild	266	270	536
	39.76%	47.62%	
Moderate	270	230	500
	40.36%	40.56%	
Severe	133	67	200
	19.88%	11.82%	
Total	669	567	1236

Table 18. Gender distribution versus severity index.

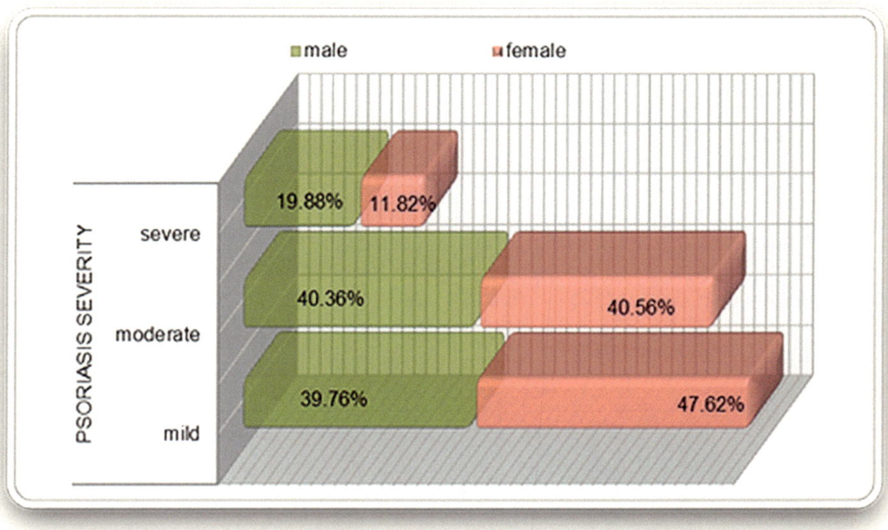

Figure 9. Gender distribution among patients involved in the study.

Our data support a male predominance in all forms of psoriasis (54.13% versus 45.87%) and greater severity in men (**Table 19**).

2.3.1.2. Age of patients at the moment of clinical examination versus severity index

The mean (medium) age of patients presents important differences reported to the severity of the disease ($F = 45.780$, $p \ll 0.01$, 95% CI) (**Figure 10**), with small values for mild cases (41.11 ± 16.07 SD) and greater values for severe cases (53.06 ± 13.82 SD) (**Table 20**).

df = 2	Chi-square χ^2	*p* 95% *confidence interval*
Pearson Chi-square—χ^2	16.70615	0.00024
M-L Chi-square	16.99982	0.00020
Correlation coefficient (Spearman Rank *R*)	−0.378898	0.00023

Table 19. Results of the study: correlations between gender distribution and the severity index.

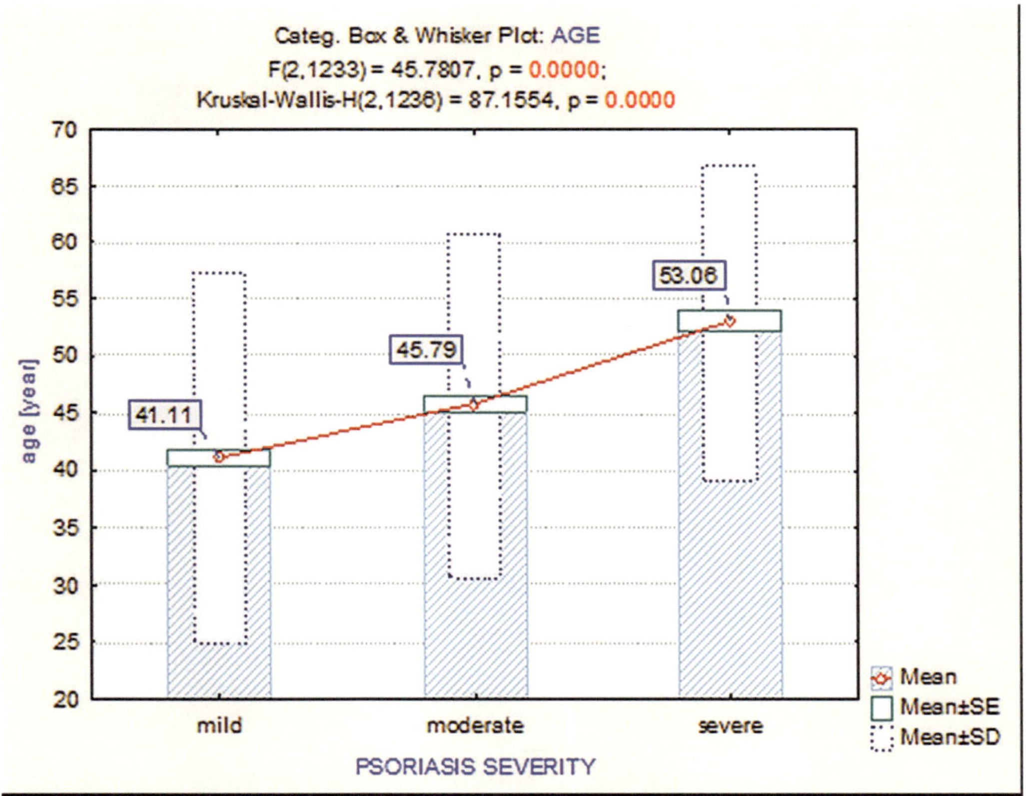

Figure 10. Mean (medium) age of patients at the moment of clinical examination.

Psoriasis is a disease of all ages but predominant around 40 years of age; early psoriasis (manifesting before 40 years of age) is associated with increased severity index, while late psoriasis (manifesting after 40 years of age) appears to be milder (**Table 21**). We do not see the peak in the age groups 20–30 and 40–50, but there is a quite uniform distribution starting with the age group 20 and ending with age group 60 years old (**Figure 11**). The most active age group 30–50 years is affected by psoriasis (**Table 22**).

Psoriasis	Media age	Media		Dev.std	Er.std	Min	Max	Q25	Median	Q75
		−95%	+95%							
Severe	53.06	51.13	54.99	13.82	0.98	12.00	88.00	43.50	53.50	63.00
Moderate	45.79	44.47	47.11	15.01	0.67	13.00	91.00	34.00	45.00	57.00
Mild	41.11	39.74	42.47	16.07	0.69	6.00	89.00	29.00	40.00	52.00
All Groups	44.94	44.05	45.82	15.84	0.45	6.00	91.00	33.00	44.00	57.00

Table 20. Age of patients at the moment of clinical examination versus severity index.

	F (95% *confidence interval*)	*p*
Levene Test of Homogeneity of Variances	3.034166	0.048474
Brown-Forsythe Test of Homogeneity of Variances	2.843525	0.058602
Test ANOVA	45.78075	0.000000

Table 21. Test ANOVA—results.

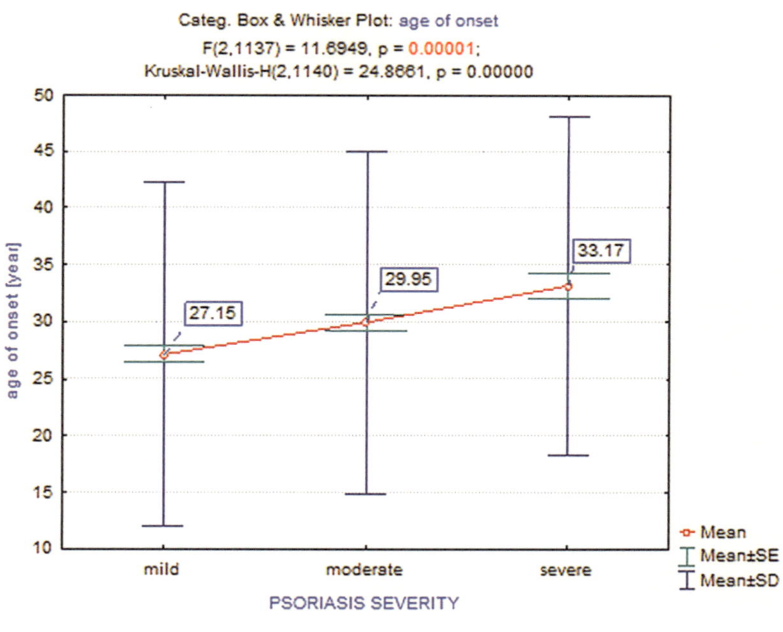

Figure 11. Mean (medium) age of patients at the onset of disease.

Unequal N HSD test	*p* (95% *confidence interval*)
Mild versus moderate	0.000025
Mild versus severe	0.000022
Moderate versus severe	0.000027

Table 22. Results of the unequal N HSD test: correlations between age of patients and the severity index.

2.3.1.3. Age of the patients at the onset of psoriasis versus severity index

The first diagnosis of psoriasis was made at the age 10–30 for the most of the patients and the percentage of psoriasis de novo falls with age (**Table 23**). This could mean that majority of patients were diagnosed previously or they do not seek special care in the older age. Our findings suggest that there is a march over time toward greater severity in the disease.

The medium of age of onset shows statistical differences related to severity of psoriasis (F = 11.69, p = 0.000009, 95% CI): for mild forms were 27.15 ± 14.92 SD (**Table 24**), for moderate cases 29.95 ± 15.07 SD, and for severe cases 33.17 ± 15.07 SD (**Table 25**).

Psoriasis	Media age	Media		Dev.std	Er.std	Min	Max	Q25	Median	Q75
		−95%	+95%							
Mild	27.15	25.79	28.52	15.20	0.70	1.00	72.00	16.00	25.00	36.00
Moderate	29.95	28.58	31.32	15.07	0.70	0.50	76.00	18.00	27.00	40.00
Severe	33.17	31.07	35.26	14.92	1.06	3.00	70.00	22.00	32.00	43.00
All groups	29.34	28.45	30.22	15.24	0.45	0.50	76.00	18.00	27.00	39.00

Table 23. Age of patients at the onset of psoriasis versus severity index.

	F (95% *confidence interval*)	*p*
Levene Test of Homogeneity of Variances	0.108982	0.896756
Brown-Forsythe Test of Homogeneity of Variances	0.060732	0.941079
Test ANOVA	11.69489	0.000009

Table 24. Test ANOVA—results.

Unequal N HSD test	*p* (95% *confidence interval*)
Mild versus moderate	0.012604
Mild versus severe	0.000029
Moderate versus severe	0.032170

Table 25. Results of the unequal N HSD test: correlations between age of patients at the onset of psoriasis and the severity index.

2.3.1.4. Distribution of cases reported to residence/location versus severity index

The present study confirms the higher prevalence of psoriasis in urban area, but mild cases were diagnosed compared with severe and untreated forms seen in people living in rural areas (**Figure 12**). Explanations can be found in reduced accessibility of people living in villages far away from a specialized medical center; long period of no treatments especially in milder forms considering the disease an esthetic problem rather than a disease; stress-less life, open air activity with many hours of sun bathing/exposure; different nutrition habits (less industrialized and processed food, less meat, and more vegetables), type of water, skin-care practices, tobacco, alcohol, smaller exposure to drugs, and other chemicals (**Table 26**).

Major association exists between index severity and residence of the patients ($r = 0.319$, $p = 0.0037$, $\chi^2 = 9.507$, $p = 0.0086$, 95% CI). Although the prevalence of psoriasis is higher in urban area, mild cases are diagnosed, severe and untreated forms are seen in people living in rural areas (**Table 27**).

2.3.1.5. Level of education versus severity index

High level of education was recognized in patients severely affected by psoriasis. Persons in worrying conditions were related to income/job such as retired people, with no income or social-assisted developed severe forms of psoriasis (**Table 28**).

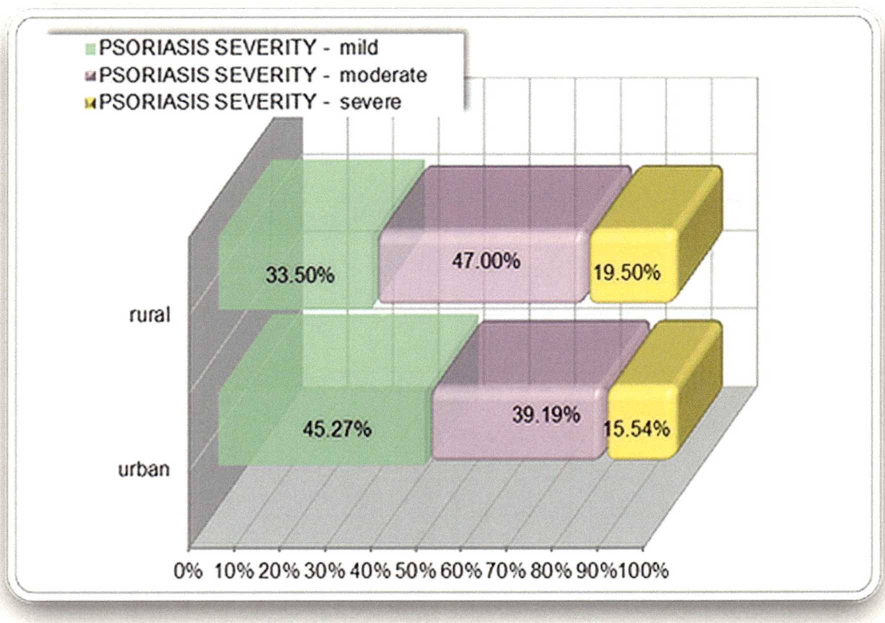

Figure 12. Residence distribution among patients involved in the study.

Psoriasis severity	Urban	Rural	Total
Mild	469	67	536
	45.27%	33.50%	
Moderate	406	94	500
	39.19%	47.00%	
Severe	161	39	200
	15.54%	19.50%	
Total	1036	200	1236

Table 26. Residence versus severity index.

df = 2	Chi-square χ^2	*p* (95% *confidence interval*)
Pearson Chi-square—χ^2	9.507847	0.00862
M-L Chi-square	9.698231	0.00784
Correlation coefficient (Spearman Rank *R*)	0.3191024	0.00317

Table 27. Results of the study: correlations between residence distribution and the severity index.

Level of education	Psoriasis severity			Total
	Mild	Moderate	Severe	
Middle school	19	23	12	54
	35.19%	42.59%	22.22%	
College	46	72	30	148
	31.08%	48.65%	20.27%	
Vocational school	13	23	12	48
	27.08%	47.92%	25.00%	
High school	124	158	63	345
	35.94%	45.80%	18.26%	
Postsecondary school	20	15	12	47
	42.55%	31.91%	25.53%	
Students	121	56	5	182
	66.48%	30.77%	2.75%	
University graduates	193	153	66	412
	46.84%	37.14%	16.02%	
Total	536	500	200	1236

Table 28. Level of education versus severity index.

Level of education points out a strong correlation with severity ($r = -0.413$, $p \ll 0.01$); patients with less than 12 years of school presented more cases with psoriasis type moderate-severe (**Table 29**). Although high educated persons, with university degree are more often diagnosed with psoriasis, cases are less severe.

Although higher education suggests a higher prevalence of psoriasis, a lower level of education correlates strongly with moderate-severe forms of psoriasis.

Education may be related to multiple confounding factors including alcohol intake, smoking, and access to specialized dermatological care.

2.3.1.6. Jobs distribution/income versus severity index

Among pupils and students, the most frequently diagnosed form of psoriasis was mild one (66.48%), severe disease being reported to only 2.75%, while persons without any occupation presented severe psoriasis 24.16%, respectively, 24% (**Table 30**). Moderate forms were seen in retired persons (43.62%) and jobless (42.4%). Jobless patients had worse severity ($\chi^2 = 66.67$, $p \ll 0.01$, 95% CI) (**Table 31**).

df = 12	Chi-square χ^2	*p* (95% *interval de încredere*)
Pearson Chi-square—χ^2	77.51211	0.00000
M-L Chi-square	85.73127	0.00000
Correlation coefficient (Spearman Rank *R*)	−0.4139638	0.00000

Table 29. Results of the study: correlations between level of education and the severity index.

Job	Psoriasis severity			Total
	Mild	Moderate	Severe	
Pupil/student	121	56	5	182
	66.48%	30.77%	2.75%	
Employee	313	316	123	752
	41.62%	42.02%	16.36%	
Retired	48	65	36	149
	32.21%	43.62%	24.16%	
Social assisted	12	10	6	28
	42.86%	35.71%	21.43%	
With no income	42	53	30	125
	33.60%	42.40%	24.00%	
Total	536	500	200	1236

Table 30. Jobs distribution versus severity index.

df = 8	Chi-square χ^2	*p* (95% *confidence interval*)
Pearson Chi-square—χ^2	66.67419	0.00000
M-L Chi-square	73.96201	0.00000
Correlation coefficient (Spearman Rank *R*)	0.3056883	0.000

Table 31. Results of the study: correlations between jobs distribution and the severity index.

2.3.2. *Correlations between clinical data and the severity index of psoriasis*

2.3.2.1. *Family history of psoriasis versus severity index*

There was a positive family history of psoriasis in 29.53% of subjects, 16.18% first-degree relatives, 9.30% second-degree, 2.91% third-degree, and 1.13% fourth-degree (**Table 32**).

A family history of psoriasis was associated with greater disease severity ($r = -0.448$, $\chi^2 = 18.32$, $p = 0.01893$, 95% CI) (**Table 33**).

2.3.2.2. *The distribution of (unique/multiple) psoriatic lesions at the moment of clinical inspection versus severity index*

The results (**Table 34**) prove the absence of an important correlation between the severity index and type of lesions at the onset of psoriasis (unique/multiple lesions) ($r = 0.0249$, $p = 0.381$, 95% CI) (**Table 35**). One can notice that in 19.27% cases of severe psoriasis, patients describe multiple lesions at the first diagnosis (**Figure 13**).

2.3.3. *Correlations between comorbidities and the severity index of psoriasis*

2.3.3.1. *Presence of general comorbidities versus index severity*

Comorbidities were present in 36.1% of patients with mild form of psoriasis, 44.05% with moderate forms, and in 19.64% of severe psoriasis (**Figure 14, Table 36**).

Psoriasis severity	Family history					Total
	Absent	First degree	Second degree	Third degree	Fourth degree	
Mild	361	95	60	14	6	536
	41.45%	47.50%	52.17%	38.89%	42.86%	
Moderate	368	79	29	19	5	500
	42.25%	39.50%	25.22%	52.78%	35.71%	
Severe	142	26	26	3	3	200
	16.30%	13.00%	22.61%	8.33%	21.43%	
Total	871	200	115	36	14	1236

Table 32. Results of the study: family history versus severity index.

df = 8	Chi-square χ^2	*p* (95% *confidence interval*)
Pearson Chi-square—χ^2	18.32477	0.01893
M-L Chi-square	19.13866	0.01414
Correlation coefficient (Spearman Rank *R*)	−0.44809	0.011536

Table 33. Results of the study: correlations between family history and the severity index.

Psoriasis severity	Onset location of psoriasis		Total
	Unique location	Multiple locations	
Mild	492	44	536
	43.66%	40.37%	
Moderate	456	44	500
	40.46%	40.37%	
Severe	179	21	200
	15.88%	19.27%	
Total	1127	109	1236

Table 34. Results of the study: distribution of psoriatic lesion(s) versus severity index.

df = 2	Chi-square χ^2	*p* (95% *confidence interval*)
Pearson Chi-square—χ^2	0.9511274	0.62154
M-L Chi-square	0.9196143	0.63141
Correlation coefficient (Spearman Rank *R*)	0.0249217	0.38135

Table 35. Correlations between the distribution of (unique/multiple) psoriatic lesions and the severity index.

The results ($r = 0.41$, $\chi^2 = 18.79$, $p = 0.00008$, 95% CI) confirm a strong association between the presence of comorbidities and severity of psoriasis (**Table 37**).

2.3.3.2. Comorbidities: appendectomy versus index severity

Appendectomy (**Table 38, Figure 15**) does not correlate with severity index of psoriasis ($r= -0.0096$, $\chi^2=0.967$, $p = 0.616$, 95% CI) (**Table 39**).

2.3.4. Correlations between evolution characteristics and the severity index of psoriasis

2.3.4.1. Risk factors: alcohol consumption versus index severity

Severe forms of psoriasis were found in patients with declared chronic alcohol intake (21.22%), while mild forms were depicted within non-consumers (47.94%) (**Table 40, Figure 16**).

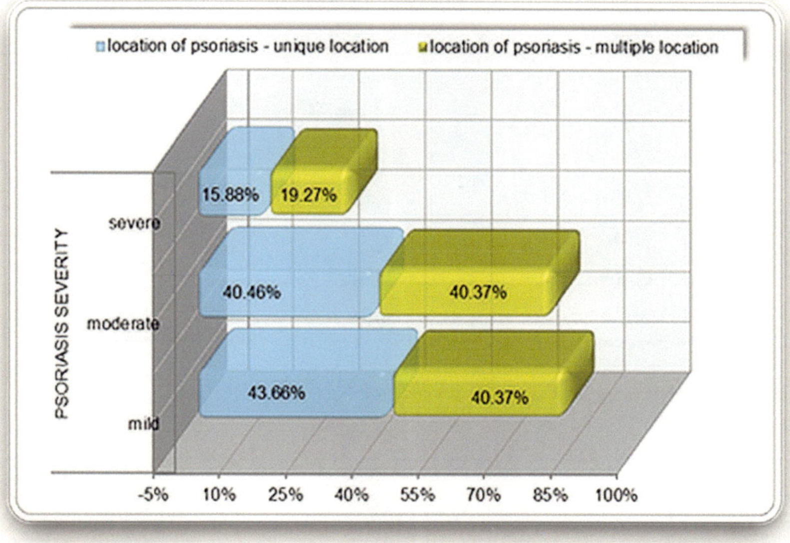

Figure 13. The distribution of (unique/multiple) psoriatic lesions among patients involved in the study.

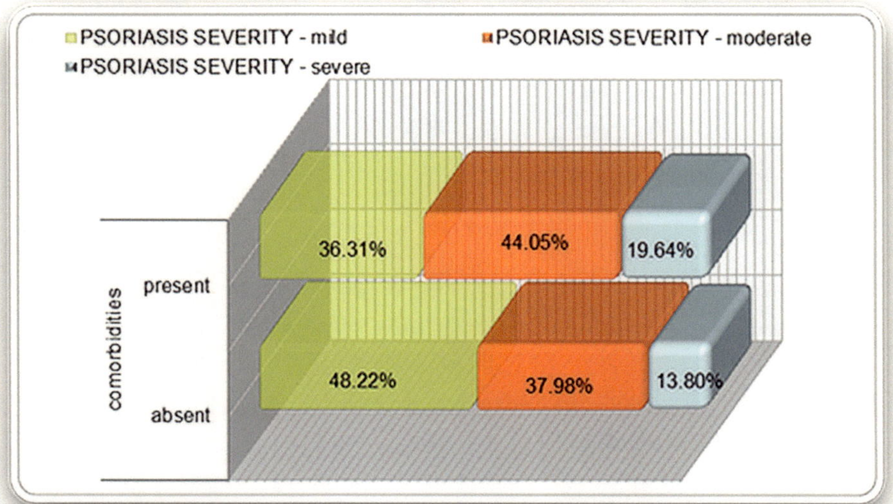

Figure 14. The distribution of comorbidities among patients involved in the study.

Psoriasis severity	Comorbidities		Total
	Absent	Present	
Mild	353	183	536
	48.22%	36.31%	
Moderate	278	222	500
	37.98%	44.05%	
Severe	101	99	200
	13.80%	19.64%	
Total	732	504	1236

Table 36. Results of the study: comorbidities versus severity index.

df = 2	Chi-square χ^2	*p (95% confidence interval)*
Pearson Chi-square—χ^2	18.79107	0.00008
M-L Chi-square	18.86543	0.00008
Correlation coefficient (Spearman Rank *R*)	0.4108901	0.00001

Table 37. Correlations between comorbidities and severity index.

Psoriasis severity	Appendectomy		Total
	Present	Absent	
Mild	106	430	536
	41.57%	43.83%	
Moderate	110	390	500
	43.14%	39.76%	
Severe	39	161	200
	15.29%	16.41%	
Total	255	981	1236

Table 38. Results of the study: (comorbidities) appendectomy versus severity index.

Statistically, a correlation between alcohol intake and index severity is proved ($r = -0.48$, $\chi^2 = 24.30$, $p \ll 0.01$, 95% CI) (**Table 41**).

2.3.4.2. Risk factors: smoking versus index severity

Smokers are prone to severe forms of psoriasis (17.7%), and non-smokers with less severe ones (**Table 42**, **Figure 17**).

Smoking and severity of psoriasis highly correlate ($r = 0.254$, $\chi^2 = 10.49$, $p = 0.00527$, 95% CI) (**Table 43**).

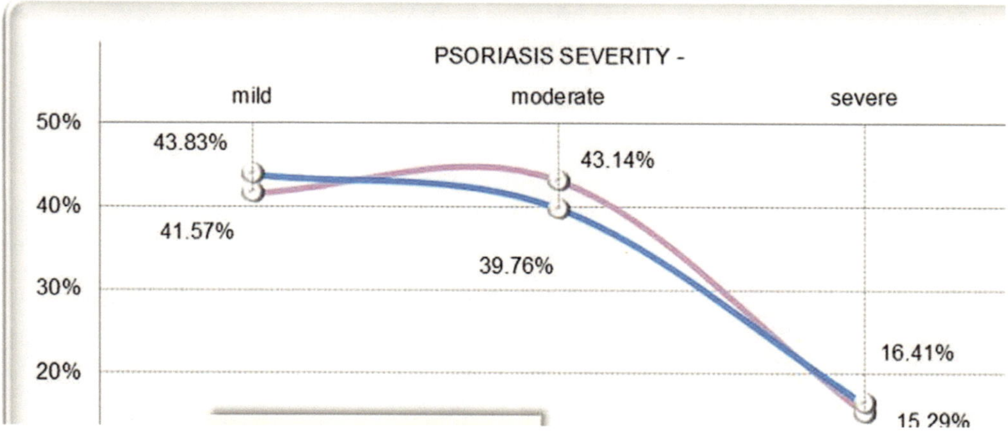

Figure 15. Number of patients with appendectomy among patients involved in the study.

df = 2	Chi-square χ^2	*p* (95% *confidence interval*)
Pearson Chi-square—χ^2	0.9677348	0.61640
M-L Chi-square	0.9633761	0.61774
Correlation coefficient (Spearman Rank *R*)	−0.009627	0.73528

Table 39. Correlations between number of patients with appendectomy and severity index.

Psoriasis severity	Alcohol consumption		Total
	Declared	Not declared	
Mild	140	396	536
	34.15%	47.94%	
Moderate	183	317	500
	44.63%	38.38%	
Severe	87	113	200
	21.22%	13.68%	
Total	410	826	1236

Table 40. Results of the study: alcohol consumption versus severity index.

2.3.5. *Multivariable analysis of factors implicated in severity of psoriasis*

In multivariate analysis, age at the moment of clinical examination (r = **0.83**, $p \ll 0.01$), age of onset (r = **−0.69**, p = 0.000053, 95% CI), education level (r = **−0.588**, p = 0.0037), residence (r = **0.688**, p = 0.0156, 95% CI), job (r = **0.671**, p = 0.0328, 95% CI), gender (r = **−0.45**, p = 0.0394, 95% CI), and smoking (r = **0.597**, p = 0.044, 95% CI) were significant factors associated with severity of psoriasis (**Table 44**).

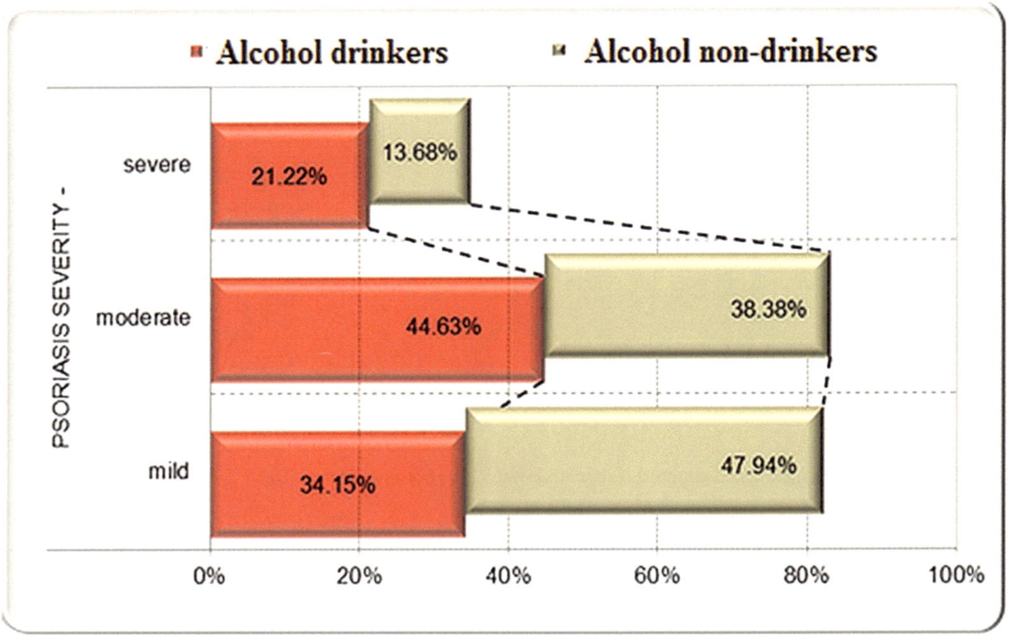

Figure 16. Alcohol consumption among patients involved in the study.

df = 2	Chi-square χ^2	*p* (95% *confidence interval*)
Pearson Chi-square—χ^2	24.30044	0.00001
M-L Chi-square	24.36224	0.00001
Correlation coefficient (Spearman Rank *R*)	−0.489582	0.000

Table 41. Correlations between alcohol consumption and severity index.

Psoriasis severity	Smoking		Total
	Nonsmoker	Smoker	
Mild	414	122	536
	46.15%	35.99%	
Moderate	343	157	500
	38.24%	46.31%	
Severe	140	60	200
	15.61%	17.70%	
Total	897	339	1236

Table 42. Results of the study: smoking versus severity index.

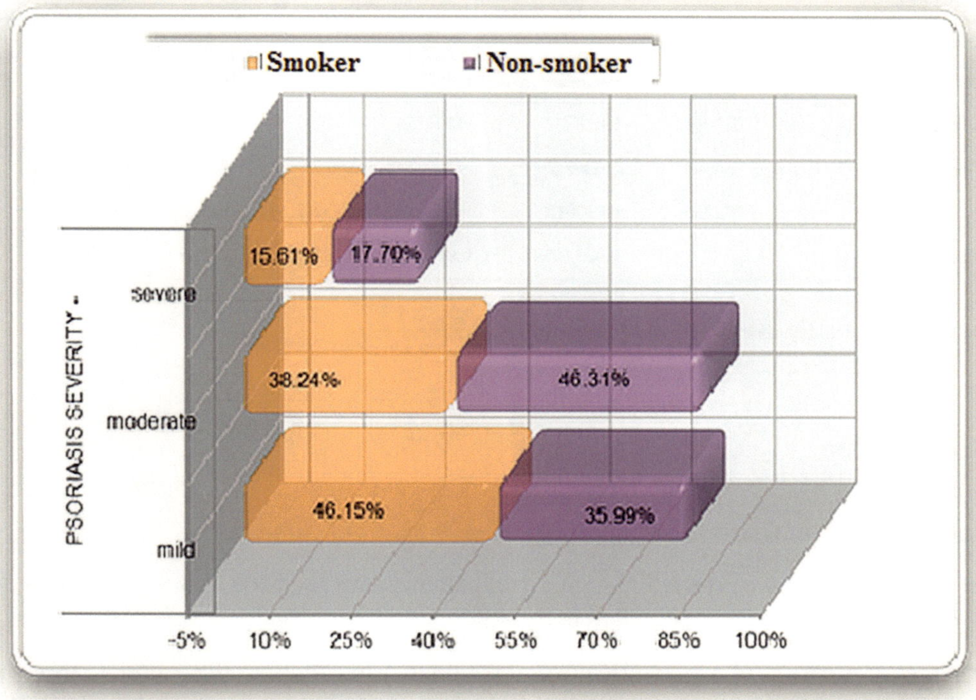

Figure 17. Smoking among patients involved in the study.

df = 2	Chi-square χ^2	*p (95% confidence interval)*
Pearson Chi-square—χ^2	10.49251	0.00527
M-L Chi-square	10.60180	0.00499
Correlation coefficient (Spearman Rank *R*)	0.252514	0.00417

Table 43. Correlations between smoking and severity index.

Partial correlation *psoriasis severity* versus	Confidence interval (Beta)	Std.Err. (Beta)	*B*	Std.Err. B	*t*	*p (95% confidence interval)*
Intercept			−4.43329	10.37951	−0.42712	0.669374
Gender	−0.45016	0.031288	−0.9429	0.04574	−2.06153	0.039482
Age at the moment of clinical examination	0.831591	0.048523	0.1777	0.00226	7.86419	0.000000
Age of onset	−0.692912	0.047558	−0.922	0.00227	−4.05634	0.000053
Multiple lesions	0.023369	0.028032	0.06017	0.07217	0.83367	0.404642
Education	−0.588659	0.030502	−0.3359	0.01156	−2.90666	0.003725
Job	0.67100	0.031403	0.4553	0.02131	2.13671	0.032836

Partial correlation *psoriasis severity* **versus**	**Confidence interval (Beta)**	**Std.Err. (Beta)**	*B*	**Std.Err. B**	*t*	*p* **(95%** ***confidence interval*****)**
Location	0.68837	0.028427	0.3510	0.05579	2.42157	0.015611
Family history	−0.013668	0.028332	−0.01158	0.02400	−0.48244	0.629586
Comorbidities	−0.034033	0.028512	−0.00023	0.00019	−1.19362	0.232876
Alcohol	−0.052250	0.033016	−0.8041	0.05081	−1.58256	0.113803
Smoking	0.59732	0.029716	0.9691	0.04821	2.01006	0.044662

Table 44. Multivariable analysis of factors implicated in severity of psoriasis.

3. Conclusion

Our study has several strengths.

First of all, the study includes a high number of patients with psoriasis followed over a period of 8 years: 1236 persons were enrolled in the study.

Second, over a period of 8 years, detailed and updated information regarding a large variety of factors throughout the cohort follow-up was collected, thus allowing data correlation between psoriasis and various factors and/or different comorbidities.

Third, correlation between psoriasis and different factors permitted the investigation of potential associations over long durations such as the analysis of the association of psoriasis with several different comorbidities, demographic data, psoriasis severity.

Some limitations of this study include the following: it was performed only on Caucasians from predominantly the same region in Romania; therefore, generalizing the results to other ethnicities may be partial.

The study was conducted in an outpatient clinic specialized for psoriasis over a period of 8 years, so an increased number of patients diagnosed with psoriasis earlier had to self-report medical history with a small proportion of missing data. Despite this retrospective characteristic, the recall and the high completion rate for all questions on psoriasis were highly accurate.

Psoriasis is a common chronic systemic disease (not a simple skin disorder), spread worldwide, with a reported prevalence varying from 0.09 to 11.43% [39]. Psoriasis can touch any age, with a great variability: from 6 to 91 years old. The number of years should not be a reason for medical advice restriction.

This complex disease, with unknown cause, has many trigger factors, unpredictable course, severe comorbidities, and a great impact on quality of life. Further research is needed to identify these comorbidities and to take into consideration when evaluating the burdens of psoriasis such as costs, impact on quality of life, and integration of psoriatic patient in the society,therefore to be able to recommend the best management and treatment.

Author details

Anca Chiriac[1], Cristian Podoleanu[2]* and Doina Azoicai[3]

*Address all correspondence to: podoleanu@me.com

1 University of Medicine and Pharmacy "Grigore T. Popa", Iasi, Romania

2 Cardiology Department, University of Medicine and Pharmacy of Târgu Mureș, Targu Mures, Romania

3 Epidemiology Department, University of Medicine and Pharmacy "Grigore T. Popa", Iasi, Romania

References

[1] Langan SM, Seminara NM, Shin DB, Troxel AB, Kimmel SE, Mehta NN, et al. Prevalence of metabolic syndrome in patients with psoriasis: A population-based study in the United Kingdom. Journal of Investigative Dermatology. 2012;**132**:556-562

[2] Langley R, Krueger G, Griffiths C. Psoriasis: Epidemiology, clinical features, and quality of life. Annals in Rheumatic Diseases. 2005;**64**:ii18–ii23

[3] Nestle FO, Kaplan DH, Barker J. Psoriasis. New England Journal of Medicine. 2009;**361**: 496-509

[4] Wade AG, Crawford GM, Young D, Leman J, Pumford N. Severity and management of psoriasis within primary care. BMC Family Practice, BMC Series. 2016;**17**:145. DOI: 10.1186/s12875-016-0544-6

[5] Nelson PA, Barker Z, Griffiths CEM, Cordingley L, Chew-Graham CA. 'On the surface': A qualitative study of GPs' and patients' perspectives on psoriasis. BMC Family Practice. 2013;**14**:158-167

[6] Mattei Peter L, Corey Kristen C, Kimball Alexa B. Cumulative life course impairment: Evidence for psoriasis. In: Linder MD, Kimball AB, editors. Dermatological Diseases and Cumulative Life Course Impairment. Current Problems in Dermatology. Vol. 44. Basel, Karger; 2013. pp. 82-90. DOI: 10.1159/000350008

[7] Brezinski EA, Dhillon JS, Armstrong AW. Economic burden of psoriasis in the United States: A systematic review. Journal of American Medical Association Dermatology. 2015;**151**(6):651-658. DOI: 10.1001/jamadermatol.2014.3593

[8] Tsai TF, Wang TS, Hung ST, Tsai PI, Schenkel B, Zhang M, Tang CH.Epidemiology and comorbidities of psoriasis patients in a national database in Taiwan. J Dermatol Sci. 2011 Jul;**63**(1):40-6. doi: 10.1016

[9] Akaraphanth R, Kwangsukstid O, Gritiyarangsan P, Swanpanyalert N. Psoriasis registry in public health hospital. Journal of the Medical Association of Thailand. 2013;**96**(8):960-966

[10] Yeung H, Takeshita J, Mehta NN, Kimmel SE, Ogdie A, Margolis DJ, Shin DB, Attor R, Troxel AB, Gelfand JM. Psoriasis severity and the prevalence of major medical comorbidity: A population-based study. Journal of American Medical Association Dermatology. 2013 Oct;**149**(10):1173-1179

[11] Callis DK, Gottlieb AB. Outcome measures for psoriasis severity: A report from the GRAPPA 2012 Annual Meeting. Rheumatology. 2013 Aug;**40**(8):1423-1424

[12] Na SJ, Jo SJ, Youn JI. Clinical study on psoriasis patients for past 30 years (1982-2012) in Seoul National University Hospital Psoriasis Clinic. Journal of Dermatology. 2013;40(9):731-735

[13] Keshavarz E, Roknsharifi S, Shirali Mohammadpour R, Roknsharifi M. Clinical features and severity of psoriasis: A comparison of facial and nonfacial involvement in Iran. Archives of Iranian Medicine. 2013;**16**(1):25-28

[14] Bahcetepe N, Kutlubay Z, Yilmaz E, Tuzun Y, Eren B. The role of HLA antigens in the aetiology of psoriasis. Medicinski Glasnik (Zenica). 2013;**10**(2):339-342

[15] Richard MA, Barnetche T, Horreau C, Brenaut E, Pouplard C, Aractingi S, Aubin F, Cribier B, Joly P, Jullien D, Le Maître M, Misery L, Ortonne JP, Paul C. Psoriasis, cardiovascular events, cancer risk and alcohol use: Evidence-based recommendations based on systematic review and expert opinion. Journal of the European Academy of Dermatology and Venereology. 2013;**27**(Suppl 3):2-11

[16] Feldman S. A quantitative definition of severe psoriasis for use in clinical trials. Journal of Dermatological Treatment. 2004;**15**:27-29

[17] Schmitt J, Wozel G. The psoriasis area and severity index is the adequate criterion to define severity in chronic plaque-type psoriasis. Dermatology. 2005;**210**:194-199

[18] Kwon HH, Na SJ, Jo SJ, Youn JI. Epidemiology and clinical features of pediatric psoriasis in tertiary referral psoriasis clinic. Journal of Dermatology. 2012 Mar;**39**(3):260-264

[19] Raychaudhuri SP, Gross J.A comparative study of pediatric onset psoriasis with adult onset psoriasis. Pediatric Dermatology. 2000 May–Jun;**17**(3):174-178

[20] Tollefson MM, Crowson CS, McEvoy MT, Maradit Kremers H. Incidence of psoriasis in children: A population-based study. Journal of the American Academy of Dermatology. 2010 Jun;**62**(6):979-987

[21] Mahé E, Maccari F, Beauchet A, Lahfa M, Barthelemy H, Reguiaï Z, Beneton N, Estève E, Chaby G, Ruer-Mulard M, Steiner HG, Pauwels C, Avenel-Audran M, Goujon-Henry C, Descamps V, Begon E, Sigal ML; GEM Resopso. Childhood-onset psoriasis: Association with future cardiovascular and metabolic comorbidities. British Journal of Dermatology. 2013 Oct;**169**(4):889-895

[22] Stefanaki C, Lagogianni E, Kontochristopoulos G, Verra P, Barkas G, Katsambas A, Katsarou A. Psoriasis in children: A retrospective analysis. Journal of European Academy of Dermatology and Venereology. 2011 Apr;**25**(4):417-421

[23] de Jager ME, de Jong EM, Meeuwis KA, van de Kerkhof PC, Seyger MM. No evidence found that childhood onset of psoriasis influences disease severity, future body mass index or type of treatments used. Journal of European Academy of Dermatology and Venereology. 2010 Nov;**24**(11):1333-1339

[24] Papadavid E, Katsimbri P, Kapniari I, Koumaki D, Karamparpa A, Dalamaga M, Tzannis K, Boumpas D, Rigopoulos D. Prevalence of psoriatic arthritis and its correlates among patients with psoriasis in Greece: Results from a large retrospective study. Journal of European Academy of Dermatology and Venereology. 2016;**30**:1749-1752. DOI: 10.1111/jdv.13700

[25] Mease P, Goffe BS. Diagnosis and treatment of psoriatic arthritis. Journal of American Academy of Dermatology. 2005;**52**:1-19

[26] Prey S, Paul C, Bronsard V, et al. Assessment of risk of psoriatic arthritis in patients with plaque psoriasis: a systematic review of the literature. Journal of European Academy of Dermatology and Venereology. 2010;**24**:31-35

[27] Estebaranz JL, Zarco MP, Samaniego ML, Garcia Calco C. Prevalence and clinical features of psoriatic arthritis in psoriasis patients on Spain. Limitations of PASE as a screening tool. European Journal of Dermatology. 2015;**25**:57-63

[28] Mease PJ, Gladmann DD, Papp KA, et al. Prevalence of rheumatologist diagnosed psoriatic arthritis in patients with psoriasis in European/North American dermatology clinics. Journal of the American Academy of Dermatology. 2013;**69**:729-735

[29] Reich K, Kruger K, Mossner R, Augustin M. Epidemiology and clinical pattern of psoriatic arthritis in Germany: A retrospective interdisciplinary epidemiological study of 1511 patients with plaque type psoriasis. British Journal of Dermatology. 2009;**160**:1040-1047

[30] Marco G, Cattaneo A, Battafarano M, et al. Not simply a matter of psoriatic arthritis: Epidemiology of rheumatic diseases in psoriatic patients. Archives of Dermatological Research. 2012;**304**:719-726

[31] Henes JJ, Ziupa E, Eisfeder M, et al. High prevalence of psoriatic arthritis in dermatological patients with psoriasis: A cross sectional study. Rheumatology International. 2014;**34**:227-234

[32] Alamanos Y, Papadopoulos NG, Voulgari PV, et al. Epidemiology of psoriatic arthritis in northwest Greece, 1982-2001. Journal of Rheumatology. 2003;**30**:2641-2644

[33] Trontzas P, Andranakos A, Miyakis S, et al. Seronegative spondyloarthropathies in Greece: A population based study of prevalence, clinical pattern, and management. The ESORDIG study. Clinical Rheumatology. 2005;**24**:583-589

[34] Chiu HY, Chang WL, Huang WF, et al. Increased risk of arrhythmia in patients with psoriatic disease: A nationwide population-based matched cohort study. Journal of the American Academy of Dermatology. September 2015;**73**(3):429-438

[35] Mehta NN, Yu Y, Pinnelas R, et al. Attributable risk estimate of severe psoriasis on major cardiovascular events. American Journal of Medicine. 2011;**124**:775.e1-775.e6

[36] Mehta NN, Azfar RS, Shin DB, Neimann AL, Troxel AB, Gelfand JM. Patients with severe psoriasis are at increased risk of cardiovascular mortality: Cohort study using the General Practice Research Database. European Heart Journal. 2010;**31**:1000-1006

[37] Bordignon V, et al. High prevalence of latent tuberculosis infection in autoimmune disorders such as psoriasis and in chronic respiratory diseases, including lung cancer. Biological Regulators and Homeostatic Agents. 2011 Apr–Jun;**25**(2):213-220

[38] Bassukas ID, Kosmidou M, Gaitanis G, Tsiouri G, Tsianos E. Patients with psoriasis are more likely to be treated for latent tuberculosis infection prior to biologics than patients with inflammatory bowel disease. Acta Dermato-Venereologica. 2011 Jun;**91**(4):444-446

[39] WHO Library Cataloguing-in-Publication Data. Global report on psoriasis.World Health Organization 2016. ISBN 978 92 4 156518 9 Available from: www.who.int

Chapter 8

Ultrasonography as a New, Non-Invasive Imagistic Technique Used for the Diagnosis and Monitoring of Psoriasis

Maria Crisan, Radu Badea, Diana Crisan,
Artur Bezugly, Horatiu Colosi, Stefan Strilciuc,
Amalia Ciobanu and Carmen Bianca Crivii

Additional information is available at the end of the chapter

http://dx.doi.org/10.5772/67812

Abstract

Psoriasis is a chronic inflammatory autoimmune disease that involves the skin, nails, joints and other organs, being a systemic disease. Regardless of the clinical form, sonography can be effectively used to complete the clinical diagnosis.

Aim: The identification of non-invasive sonographic markers for the assessment of the severity of the disease and the efficacy of various therapies. Our study involved two research directions: (a) clinical and imagistic assessment of the skin and nail psoriasis lesions and (b) the imagistic evaluation of the therapeutic efficacy in psoriasis plaques and nail psoriasis by acquirement of sonographic images prior and after various therapies.

Methods: In our prospective study, we used a multimodal evaluation of the disease, based on a non-invasive approach: clinical exam, dermoscopy, conventional and high frequency sonography, Doppler, power Doppler and elastography.

Conclusions: Ultrasonography is an important tool for the non-invasive assessment of psoriatic lesions. It offers specific markers related to morphology, elasticity and blood supply of the lesions, improving the diagnosis and monitoring of the skin and nail lesions.

Keywords: psoriasis, ultrasound, skin, nails, therapy

1. Introduction

Sonography is a routine method used in clinical medicine in fields such as internal medicine, gastroenterology and gynaecology. In the past 2–3 decades, sonography has extended its utility to the field of clinical dermatology. This non-invasive method offers in '*real time*' morphological details about the skin structure and its specific conditions. It is important to mention that histology still remains the gold standard for the assessment of the skin structure and diagnosis of its associated pathology. Despite this, researchers are permanently looking for new non-invasive methods for the skin assessment, which can offer similar, identical or new markers to the histological ones, in order to improve the clinical and differential diagnosis, as well as to optimize the evaluation of the efficacy of various therapies. There is a wide range of ultrasound devices with frequencies ranging from 5 to 100 MHz. In the range of 5–10 MHz, real-time B-mode sonography is successfully applied as a non-invasive diagnostic tool in internal medicine. High-frequency ultrasound (HFU) systems using frequencies ranging from 20 to 100 MHz can be used for the study of the integumentary system and for research purposes [1–3]. High-frequency sonography devices can vary from a resolution of 72 μm and a penetration depth of 35 mm up to a resolution of 15 μm and a penetration depth of 0.8–1.5 mm [4].

These examination techniques can provide the clinician with important information about the axial and lateral extension of tumoural and inflammatory processes of the skin and the subcutaneous fatty tissue and are therefore of special interest in the diagnosis and monitoring of skin conditions under various therapies [5, 6].

1.1. Sonography: general considerations

Sonography has proven to be a useful non-invasive imaging method for the study of the skin [1]. The recent development of high-frequency ultrasound (HFU) transducers has led to a vast range of applications in dermatology, such as the evaluation of inflammatory diseases (psoriasis, scleroderma), tumours and skin ageing and so on [7]. Several studies have proven similarities between ultrasound (US) and histological sections [8]. The inclusion of ultrasound among the procedures used for the dermatological diagnosis is an attempt to replace the invasive procedures such as biopsies, with non-invasive ones as much as possible. The motivation for the extensive use of HFU derives from its ability to reveal the skin components in detail, up to 1.5 cm in depth, to assess the axial and lateral extension of various lesions, the inflammatory processes, as well as the efficacy of different local therapies [9].

The main ultrasonographic techniques used in dermatology in present times are conventional ultrasound (CUS) and high-frequency ultrasound (HFU) [10, 11]. The integumentary system can be explored both with conventional imagistic equipments and specialized dermatological devices.

The *conventional ultrasound* (CUS) skin examination can be performed with 7.5–13 MHz transducers offering an axial and lateral resolution of 0.2 mm and an ultrasonic depth of up to 5–7 cm. The B-mode is the recommended method for profound structures, but it can also identify skin and nail structures under specific conditions. The *Doppler* or *power Doppler* examination is important for the identification of blood vessels, an important feature for the discrimination

http://dx.doi.org/10.5772/67812

between inflammatory or tumoural lesions. The *Doppler technique* can identify the presence of vascular signal, describes the distribution and characterizes the microcirculation (speed of the blood, pulsatile index, resistivity index). *Power Doppler* has a higher sensitivity than colour Doppler allowing the detection of smaller velocities. The method is particularly useful for the examination of superficial structures [12]. *Spectral Doppler* techniques allow the differentiation between venous and arterial flow and the measurements of specific parameters '*in real time*', such as velocity (V), pulsatile index (IP) or resistive index (IR). Combining greyscale ultrasound with Doppler ultrasound allows the assessment of skin and skin lesions including morphology, size, shape, margins, macrocirculation, microcirculation and elasticity [13].

High-frequency ultrasound (HFU) with more than 13 MHz transducers can characterize the integumentary system with greater precision [14]. According to literature data and our own experience, HFU has multiple applications both in the clinical and research field:

- Identification of the histological skin layers (epidermis, dermis, hypodermis).
- Histology of the nails and identification of its components (nail plate, nail bed).
- Assessment of the interphalangeal joint structures involved in inflammatory diseases.
- Identification, qualitative and quantitative monitoring of the cutaneous alterations induced by the senescence process.
- Monitoring of various chronic inflammatory skin conditions and the efficacy of different local therapies [15–17].

Optimising the sonographic diagnosis requires modern techniques and devices, which is why ultrasonography is constantly evolving in a number of directions. For example, HFU with 100 MHz transducers, currently used only for research purposes, has an axial resolution of 11 μm, a lateral resolution of 30 μm and allows visualisation up to a depth of 2 mm [9].

Elastography is a technique, which can assess the elasticity of soft tissues during application of mechanical compression. Because tumours are 5–28 times stiffer than normal surrounding tissue, qualitative elastography or strain ratio elasticity are techniques that may improve the diagnostic accuracy or monitoring of treatment efficacy [18, 19].

Sonoelastography (SE) may depict the stiffness of the tissues. Compared with manual palpation, SE is considered as a semi-quantifiable method using a visual scale score to evaluate the focal lesion [20].

The *strain-ratio* technique compares the strain of a region of interest in a focal lesion with the strain of the surrounding tissue. The strain ratio elastography measures the axial displacement of tissue caused by mechanical stress in real time. The elastogram may be displayed as a colour overlay on the B-mode picture [21].

The newest *shear wave elasticity* (SWE) or *transient elastography* is similar to strain elastography, but instead of using the transducer pressure to compare the stiffness in an ultrasound image measuring changes in strain, a higher intensity pulse is transmitted to produce shear waves, which extend laterally from the insonated structure [22]. This stiffness is believed to start from the early stages of cancer development. Visualization of stiffness data could enable early stage differentiation of benign and malignant tissue. In addition, the elasticity of the tissue varies significantly under the influence of inflammation or congestion. Therefore, elastography is a reliable method for assessing the level of inflammation and congestion in various skin disorders and monitoring of the therapeutic efficacy; that is why ultrasonography may also be considered as a virtual knife, a stethoscope and a palpation device in the hand of a dermatologist.

Because in dermatology, most of the diagnoses are made by visual inspection and palpation of the skin, the sonographic assessment of the patients diagnosed with *psoriasis* represents a new approach of the disease, offering new, specific and non-invasive additional information [23, 24].

2. Sonographic anatomy of the skin and nails

2.1. The healthy skin

The skin is the most superficial organ of the body. It represents an area of relating to the exterior world. Along with its appendages (hair follicles, nails), the cutaneous organ represents a great morphological and functional complex structure, displaying particular and unique ultrasonographic features.

Skin disorders have a highly characteristic distribution pattern, which reflects regional differences related to structure, topography, blood supply and distribution of appendages. From histological point of view, the skin consists of three well-defined structures named epidermis, dermis and hypodermis, which can be separated into sonographic equivalents. **Figure 1** shows sonographic images taken with transducers of different MHz.

The epidermis is a stratified squamous keratinized epithelium which appears as a *continuous hyperechoic* line with homogeneous thickness, or as a bilaminar hyperechoic parallel line in the thicker palmar and plantar areas [25].

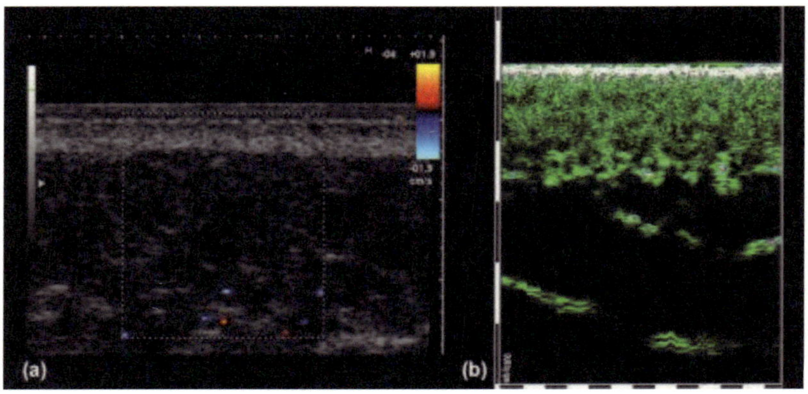

Figure 1. Sonographic diagram of the skin. (a) Skin sonography taken with an 18-MHz transducer and (b) skin sonography taken with a 22-MHz transducer (skin-scan).

The dermis is represented by a dense connective tissue, situated between the epidermis and hypodermis. With a variable thickness of 0.6–2 μm in the palms and soles, the dermis is the structure, which induces the thickness of the epidermis. Dermis is a connective tissue rich in collagen and elastic fibres, which are responsible for the echogenicity of the structure. It appears as an *echogenic band* subdivided into two regions: the papillary superficial dermis located beneath the epidermis appears less echogenic due to a decreased amount of collagen fibres and the reticular dermis, more echogenic due to the higher amount of collagen fibrils assembled in mature collagen fibres [25, 26].

The hypodermis is the subcutaneous cellular tissue consisting of adipocytes organized in lobules and separated by connective tissue septa. In ultrasound, it appears as a *hypoechoic* structure separated by *hyperechoic* fibrous septa.

The blood vessels are represented by thin (<1 mm) and easily compressible venules and arterioles situated in the hypodermis or in the deep dermis. These small vessels appear as thin anechoic tubular structures in conventional ultrasonography. In the normal healthy thin skin, the superficial vessels are identified by power Doppler as small colour dots [27].

2.2. The healthy nail unit

The nails, located on the distal phalanx of each finger, are composed of plates of heavily compacted, highly keratinized cells termed nail plate (NP), lying on the dermis, termed nail bed (NB). The nails develop from cells of the *nail matrix*, situated beneath the proximal nail fold. The stratum corneum of the proximal nail fold forms the eponychium or cuticle, which extends from the proximal end up onto the nail for about 1 mm. The distal end of the nail plate is not attached to the nail bed which becomes continuous with the skin of the finger. Near this junction there is an accumulation of keratinised cells, named hyponychium [28]. All these components display characteristic sonographic images are illustrated in **Figure 2**.

The nail plate (*NP*) appears as two hyperechoic parallel lines, displaying in between a thin virtual hypoechoic line (dark grey) called interplate space. *The nail bed* (*NB*) and the matrix are hypoechoic, usually turning slightly hyperechoic in the proximal region beneath the nail

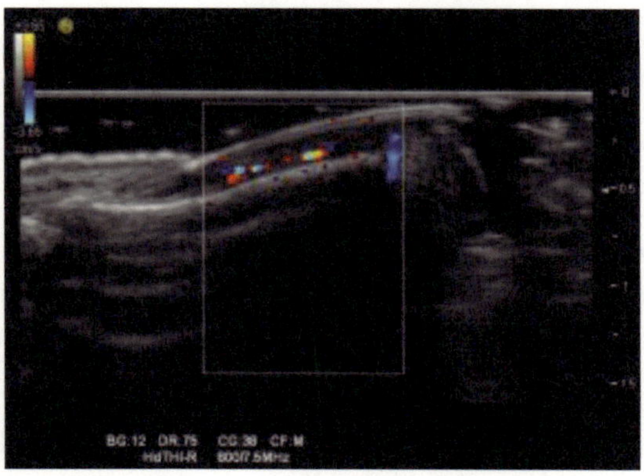

Figure 2. Ultrasonographic image of the healthy nail. Nail sonogram (18 MHz), showing the superficial hyperechogenic NP and the underlying hypoechogenic NB containing blood vessels.

matrix. *The nail folds* present the same ultrasonographic skin features with less adipose lobules in the subcutaneous tissue. *The bone margin* appears as a distinct hyperechoic line and corresponds to the dorsal bony margin of the distal phalanx. Doppler ultrasound or power Doppler detects the presence of *low-velocity* blood flow in the nail bed [13, 29].

According to Essayed et al., in nail psoriasis, the distal loss of the nail interplate space is more frequent, when compared to onychomycosis where the proximal loss of the interplate space is more frequent. In addition, they found a NB thickness greater than 1.85 mm at thumb level, which could be used to discriminate patients with psoriatic nails from onychomycosis with an accuracy, sensitivity and specificity of 73, 64 and 72%, respectively. According to the same group, the presence of three lines at the level of the nail plate could be an important ultrasonographic sign which may help in differentiating between psoriatic nail and onychomycosis [30].

3. Psoriasis

Psoriasis presents with a large spectrum of clinical features and evolution. According to literature data, about 1/3 of the patients have moderate to severe disease (PASI index >10) involving more than 10% of the body surface [31]. With a prevalence of 1–3%, the condition can occur in all age groups; however, it primarily arises in adulthood, with no gender predilection [32]. Psoriasis can also affect the nails, entheses and joints, leading to the development of a destructive inflammatory arthropathy seen in 25–34% of patients with psoriasis, named psoriasis arthritis (PsA) [33]. The pathogenesis of psoriasis is multifactorial and still not fully understood. Several lifestyle factors have also been associated with morbidity in psoriasis.

3.1. Classification and morphology of psoriasis

Psoriasis can be classified by morphology and by the pathogenetic mechanism. The commonest form of disease is *plaque psoriasis*, affecting about 80% of the patients [34]. It is characterized by thick, erythematous plaques with silvery, shiny deposits of scales. In this case, the erythematous scaly plaques tend to remain stationary or to progressively enlarge, affecting especially scalp, knees, elbows or lower back [35]. The clinical aspect of the psoriasis skin plaque is illustrated in **Figure 3**.

Inverse psoriasis usually affects the skin folds, especially the regions under the armpits, the abdominal skin fold, the breast area or the gluteal cleft; in this situation, the plaques are thinner and there is no or minimal scaling.

Guttate psoriasis usually emerges acutely following a bacterial or viral infection of the upper ways. It usually presents with small round scaly plaques scattered across the entire skin surface; it either resolves with infection or progresses to the development of psoriasis vulgaris [37].

Pustular psoriasis is characterized by a disseminated outburst of sterile pustules, accompanied sometimes by recurrent episodes of fever. It constitutes a less frequent clinical pattern. If the entire integument is affected, the condition is called 'generalized (von Zumbusch) type'. *Acrodermatitis continua of Hallopeau* is a rare, localized form of palmoplantar pustular psoriasis, often unresponsive to treatment. It usually emerges with pustules on erythematous,

http://dx.doi.org/10.5772/67812

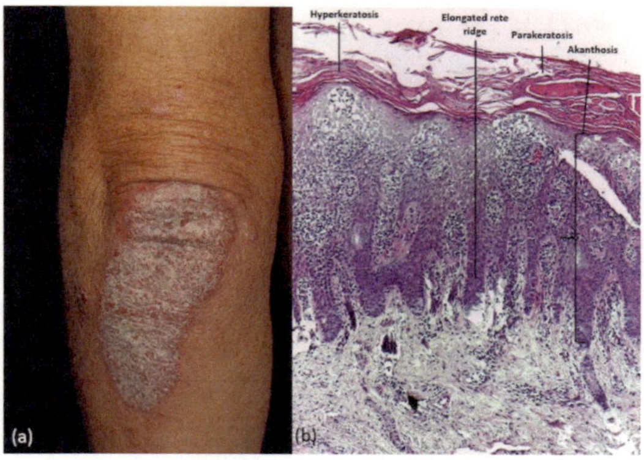

Figure 3. Clinical and histological features of psoriasis plaques. (a) Clinical aspect of a well-demarcated erythematous psoriatic plaque covered with 'silvery' scales (University Clinic Ulm, Clinic for Dermatology and Allergic diseases); (b) schematic structure of psoriasis-affected skin with thickened stratum corneum due to a differentiation disturbance of keratinocytes, elongated rete ridges due to the hyperproliferation of the stratum spinosum, parakeratosis (no loss of nuclei of keratinocytes in the stratum corneum) and acanthosis (thickening of the epidermis) [36].

scaly patches of the distal phalanges of fingers and toes. The frequent involvement of the nail bed and matrix leads to severe nail dystrophy [38].

Erythrodermic psoriasis is the generalized form of the disease, where the entire integument is highly erythematous and covered by superficial scales. Patients usually also develop fatigue, myalgia, fever and chills.

Nail psoriasis emerges in about 61% of cases of cutaneous psoriasis. In less than 5% of cases, the involvement of the nails may appear without cutaneous plaques. The classical manifestations of the nail apparatus include pitting, trachyonychia, leukonychia, Beau 's lines and transverse grooves. The nail bed and hyponychium can present with onycholysis, oil drops, subungual hyperkeratosis and at the distal nail bed splinter haemorrhages may occur [34]. The clinical aspect of nail psoriasis is illustrated in **Figure 4**.

Psoriatic arthritis is an inflammatory disease in which the cutaneous psoriasis plaques coexist with arthritis usually in the absence of rheumatoid factor [39]. The estimated prevalence of psoriatic arthritis among patients with psoriasis is 4–42% (typically) and 80% of patients with psoriatic arthritis present nail psoriasis.

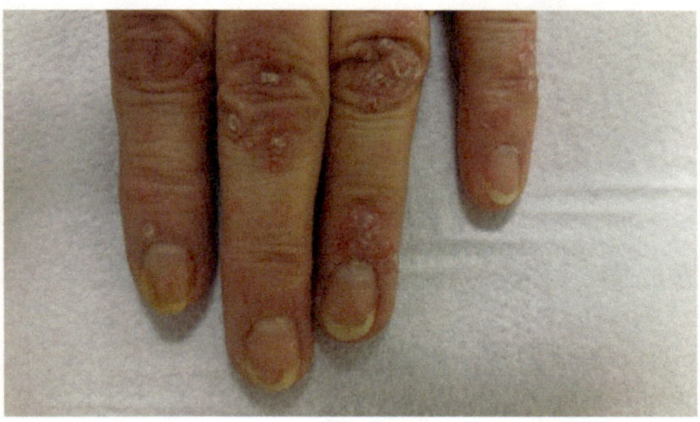

Figure 4. Clinical aspect of nail psoriasis. Pitting, onycholysis, discoloration, periungual lesions.

3.2. Sonography of the psoriasis plaque

Sonography of the psoriasis plaque reveals different features accordingly to the inflammatory process in psoriasis (**Figures 5** and **6**):

- Thickening of the epidermis (hyperechogenic band) and dermis (echogenic or hypoechogenic band) as one of the most common features.
- Hypoechoic band in the upper dermis, particularly detectable in the most active stages of the disease; the hypoechoic band corresponds to the thicker stratum corneum of the epidermis of the psoriasis plaque and is associated with the local inflammatory reaction.
- Increased dermal blood flow (vasodilatation) within the lesion (colour Doppler, power Doppler) due to the local inflammatory process.
- Reduction of epidermal and dermal thickness and the thinning/disappearance of the hypoechoic band at the superficial dermis level as indicators of therapeutic efficacy.
- Slightly increased tissue stiffness (elastography) compared to the surrounding healthy skin (induced by the inflammatory reaction) and a decrease of the lesion stiffness after topical or oral therapies; the tissue stiffness increases in inflammatory processes; it is not specific to psoriasis, can be however of great value for the assessment of the anti-inflammatory therapy in psoriasis [21].

The clinical and sonographic features of active and chronic stationary psoriasis lesions are illustrated in **Figure 5**.

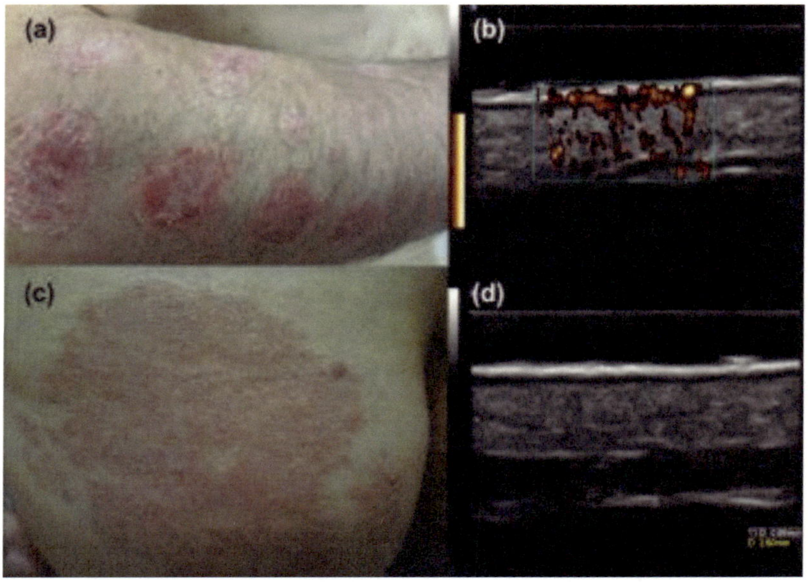

Figure 5. Clinical and sonographic images of active inflammatory and chronic stationary psoriasis plaques. (a) Active inflammatory, infiltrated red plaques covered by silvery scales; (b) thick hyperechoic epidermis, thin hypoechoic band in the upper dermis, thick echogenic and hypervascularised dermis; (c) pale red and less infiltrated stationary psoriasis plaque; (d) thickening of the epidermis and dermis with a thin hypoechoic subepidermal band and no blood vessels identified by Doppler.

http://dx.doi.org/10.5772/67812

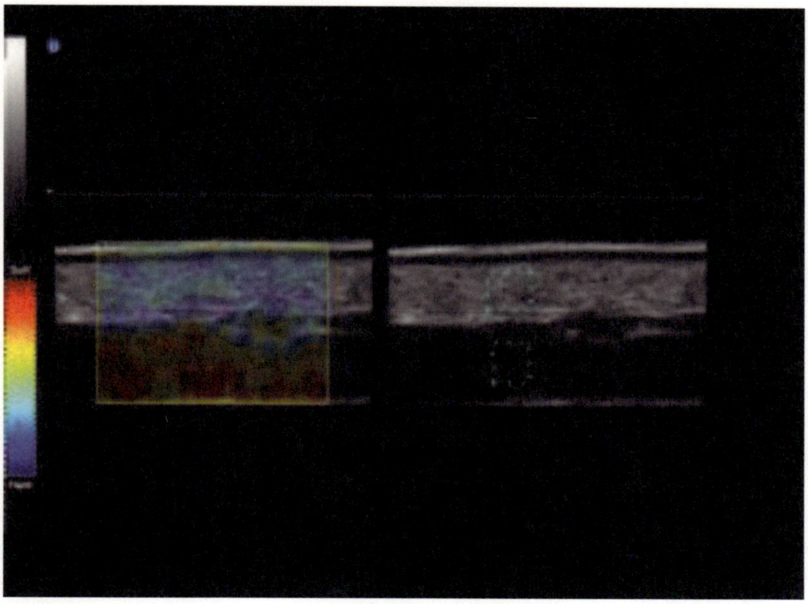

Figure 6. Sonoelastographic appearance of a psoriasis plaque. Slightly blue appearance of the skin lesion, codifying the increase in the stiffness due to the local inflammatory process, compared to the healthy surrounding skin.

The local changes of the tissue elasticity corresponding to a psoriasis plaque are revealed in **Figure 6**.

Related to the therapeutic approach in psoriasis patients, our group used high-frequency ultrasound to investigate the skin reaction after topical therapy with *low potency steroids* (cortisone) and natural extracts of *cranberry* and *black elderberry*, showing that ultrasound can evaluate with great accuracy the changes in psoriasis plaques induced by various topical therapies [16, 17]. We assessed in a comparative manner the anti-inflammatory effect of the natural extracts of cranberry and black elderberry and of cortisone with control lesions only treated with emollients. We could demonstrate by using high-frequency ultrasound a significant improvement of the psoriasis lesions following local therapy with the above-mentioned products. Our results showed a significant decrease of the dermal echogenicity as well as a decrease of the dermal thickness at the level of the treated plaques, due to the decrease of the local inflammatory infiltrate.

3.3. Sonography of nail psoriasis

Psoriatic onychopathy can be the single manifestation of psoriasis or precede the psoriatic plaques in the skin. About 80% of patients with psoriatic arthritis present nail psoriasis [40]. Ultrasound can identify nail changes in psoriasis; however, the finding varies according to the phase of activity of the disease, going from the early inflammatory phase to the late fibrous phase [30]. The most common sonographic features revealed by sonography in nail psoriasis are as follows:

- increased thickness and decreased echogenicity of the NB (**Figure 7**);
- focal hyperechoic spots in the ventral plates;

- loss of definition of the dorsal and ventral nail plate;
- wavy plates and thickening of the dorsal and ventral plates;
- increased blood flow in the proximal NB with low flow arterial vessels especially during the active phases of disease;
- decreased blood flow in the late phase especially in the middle and distal NB;
- preserved distal interplate space of the NP (loss of interplate space proximally in onychomycotic nails);
- thickening of the nail bed (NB thickness > 2 mm as a cut-off value to differentiate between psoriatic nails and healthy nails) [30].

3.4. Sonography of the distal nail joints in psoriasis

In patients with psoriasis arthritis (PsA), the immunological process at joint level is very similar to that in the skin [39]. The process occurs in the deep layer of the synovial membrane whose cells begin to proliferate. The histology of PsA reveals a more intense hyperaemia when compared to rheumatoid arthritis (RA). Inflammatory lesions of tendon and ligament entheses are common in PsA [39]. Five clinical manifestations of PsA were described by Gladman et al. considering that the clinical manifestations are quite distinctive and different from rheumatoid arthritis (RA) [41].

PsA spinal lesions and sacroiliac joint lesions are asymmetric. Involvement of the smaller joints of the hands and feet, especially of the distal interphalangeal joints, seems to be a characteristic feature. According to the same authors, the lesions are accompanied by proliferative lesions of bone tissue located at erosion margins, a very characteristic sonographic sign [42].

The sonographic features of PsA were described by using different equipments: greyscale ultrasound, colour Doppler; power Doppler (power Doppler technique visualizes slow flow in soft tissue, but unlike colour Doppler it does not provide the direction and velocity of blood

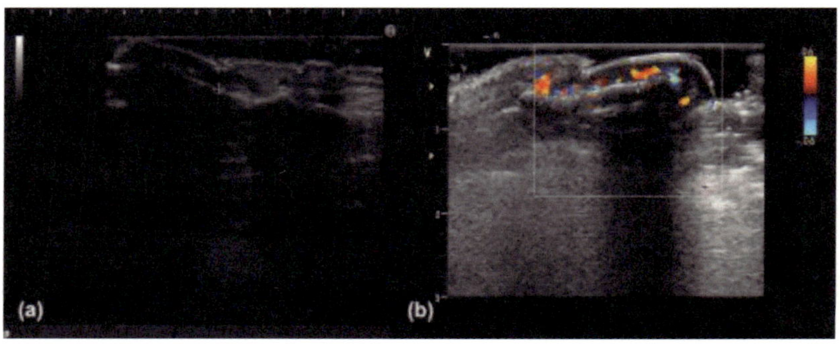

Figure 7. Sonography in nail psoriasis. (a) Nail psoriasis and psoriatic arthropathy with thickening of the NB, irregular wavy nail plates, hyperechoic spots in the nail plate, prominent synovium, anechoic fluid (greyscale). (b) Nail psoriasis with irregular nail plate (NP) and intense Doppler signal in the NB.

http://dx.doi.org/10.5772/67812

flow); contrast agents show the microcirculation in real time, providing a dynamic assessment of lesion vascularity [43].

The most common sonographic features of PsA are as follows:

- prominent synovium, as a form of an intra-articular mass with echogenicity comparable to soft tissues and non-compressible;
- anechoic fluid;
- periarticular erosions commonly in the interphalangeal joints, appearing as tiny discontinuities of regular bone margins;
- tendinopathy as hypo or heterogeneous echogenicity at the insertion sites of the tendinous even in subclinical stages;
- increased blood flow in the synovium on colour Doppler imaging in active phases [44].

Various sonographic techniques can therefore be effectively used in order to compare different sonographic parameters as an evaluation marker of therapeutic effectiveness. Power Doppler is important for allowing the slow flow detection allowing the visualisation of increased vascularity within inflamed tissue. The method has been used for the semi-quantitative assessment of inflammatory processes (synovial hyperemia) [45].

By means of Doppler, the number of coloured pixels before and after therapy can be evaluated as an indicator of therapy efficacy. The evaluation of treatment effectiveness by spectral Doppler is based on assessing different parameters of which the peripheral flow resistance quantified as resistive index (RI) is more important.

According to literature data, normal peripheral blood flow in the osteoskeletal system is characterised by high values of the IR and the diastolic phase of blood flow is not observed (RI = 1) [39]. The blood flow resistance within inflamed synovium decreases. By contrast, a normalisation of the RI values appears following therapy [24]. The flow in normal synovial membrane, tendons and entheses remain undetectable [39].

4. Study

4.1. Objective

The aim of our study is to identify non-invasive sonographic markers for the assessment of chronic stationary psoriasis plaques and nail psoriasis and for the evaluation of the therapeutic efficacy of various local treatments. We have focused on this issue taking into consideration the research done in the field of imagistic skin assessment as well as our own experience. Thus, during the past 2–3 years, our work involved two research directions:

- A clinical and imagistic assessment of patients suffering from chronic stationary plaque psoriasis and nail psoriasis.
- An imagistic evaluation of the therapeutic efficacy by acquirement of sonographic images before and after different topical therapies.

4.2. Methods

In our prospective controlled study, we used a multimodal evaluation of the disease, based on a non-invasive approach: clinical examination, dermoscopy, conventional and high-frequency ultrasound, colour Doppler, spectral Doppler, power Doppler and elastography.

The study included a total of 74 patients, 46 females and 28 males, aged between 19 and 63 years, with a duration of disease of 6–39 months before admission to the study. The diagnosis of plaque psoriasis with or without nail involvement was made by an experienced dermatologist based on clinical findings. Another group of 30 healthy subjects, 13 females and 17 males, aged 18–59 years, were included as the control group. Patients suffering from autoimmune diseases, diabetes, onychomycosis smokers were excluded from the study, since these conditions might have an influence on the peripheral circulation especially at nail bed level.

All subjects, patients and healthy control participants underwent a sonographic examination, performed by an experienced sonographer, using transducers ranging from 13 to 20 or 40 MHz, in order to better identify structural details.

Sonographic images were taken from the psoriatic skin lesion, healthy surrounding skin, healthy and psoriatic nails. In the healthy control group, the sonographic images of the nails were taken from the same fingers: the thumb and index. On the psoriasis plaque, the centre and the margin of the lesion together with the surrounding normal skin were examined before and after therapy. In the psoriasis group, sonograms were taken from nails with clinical signs of psoriasis as well as apparently healthy nails.

In all our examinations, the ultrasound probe was perpendicularly placed over the region of interest, covered with a large amount of gel in order to provide the best acoustic interface. Each area was examined in greyscale mode in order to identify the morphological and structural parameters, with Doppler techniques and elastography. Part of our work concerning the role of ultrasound in the assessment of the therapeutic efficacy in plaque psoriasis patients was already published [16, 17, 21]. Therefore, in this study, we focused on the examination of the nail apparatus. The parameters of interest were the morphology of the nail unit, the thickness of the nail plate and nail bed, the blood flow distribution, the measurement of the resistive index (IR) and pulsatility index (IP). Data description and data analysis were performed using Microsoft Excel and PSPP 0.10.2. The hypothesis testing was performed by means of *t*-tests for independent samples, with Bonferroni correction for multiple comparisons. Informed consent was obtained from each patient included in our study. The study protocol was approved by the Ethical Committee of the institution.

4.3. Results and discussion

The sonograms of the skin showed differences between healthy skin and the psoriasis plaque. The sonography of the psoriasis plaques revealed: a thicker epidermis, a thicker dermis, with detectable blood vessels only in the active lesions as well as a focal hypoechoic band in the upper dermis compared to the healthy skin. Active lesions are the erythematous infiltrated psoriasis patches appeared for less than 6 months, covered with thinner scales, allowing a better penetration of the ultrasound.

No blood vessels were identified in the healthy skin. Similar aspects were described by other authors [24]. According to literature data, our work revealed that the thickness of the epidermis and dermis, the presence and the intensity of the Doppler signal and the presence of the hypoechoic subepidermal band are imagistic markers, which characterize the psoriasis plaque and allow an effective monitoring of the therapeutic efficacy. The ultrasonographic evaluation in psoriasis completes the clinical diagnosis, being sometimes essential for the differential diagnosis of various dermatoses (eczema, scleroderma, erythematous lupus, etc.).

The sonograms of psoriatic nails revealed an increased thickness of the NP and NB in psoriasis onychopathy, compared to healthy control nails, but with no statistical significance. The same observations were communicated by Essayed et al. [29]. According to literature data, the thickness of the nail bed could be a morphologic marker for a subclinical nail involvement and a good parameter for the evaluation of the therapeutic efficacy [46].

The blood supply of the nail bed as well as blood velocity (V), pulsatility index (PI) and resistive index (RI) were investigated by colour Doppler, spectral and power. We found an interesting distribution of the blood vessel parameters in the NB according to the local inflammatory process. We measured all data mentioned above and established the mean values for each of them in every group of interest.

In the control group, all parameters mentioned were taken from the same fingers (thumb and index). We noticed that the thickness of the nail plate has an average of 0.55 mm, being slightly higher in men (statistically not significant). The average thickness of the nail bed was slightly higher in left-handed persons. This can be explained by the fact that left-handed people, using mainly their left hand for daily activities, can develop a local hypervascularity state at the level of the nail bed, leading to a structural reorganization and consequent thickening of the nail matrix.

Concerning the distribution of the blood vessels at nail bed level, we identified following aspects:

- In *healthy nails*, we identified few thin blood vessels especially in the middle part and distal extremity of the NB; power Doppler revealed tiny vascular spots in the whole NB.
- In *psoriasis patients without clinical nail involvement*, we identified larger colour spots corresponding to dilatation of blood vessels according to the local inflammation status.
- In 21 *psoriasis patients with nail involvement having clinical changes* and an evolution longer than 19 months, the blood supply was reduced and present especially at the proximal NB region.

The variation of the mean values of the sonographic parameters is presented in **Table 1**.

Concerning the IP parameter, we found a discrete increase in psoriasis patients without nail involvement (due to a minimal local inflammatory process) and almost double values in patients with nail involvement. The highest values were observed in patients having changes in the associated distal interphalangeal joints. The data is displayed in **Figure 8**.

The IP index is known to display increased values in the periphery due to the presence of the pre-capillary sphincters, as it is the first parameter to undergo a change at the beginning of

	Average values in control group		Psoriasis patients without nail changes		Psoriasis patients with nail changes	
Vm average	4.49	[1.3–8.49]	5.28	[1.3–10.23]	5.99	[0.9–13.48]
IP average	1.34	[0.52–2.79]	1.31	[0.39–2.04]	2.36	[1.44–3.98]
IR average	0.66	[0.41–1.12]	0.64	[0.28–0.79]	0.98	[0.83–1.75]

Table 1. Average values of blood velocity, IP and IR in the control group, patients with psoriatic nail changes and without nail changes.

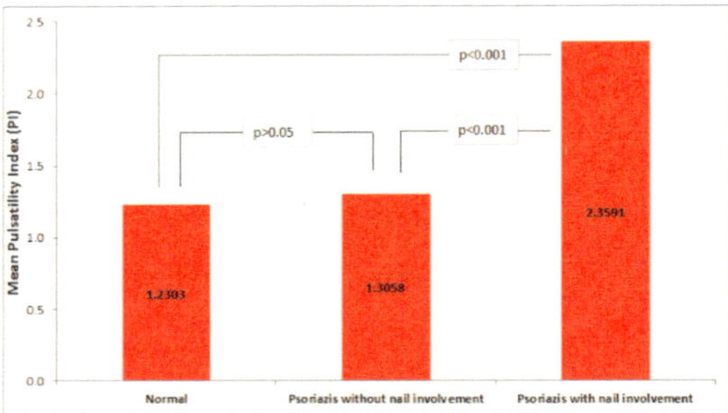

Figure 8. The evolution of IP parameter during the clinical stages of the psoriasis. The pulsatile index (IP) measured at the nail level increases slightly in patients with skin plaque psoriasis and reach high values in patients with clinical nails involvement.

the local inflammatory process. Therefore, a slight increase of the IP is noticed at the level of the nail bed, due to the existence of a subclinical inflammatory process. In chronic situations where fibrosis settles in, IP continues to increase reaching almost double values. IP values above 2 can be seen in patients displaying the involvement of the distal interphalangeal joints (synovitis, articular erosions). Therefore, the IP index can be considered a predictor marker for the progression of the disease towards nail psoriasis and involvement of the distal interphalangeal joint.

Concerning the IR parameter, the value slowly decreases from 0.66 to 0.64 in patients without nail involvement and increases in patients with clinical nails changes to 0.98 (**Figure 9**).

IR, IP and the blood velocity are imagistic markers, which can quantify the microcirculation at the level of the nail bed. In psoriasis patients with no nail involvement, a subclinical inflammatory status can be identified at the level of the nail bed, quantified by an increase of the IP value and a decrease of the IR. Clinical nail changes in psoriasis represent the morphological expression of an intense inflammatory process (IP > 1.3), which induces a local fibrosis of the tissue with a slow increase of the IR (IR > 0.64). According to Ovistgaard et al., inflammatory processes also involving the inflammation of the joint synovia display a decreased IR, which tends to normalize after therapy [47].

Further clinical, imagistic and histological studies are required to better characterize the accuracy and relevance of the studied parameters as potential signs of disease progression, risk of complications' development and efficacy of various therapies in psoriasis.

http://dx.doi.org/10.5772/67812

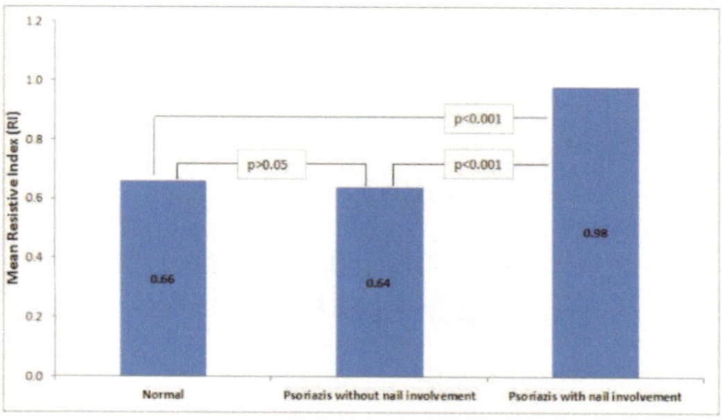

Figure 9. The evolution of the IR parameter according to the clinical stages and local inflammation process of disease.

To our knowledge, this is the first imagistic study quantifying the microcirculation at nail bed level in psoriasis, by measuring the values of the vascular parameters (IP, IR). We consider IP and IR as two imagistic parameters which can be objectively used for the diagnosis as well as for the long-term evaluation of various therapies.

5. Conclusions

Ultrasonography is an important non-invasive tool, which completes the clinical diagnosis in skin pathology. It offers new and specific 'real time' markers, which allow the assessment of the extension, evolution, risks and long-term therapeutic efficacy in inflammatory skin disorders such as psoriasis. Ultrasound has become an invaluable tool for dermatologists for daily clinical practice, offering at the same time multiple new research perspectives.

Acknowledgements

We are indebted to Prof. Sorin Dudea for providing us with the ultrasonographic images

Author details

Maria Crisan[1]*, Radu Badea[1], Diana Crisan[2], Artur Bezugly[4], Horatiu Colosi[1], Stefan Strilciuc[3], Amalia Ciobanu[1] and Carmen Bianca Crivii[1]

*Address all correspondence to: mcrisan7@yahoo.com

1 University of Medicine and Pharmacy "Iuliu Hatieganu", Cluj-Napoca, Romania

2 University Ulm, Ulm, Germany

3 Department of Public Health, Babeș-Bolyai University, Cluj-Napoca, Romania

4 Scientific-Practical Center of Dermatology Dept. of Clinical Deramatology and Cosmetology-Moscow, Russia

References

[1] Zanzoni A, Montecchi-Palazzi L, Quondam MX. Mint: A molecular interaction database. FEBS Lett. 2002;**513**:135-140. DOI: 10.1016/s0014-5793.

[2] Schmid-Wendtner M, Burgdorf W. Ultrasound scanning in dermatology. Arch Dermatol. 2005;**141**:217-224. DOI:10.1001/archderm.141.2.217.

[3] Lasagni C, Seidenari S. Echographic assessment of age dependant variations of skin thickness: a study on 162 subjects. Skin Res Technol. 1995;**1**:81-85. DOI: 10.1111/j.1600-0846.1995.tb00022.x.

[4] Tsukhara K, Takema Y, Moriwaki S, Fujimura T, Kitahara T, Immokava G. Age related alterations of echogenicity in Japanese skin. Dermatology. 2000;**200**:303-307. DOI: 18392.

[5] Lucas VS, Burk RS, Creehan S, Grap MJ. Utility of high-frequency ultrasound: moving beyond the surface to detect changes in skin integrity. Plast Surg Nurs. 2014;**34**(1):34-38. DOI: 10.1097/PSN.0000000000000031.

[6] Cammarota T, Pinto F, Magliaro A, et al. Current uses of diagnostic high frequency ultrasound in dermatology. Eur J Radiol. 1998;**27**(2):215-223.

[7] Szymanska E, Nowicki A, Mlosek K, et al. Skin imaging with high frequency ultrasound-preliminary results. Eur J Ultrasound. 2000;**12**:9-16.

[8] Mandava A, Ravuri PR, Konathan R. High-resolution ultrasound imaging of cutaneous lesions. Indian J Radio Imaging. 2013;**23**(3):269-277. DOI: 10.4103/0971-3026.120272.

[9] Barcaui E de O, Carvalho ACP, Piñeiro-Maceira J, Barcaui CB, Moraes H. Study of the skin anatomy with high-frequency (22 MHz) ultrasonography and histological correlation. Radiol Bras. 2015;**48**(5):324-329. DOI: 10.1590/0100-3984.2014.0028.

[10] Badea R, Crişan M, Lupşor M, Fodor L. Diagnosis and characterization of cutaneous tumors using combined ultrasonographic procedures (conventional and high resolution ultrasonography). Med Ultrasound. 2010;**12**(4):317-322.

[11] Crișan D, Badea AF, Crișan M, Rastian I, Solovastru LG, Badea R. Integrative analysis of cutaneous skin tumours using ultrasonogaphic criteria. Preliminary results. Med Ultrasound. 2014;**16**(4):285-290.

[12] Jemec GB, Gniadecka M, Ulrich J. Ultrasound in dermatology Part I. High frequency ultrasound. Eur J Dermatol. 2000;**10**:492-497.

[13] Toprak H, Kilic E, Serter A, Kocakoc E, Ozgocmen S. Ultrasound and Doppler US in evaluation of superficial soft-tissue lesions. J Clin Imaging Sci. 201;**4**:12. DOI: 10.4103/2156-7514.127965.

[14] Gaitini D. Wortsmax X, Jemec GBE. Dermatologic ultrasound with clinical and histologic correlations. Introduction to color Doppler ultrasound of the skin. New York: Springer; 2013, pp. 3-14.

[15] Barcaui E de O, Carvalho ACP, Lopes FPPL, Piñeiro-Maceira J, Barcaui CB. High frequency ultrasound with color Doppler in dermatology. An Bras Dermatol. 2016;**91**(3):262-273. DOI: 10.1590/abd1806-4841.20164446.

[16] Crisan M, David L, Moldovan B, Vulcu A, Dreve S, Perde-Schrepler M, Tatomir C, Filip AG, Bolfa P, Achim M, Chiorean I, Kacso I, Berghian Grosan C, Olenic L. New nanomaterials for the improvement of psoriatic lesions. J Mater Chem B. 2013;**1**:3152-3158.

[17] David L, Moldovan B, Vulcu A, Olenic L, Perde-Schrepler M, Fischer-Fodor E, et al. Green synthesis, characterization and anti-inflammatory activity of silver nanoparticles using European black elderberry fruits extract. Colloids Surf B Biointerfaces. 2014;**122**:767-777. DOI: 10.1016/j.colsurfb.2014.08.018.

[18] Sait M, Duymus M, Avcu S. Sonographic elastography of the thyroid gland. Pol J Radiol. 2016;**81**:152-156. DOI: 10.12659/PJR.896178.

[19] Cantisani V, Grazhdani H, Drakonaki E, D'Andrea V, Di Segni M, Kaleshi E, Calliada F, Catalano C, Redler A, Brunese L, Drudi FM, Fumarola A, Carbotta G, Frattaroli F, Di Leo N, Ciccariello M, Caratozzolo M, D'Ambrosio F. Strain US elastography for the characterization of thyroid nodules: advantages and limitation. J Endocrinol. 2015;**2015**:908575. DOI: 10.1155/2015/908575.

[20] Evans A, Patsy W, Kim T, McLean D, Brauer K, Purdie C, et al. Quantitative shear wave ultrasound elastography: initial experience in solid breast masses. Breast Cancer Res. 2010;**BCR 12**(6):R104.

[21] Cucos M, Crisan M, Lenghel M, Dudea M, Croitoru R, Dudea SM. Conventional ultrasonography and elastography in the assessment of plaque psoriasis under topical corticosteroid treatment. Med Ultrasound. 2014;**16**:107-113.

[22] Dasgeb B, Morris MA, Mehregan D, Siegel EL. Quantified ultrasound elastography in the assessment of cutaneous carcinoma. Br J Radiol. 2015;**88**(1054):20150344. DOI: 10.1259/bjr.20150344.

[23] Arda K, Ciledag N, Aktas E, Aribas BK, Köse K. Quantitative assessment of normal soft-tissue elasticity using shear-wave ultrasound elastography. Am J Roentgenol. 2011;**197**(3):532-536.

[24] Gutierrez M, Wortsman X, Filippucci E, De Angelis R, Filosa G, Grassi W. High-frequency sonography in the evaluation of psoriasis: nail and skin involvement. J Ultrasound Med. 2009;**28**(11):1569-1574.

[25] Lacarrubba F, Nardone B, Musumeci ML, Micali G. Ultrasound evaluation of clobetasol propionate 0.05% foam application in psoriatic and healthy skin: a pilot study. Dermatol Ther. 2009;**22**(1):19-21. DOI: 10.1111/j.1529-8019.2009.01267.x.

[26] Crisan D, Lupsor M, Boca A, Crisan M, Badea R. Ultrasonographic assessment of skin structure according to age. Indian J Dermatol Venereol Leprol. 2012;**78**(4):519. DOI: 10.4103/0378-6323.98096.

[27] Serup J, Keiding J, Fullerton A, Gniadecka M, Gniadecki R. High-frequency ultrasound examination of skin: introduction and guide. In: Serup J, Jemec GB, editors. In vivo

examination of the skin: handbook of non-invasive methods. Boca Raton FL: CRC Press; 1995. pp. 239-256.

[28] Torp-Pedersen ST, Terslev L. Settings and artefacts relevant in colour/power Doppler ultrasound in rheumatology. Ann Rheum Dis. 2008;**67**(2):143-149. DOI: 10.1136/ard.2007.078451.

[29] Perrin C. The 2 clinical subbands of the distal nail unit and the nail isthmus. Anatomical explanation and new physiological observations in relation to the nail growth. Am J Dermatopathol. 2008;**30**(3):216-221. DOI: 10.1097/DAD.0b013e31816a9d31.

[30] Essayed SM, al-Shatouri MA, Nasr Allah YS, Atwa MA. Ultrasonographic characterization of the nails in patients with psoriasis and onychomycosis. Egyptian J Radiol Nucl Med. 2015;**46**:733-739.

[31] Salgo R, Thaçi D. Treatment of moderate-to-severe plaque psoriasis. G. Ital Dermatol Venereol. 2009;**144**:701-711.

[32] Parisi R, Symmons DP, Griffiths CE, Ashcroft DM. Identification and Management of psoriasis and associated comorbidity (IMPACT) project team. Global epidemiology of psoriasis: a systematic review of incidence and prevalence. J Invest Dermatol. 2010;**133**:377-385.

[33] Gladman DD. Psoriatic arthritis. Dermatol Ther. 2004;**17**:350-363.

[34] Ayala F. Clinical presentation of psoriasis. Reumatismo. 2007;**59**:40-45.

[35] Christophers E. Psoriasis epidemiology and clinical spectrum. Clin Exp Dermatol. 2001; **26**:314-320.

[36] Crisan D. Anti-inflammatory effect of metallic silver and gold nanoparticles complexed with polyphenolic compounds in human chronic stationary plaque psoriasis. Open Access Repositorium der Universität Ulm. Dissertation; 2016; http://dx.doi.org/10.18725/OPARU–3962.

[37] Vence L, Schmitt A, Meadows CE, Gress T. Recognizing guttate psoriasis and initiating appropriate treatment. W V Med J. 2015;**111**:26-28.

[38] Oji V, Luger TA. The skin in psoriasis: assessment and challenges. Clin Exp Rheumatol. 2015;**33**:14-19.

[39] Sankowski AJ, Łebkowska UM, Ćwikła J, Walecka I, Walecki J. Psoriatic arthritis. Polish J Radiol. 2013;**78**(1):7-17.

[40] Al-Heresh AM, Proctor J, Jones SM et al. Tumour necrosis factor-alpha polymorphism and the HLA-Cw 0602 allele in psoriatic arthritis. Rheumatology. 2002;**41**:525-530.

[41] Gladman D, Antoni C, Mease P, Clegg D, Nash P. Psoriatic arthritis: epidemiology, clinical features, course, and outcome. Ann Rheumatic Dis. 2005;**64**:ii14–ii17.

[42] Kaeley GS. Review of the use of ultrasound for the diagnosis and monitoring of enthesis in psoriatic arthritis. Curr Rheumatol Rep. 2011;**13**:338-345. DOI: 10.1007/s11926-011-0184-8.

[43] Greis C. Ultrasound contrast agents as markers of vascularity and microcirculation. Clin Hemorheol Microcirc. 2009;**43**(1-2):1-9. DOI: 10.3233/CH-2009-1216.

[44] Delle Sedie A, Riente L. Psoriatic arthritis: what ultrasound can provide us. Clin Exp Rheumatol. 2015;**33**:S60–S65.

[45] Koski JM et al. Power Doppler ultrasonography and synovitis: correlating Ultrasound imaging with histopathological findings and evaluating the performance of ultrasound equipment. Ann Rheum Dis. 2006;**65**:1590-1595.

[46] Schons KRR et al. Nail psoriasis: a review of the literature. An Bras Dermatol. 2014; **9**:312-317.

[47] Ovistgaard E. Rogind H, Torp-Pedersen S et al. Quantitative ultrasonography in rheumatoid arthritis of inflammation by Doppler technique. Ann Rheum Dis. 2001;**60**:690-693.

Section 3

Treatment

Chapter 9

Pharmacogenetics of Psoriasis Treatment

Sara Redenšek and Vita Dolžan

Additional information is available at the end of the chapter

http://dx.doi.org/10.5772/intechopen.68185

Abstract

Psoriasis is a chronic systemic, immune-mediated disorder of unknown aetiology, usually presenting with typical inflammatory skin lesions and/or joint manifestations, but systemic inflammation that may lead to the development of co-morbidities may also be present. First-line therapy encompasses local cutaneous treatment and phototherapy, but with more severe symptoms or systemic course, systemic treatment with methotrexate (MTX), immunosuppressant cyclosporine, retinoid acitretin or biologicals may be used. Treatment response varies between patients in terms of efficacy and/or toxicity, which could, among other reasons, be due to genetic differences between patients. Approximately 10–30% of patients experience adverse drug reactions with MTX treatment, leading to discontinuation of MTX mostly due to hepatotoxicity. Around 15% of patients experience adverse events when treated with biologicals; however, the most frequent reason for discontinuation is inefficacy or loss of the initially favourable response over time. Inefficacy or occurrence of adverse drug reactions cannot be predicted, so genetic biomarkers of drug response in combination with clinical data could be helpful in treatment planning. Several polymorphic genes have already been associated with treatment outcome, most of them involved in drug metabolism, transport and target pathways. Genetic biomarkers could be helpful in personalized care of psoriasis patients in order to prevent adverse events or predict inefficacy of a certain drug.

Keywords: psoriasis, pharmacogenetics, genetic polymorphisms, personalized medicine, methotrexate, biologic agents

1. Introduction

Psoriasis is a chronic systemic immune-mediated disorder of which etiopathogenesis is not yet fully understood, though there is evidence of genetic, immunologic and environmental factors playing a role in the development and the severity of the disease. The most common symptoms involve typical inflammatory skin lesions, but systemic inflammation may also be present [1, 2]. Psoriatic arthritis (PsA) is the most frequent systemic manifestation that can accompany the skin lesions and occurs in up to 40% of patients [3]. Systemic inflammation is also one of the reasons for the occurrence of many other comorbidities in patients with psoriasis, such as metabolic syndrome which includes obesity, type 2 diabetes, hypertension and dyslipidaemia, cardiovascular diseases, chronic inflammatory bowel disease and also cancer in some cases [4]. Furthermore, lower quality of life and psychological disorders are also more frequent among psoriasis patients as compared to general population [5, 6]. It is proven that lifestyle, including diet, smoking and alcohol consumption, influences the occurrence and the course of psoriasis and the comorbidities [7]. Elevated body mass index and visceral fat can also increase the probability of more progressive course of the disease [7].

The severity of the disease is evaluated by the Psoriasis Area and Severity Index (PASI) score that takes into account the area of the affected skin, the thickness of skin plaques and the severity of inflammation. PASI score is calculated before the treatment strategy is chosen and is also used to monitor the treatment response. The response to treatment is considered to be good when PASI has decreased for at least 75% from the baseline score in 3–6 months after the first dose was administered (PASI75) [8]. The minimum treatment goal is usually set at PASI decreasing for at least 50% from the baseline score (PASI50). If PASI50 is not met, the treatment plan is usually changed [9]. However, PASI only evaluates the dermatological manifestations of the disease and neglects the psychological aspect. Therefore, Dermatology Life Quality Index (DLQI) is also assessed with a questionnaire to evaluate the impact of psoriasis on a patient's physical, psychological and social well-being. The treatment goal is to achieve DLQI of zero to one after 2–4 months of treatment, but if this cannot be achieved, at least DLQI below five should be aimed for [9].

The patient's response to systemic psoriasis treatment cannot be predicted. Furthermore, the interindividual variability in the treatment response is quite extensive and adverse events occur frequently [6]. A study conducted 3 years ago discovered that approximately 75% of traditional systemic drugs are discontinued after 143 days of treatment ($p < 0.0001$), mostly because of adverse events ($p < 0.001$) [8]. Besides the choice and the dose of the drug and patient's compliance to treatment, many other factors may influence the treatment response, such as patient's demographic characteristics (age, gender, body mass, ethnicity), the severity of the disease, concomitant treatment with other drugs, patient's diet, alcohol consumption, cigarette smoking as well as comorbidities. However, a lot of attention has been lately focused on the role of genetic factors that may influence the course of the disease and treatment response [10, 11]. Several pharmacogenetics studies were performed to assess the influence of genetic factors on treatment response, mainly investigating the interindividual variability in genes involved in drug metabolism, transport and mechanisms of action and the association between genetic variability and the efficacy of treatment and the occurrence of adverse events [7, 12].

1.1. Genetic factors are associated with treatment response

Our genetic characteristics are encoded in our genome [13]. Interindividual differences between people are due to differences in less than 1% of genomic DNA sequence between unrelated individuals. Different variants of the same gene or genetic locus are called alleles. A variant is called a polymorphism when there are at least two alleles present in the population and the frequency of the less prevalent allele is more than 1%. A great majority of variants are due to single nucleotide polymorphisms (SNPs), which means that alleles differ only in one nucleotide. In addition to SNPs, deletions, insertions, duplications of nucleotides or longer sequences, microsatellites, changes in variable number of tandem nucleotide repeats (VNTR) and others may account for genetic polymorphism. Genetic polymorphisms may influence the process of transcription, translation and/or function of proteins. If variants change the binding site for different regulatory proteins, transcription may be altered. Amino acids are encoded as a sequence of three nucleotides, called codons. If a polymorphism changes a codon, another amino acid can be incorporated into a protein, which can change the characteristics and function of a protein. Insertion of only one nucleotide causes frame shift, which results in a premature stop codon and non-functional protein. The same happens after a stop codon is formed in the middle of an exon or when SNPs alter mRNA splicing. Gene deletions may cause depletion of proteins while, on the other hand, gene duplications lead to excess of the encoded protein [14].

Genetic polymorphisms may also influence expression and function of proteins involved in drug metabolism and transport as well as drug targets and their effector pathways. Because of that, genetic polymorphisms may influence patients' response to drugs and the occurrence of adverse effects. Pharmacogenetics studies the associations between genetic polymorphisms and the course of disease and response to treatment. The aim of this chapter is to summarize the current knowledge on pharmacogenetic polymorphisms that may influence the response to systemic treatment in patients diagnosed with psoriasis. Such polymorphisms have been investigated as predictive biomarkers of treatment response that would support personalized treatment approaches in patients with psoriasis.

2. Pharmacogenetics of systemic psoriasis treatment

2.1. Low-dose methotrexate

Methotrexate (MTX) is an immunomodulatory drug that is widely used in the treatment of psoriasis and PsA and is frequently the first-line systemic treatment for these two indications. It is usually orally administered once per week in doses of 7.5–30 mg [9]. Good response to treatment is achieved in approximately 50% of cases [8]. On the other hand, from 10 to 30% of patients have to discontinue the treatment because of adverse drug reactions. These include nausea, malaise, gastrointestinal ulcers, depression, infections, nephrotoxicity and most importantly hepatotoxicity and bone marrow suppression [9]. Adverse events are usually mild and can be eliminated by dose reduction. However, some adverse events may be severe or even life-threatening and cannot be predicted. This is the reason why patients treated with MTX are monitored very closely, and liver and kidney functions and blood status have to be checked regularly [8]. With the low doses used for psoriasis treatment, MTX plasma concentrations are too low to be measured, so drug monitoring cannot be used to predict the occurrence of adverse events. It has been therefore proposed that genetic polymorphisms should be investigated as predictors of response to treatment, either efficacy or toxicity [15–17].

MTX is a folate analogue and as such inhibits folic acid metabolism. Folic acid is a donor of methyl group in the process of deoxythymidylate synthesis that is required for DNA synthesis and cell proliferation as well as donor of methyl groups for methionine synthesis that directs the methyl group towards methylation reactions [18].

MTX enters the cell through the reduced folate carrier SLC19A1 and is activated by folylpolyglutamate synthase that adds glutamate moieties to the molecule. MTX polyglutamate primarily inhibits dihydrofolate reductase (DHFR), thus inhibiting also thymidylate synthase (TYMS) reaction, which results in inhibition of DNA synthesis. Indirectly it inhibits also other enzymes of folate metabolic pathway and methylation reactions, such as methylentetrahydrofolate dehydrogenase (MTHFD1), methylentetrahydrofolate reductase (MTHFR), methionine synthase (MS) and methionine-synthase reductase (MSR) (**Figure 1**) [19].

MTX is also adenosine pathway inhibitor. It inhibits the enzyme 5-aminoimidazole-4- carboxamide ribonucleotide (AICAR) transformylase (ATIC), which results in elevated levels of AICAR. AICAR inhibits adenosine deaminase (ADA) and this consequently leads to higher intercellular concentrations of adenosine. Adenosine is released into circulation, and its binding to adenosine receptors on the target cells contributes significantly to the anti-inflammatory effects of MTX (**Figure 1**) [18].

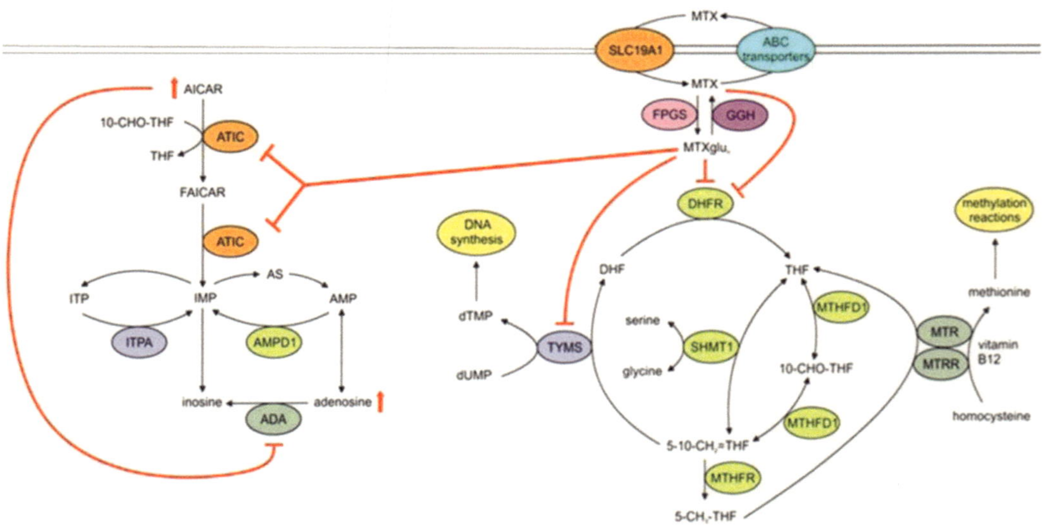

Figure 1. Schematic view of MTX mechanism of action on folate and adenosine pathway. SLC19A1—reduced folate carrier, MTX—methotrexate, ABC—ABC transporters (ATP dependent), FPGS—folypolyglutamate synthase, GGH—gamma-glutamyl hydrolase, MTXglu—methotrexate polyglutamate, DHFR—dihydrofolate reductase, THF—tetrahydrofolate, MTHFD1—methylentetrahydrofolate dehydrogenase, SHMT1—serine hydroxymethyltransferase, MTHFR—methylentetrahydrofolate reductase, MTR—methionine synthase, MTRR—methionine synthase reductase, TYMS—thymidylate synthase, DHF—dihydrofolate, dTMP—deoxythimidine monophosphate, dUMP—deoxyuridine monophosphate, AICAR—5-aminoimidazole-4-carboxamide ribonucleotide, ATIC—AICAR transformylase, THF—tetrahydrofolate, FAICAR—5-formamidoimidazole-4-carboxamide ribotide, ITP—inosine triphosphate, IMP—inosine monophosphate, AMP—adenosine monophosphate, AS—adenylosuccinate, AMPD1—AMP deaminase, ITPA—inosine triphosphatase, ADA—adenosine deaminase.

http://dx.doi.org/10.5772/intechopen.68185

Cells are protected from toxic effects of MTX by transmembrane transporters ABC (ATP-binding cassette), especially ABCB1, ABCC2 and ABCG2. They are ATP dependent, and they actively pump MTX out of the cell. On the other hand, solute carriers (SLC), such as SLC19A1 and SLCO1B1, facilitate MTX transport in the direction of the concentration gradient (**Figure 1**) [19].

Most of the genes coding for the enzymes in folate and adenosine pathway as well as for folate and MTX transporters are polymorphic. As genetic polymorphisms may lead to differences in expression and activity of enzymes, polymorphisms in the genes coding for the above mentioned proteins (transporters and enzymes) contribute to interindividual variability in therapeutic response and toxicity profile of drugs among patients. Several of the above mentioned polymorphic genes were already studied in relation to MTX treatment response in rheumatoid arthritis (RA) and cancer, but studies regarding psoriasis are scarce. Studies pointing out positive associations between polymorphisms and response to MTX in psoriasis and PsA are listed in **Table 1**.

Genes	Variants	*p*-value	Predicted effect	Reference
Efficacy				
TYMS	rs34743033 28-bp repeat	0.048	Carriers of the 3R allele susceptible to poor response to MTX	[20]
ABCC1	rs35592 c.1219-176T>C	0.008	Homozygotes for the major allele respond better to MTX	[25]
	rs2238476 c.3391-1960G>A	0.02		
	rs28364006 c.4009A>G	0.02		
ABCG2	rs13120400 c.1194+928A>G	0.03	Minor allele associated with better response to MTX	[25]
	rs17731538 c.204-1592C>T	0.007	Major allele associated with better response to MTX	
DHFR	rs1232027 g.80619201G>A	0.02	Minor allele associated with better response to MTX	[15]
Toxicity				
SLC19A1	rs1051266 c.80A>G	0.025	A allele associated with occurrence of adverse events	[20]
		0.03	A allele associated with toxicity	[25]
MTHFR	rs1801131 c.1298A>C Glu429Ala	0.042	C allele associated with lower risk of hepatotoxicity	[20]
	rs1801133 c.677C>T Ala222Val	0.04	Homozygotes for the minor allele more susceptible to liver toxicity	[15]

Genes	Variants	*p*-value	Predicted effect	Reference
TYMS	rs34489327 nt.1494del6	0.015	Polymorphism increases the risk for hepatotoxicity	[20]
	rs34743033 28-bp repeat	0.0025	3R allele increased risk for adverse events in patients without folic acid supplementation	
ATIC	rs2372536 c.347C>G	0.038	G allele associated with increased risk for MTX discontinuation due to adverse events	[20]
		0.01	Homozygotes for the major allele more susceptible to MTX toxicity	[22]
	rs4672768 c.1660-135G>A	0.02	Homozygotes for the major allele more susceptible to MTX toxicity	[22]
ABCC1	rs2238476 c.3391-1960G>A	0.01	Homozygotes for the major allele more susceptible to toxicity	[25]
	rs3784864 c.616-1641G>A	0.03	Carriers of at least one major allele more susceptible to toxicity	
	rs246240 c.616-7942A>G	0.0006	Homozygotes for the major allele more susceptible to toxicity	
	rs3784862 c.615+413G>A	0.002	Homozygotes for the major allele more susceptible to toxicity	
	rs1967120 c.489+409G>A	0.01	Carriers of at least one major allele more susceptible to toxicity	
	rs11075291 c.49-3198G>A	0.008	Carriers of at least one major allele more susceptible to toxicity	
ADORA2A	rs5760410 g.24815406G>A	0.03	Homozygotes for the major allele more susceptible to toxicity	[25]

Table 1. Genetic polymorphisms in folate and adenosine pathway and MTX transporters associated with MTX treatment outcome in patients with psoriasis or psoriatic arthritis.

2.1.1. Genetic variability in folate pathway and MTX treatment

The direct target of MTX within folate pathway is DHFR that converts dihydrofolic acid into tetrahydrofolic acid (**Figure 1**). It is therefore surprising that the impact of *DHFR* polymorphisms on the efficacy and toxicity of treatment of cutaneous psoriasis have not been studied yet. However, a study that included 281 patients with PsA showed association between the minor allele of the rs1232027 polymorphism (35289G>A) and MTX efficacy ($p = 0.02$; OR = 2.99). Patients with rs1232027 A allele had a statistically significant better response to MTX [15].

TYMS is one of the key enzymes providing deoxythymidylate for DNA synthesis, thus enabling cell proliferation. Two common functional polymorphisms in *TYMS* gene could influence therapeutic response to MTX [20]. rs34743033 polymorphism in the promoter region (5′UTR) is due to a double or triple tandem 28 bp repeat (2R and 3R). Because the 3R allele is associated with increased transcription/translation of the gene, rs34743033 may contribute to elevated activity of the enzyme and lead to depletion of the substrate for homocysteine methylation (**Figure 1**). The second most studied *TYMS* polymorphism, rs34489327, is due to a 6 bp deletion at nucleotide 1494 in the 3′UTR (3′UTR 6bp del) and leads to decreased TYMS formation [21]. The presence of 3R allele (homozygous or heterozygous variant genotype) was significantly related to poor response to treatment (OR = 2.96; $p = 0.048$), in fact carriers of 3R allele were three times less likely to respond to MTX. Furthermore, among psoriasis patients, the 3R allele was significantly ($p = 0.029$) more frequent in non-responders (64%) compared to responders (50%). On the other hand, 3′UTR 6bp del allele did not show any association with MTX efficacy. After including only patients not receiving folic acid supplementation, both 5′UTR 3R and 3′UTR 6bp del alleles were more frequent in non-responders compared to responders, but association with treatment response was not significant [20]. The *TYMS* 3′UTR 6bp del polymorphism showed significant association with occurrence of adverse events ($p = 0.025$), irrespective of folic acid supplementation. When researchers excluded patients who received folic acid supplementation, both polymorphisms (2R/3R repeat and 6 bp deletion) appeared to influence adverse events occurrence. Patients with *TYMS* 5′UTR 3R/3R genotype had 13-fold (OR = 13.2) higher chance of experiencing any adverse event, 15-fold (OR = 15.75) higher chance of developing hepatotoxicity and 12-fold (OR = 11.8) higher chance of experiencing a symptomatic adverse event compared to patients with other genotypes. *TYMS* 5′-UTR 3R allele also conferred risk for MTX discontinuation ($p = 0.033$) in this group of patients. The 3′UTR 6bp del was more frequent in patients experiencing adverse events or symptomatic adverse events, which may be due to the reduced mRNA expression caused by this polymorphism. Among patients with no concomitant folate supplementation, carriers of 3′UTR 6bp del polymorphism had an eight-fold (OR = 8.4) increased risk of developing elevated ALT levels [20]. Folic acid supplementation during MTX treatment is thus important for decreasing the risk of adverse events.

MTHFR is the central enzyme in folate pathway as it is responsible for the conversion of 5,10-methylentetrahydrofolate, which is a substrate for TYMS, to 5-methyltetrahydrofolate, which is a substrate for homocysteine remethylation (**Figure 1**). The most studied polymorphisms in *MTHFR* gene are rs1801133 (c.677C>T, p.Ala222Val) and rs1801131 (c.1298A>C, p.Glu429Ala), which cause reduced activity of the enzyme. Homozygous (TT) or heterozygous (CT) genotypes of the MTHFR 677C>T decrease the enzyme's activity by 70 or 40%, respectively. Furthermore, a homozygous (CC) genotype of the 1298A>C polymorphism decreases the enzyme's activity for 40%. Due to decreased enzyme activity, patients heterozygous for these polymorphisms could be more susceptible to MTX-induced adverse events [21]. In the first pharmacogenetic study of psoriasis patients that included 203 patients followed for 3 months after the initiation of treatment, 104 patients experienced at least one adverse event and, out of those, 67 patients (33%) had to discontinue the therapy. The most common adverse event was nausea (35%), closely followed by abnormal transaminase levels (30%). This study reported lower risk of developing hepatotoxicity in patients with 1298C allele ($p = 0.042$) and in patients with double heterozygosity 677CT/1298AC not receiving folic acid supplementation [20]. On the other hand, the frequency of *MTHFR* polymorphisms did not differ significantly between responders and non-responders [20]. Similarly, no association was found between *MTHFR* 677T allele and MTX efficacy in another study that included 330 patients, of which 250 were classified as responders and 80 as non-responders [22]. PsA patients carriers of *MTHFR* 677TT genotype suffered higher risk for hepatic adverse events compared to non-carriers (OR = 2.53; $p = 0.04$) [15].

Polymorphisms in *MTHFD1, MTR* and *MTRR* genes were not studied in psoriasis patients yet, although they were associated with MTX toxicity in RA patients in some of the studies [19, 23].

2.1.2. Genetic variability in adenosine pathway and MTX treatment

MTX directly inhibits ATIC, the key enzyme in the adenosine pathway (**Figure 1**). The consequent accumulation of AICAR indirectly leads to accumulation of adenosine in circulation, which acts as an anti-inflammatory factor. The most studied genetic polymorphism in *ATIC* is rs2372536 (c.347C>G, p.Thr116Ser), which changes the codon, so serine is incorporated into the protein instead of threonine. According to various studies, this polymorphism does not affect patient's response to MTX, and its frequency does not differ between responders and non-responders, but it did have a slight influence on the occurrence of adverse events, especially nausea, elevated alanine and aminotransferase levels. Patients who discontinued the MTX therapy had a higher frequency of the 347G allele ($p = 0.038$), but genotype distribution was not significantly different. Carriers of *ATIC* 347G allele had 1.6-fold increased risk of discontinuing the treatment because of adverse events [10, 20]. A study by Warren et al. investigated several *ATIC* polymorphisms and also found association with the outcome of MTX therapy. Two polymorphisms, in particular, rs2372536 and rs4672768, were associated with MTX toxicity ($p = 0.01$ and $p = 0.02$, respectively) [22].

ADA is the enzyme inhibited because of accumulation of AICAR following MTX treatment. A functional polymorphism *ADA* rs73598374 (c.22G>A, p.Asp8Asn) lowers the enzyme activity and may be thus associated with higher efficacy of MTX. The association between this polymorphism and toxicity and efficacy of MTX was, however, not confirmed in psoriasis patients [20].

No other polymorphic genes in adenosine metabolic pathway were investigated in psoriasis patients. However, in Slovenian patients with RA, several other genes in adenosine pathway were studied. *AMPD1* rs17602729 (c.34C>T, p.Gln45Ter) polymorphism was associated with better response to MTX. On the contrary, *ITPA* rs1127354 polymorphism (c.94C>A, p.Pro23Thr) that may decrease the release of adenosine into the circulation was associated with poor response to MTX [24].

The anti-inflammatory effect of adenosine is directly related to its binding to the adenosine receptors (ADORA). Only one pharmacogenetic study investigated adenosine receptors so far and included 374 patients with chronic plaque psoriasis, who had been treated with MTX for at least 3 months. No significant association was detected between polymorphisms in *ADORA1* gene for adenosine receptor A1 and *ADORA2A* gene for adenosine receptor A2a and the efficacy of MTX. However, there was one polymorphism, *ADORA2A* rs5760410, that was associated with higher probability of adverse events ($p = 0.03$) [25].

2.1.3. Genetic variability in folate and MTX transport and MTX treatment

Polymorphisms in transporters may influence intracellular MTX levels and, thus, also influence therapeutic effect. SLC19A1 (RFC1) is a reduced folate carrier, which facilitates the MTX transport into the cell. Many studies investigated the most common functional polymorphism in *SLC19A1* (RFC1) gene, rs1051266 (c.80G>A, p.His27Arg) and its influence on MTX treatment outcome. According to some studies, this polymorphism influences toxicity but has no effect on efficacy [20, 25]. On the contrary, studies in RA patients showed a better response to MTX in carriers of 80AA genotype [21]. Psoriasis patients with documented adverse events had a higher frequency of 80A allele ($p = 0.025$) in either homozygous or heterozygous state, so the effect was dominant ($p = 0.049$). When specific adverse events were analysed, SLC19A1 (RFC1) 80A allele was associated with higher risk for hepatotoxicity ($p = 0.053$) and symptomatic side effects ($p = 0.043$). Also, an epistatic effect of the loci, *RFC1* and *TYMS*, was observed. Two-loci genotype *RFC1* 80A/TS 3′-UTR 6bp del increased the risk of symptomatic side effects nearly three-fold (OR = 2.86). In addition, two-loci genotype *RFC1* 80A/*ATIC* 347G increased the risk for MTX discontinuation ($p = 0.0076$). Even the *RFC* 80A allele alone increased the risk of discontinuation in patients not receiving folic acid supplementation [20]. A weak association of this polymorphism to the onset of toxicity ($p = 0.03$) was shown in the study by Warren et al. [25]. However, in PsA, rs1051266 polymorphism was related neither to efficacy nor to toxicity of MTX [15].

On the other hand, polymorphisms in genes coding for the efflux ABC transporters showed association with efficacy as well as toxicity. In the study by Warren et al., two polymorphic transporter genes were investigated in psoriasis patients: *ABCC1* and *ABCG2*. In *ABCC1*, 40 polymorphisms were tested and three of them were associated with MTX efficacy. The most significant one was rs35592 ($p = 0.008$), the other two were rs2238476 ($p = 0.02$) and rs28364006 ($p = 0.02$). For all the three polymorphisms, the homozygosity for wild-type (major) allele was associated with better response to MTX. They also tested 12 *ABCG2* SNPs and two of them, rs17731538 and rs13120400, were associated with response to MTX although the effect was very small. In the case of rs17731538, the wild-type (major) allele was associated with better response ($p = 0.007$; OR = 2.1), whereas in the case of rs13120400 the minor allele was associated with better response ($p = 0.03$; OR = 1.8) [25]. When investigating the influence on toxicity, six *ABCC1* SNPs were found to be associated with MTX adverse events. The strongest correlation was found with polymorphisms rs246240 ($p = 0.001$; OR = 2.2) and rs3784862 ($p = 0.002$; OR = 2.1), in both cases homozygotes for the major allele were at increased risk for toxicity. Carriers of these polymorphisms had up to two-fold higher risk of experiencing an adverse drug reaction, irrespective of the type of the adverse event. Furthermore, the correlation between the onset of toxicity and rs2238476 was also observed. Carriers of two copies of the rs2238476 major allele had a higher chance of experiencing adverse events ($p = 0.01$; OR = 2.49). On the other hand, the investigated polymorphisms in *ABCG2* gene were not associated with toxicity [25].

2.2. Cyclosporine

Cyclosporine is an orally administered systemic immunosuppressive drug that may be used to treat the most resistant forms of psoriasis, especially the plaque-type diseases [9]. It inhibits the first phase of T-lymphocyte activation, thus decreasing the levels of inflammatory cytokines, among them interleukin-2 (IL2) and interferon- gamma (IFNG) [26]. It is usually administered in doses of 2.5–5 mg/kg of body weight/day [9]. The current knowledge on cyclosporine pharmacogenetics comes from studies in recipients of solid organ transplants. Bioavailability and clearance of the drug are influenced by polymorphic P-glycoprotein (ABCB1) in gastrointestinal tract and CYP3A4 and CYP3A5 in the liver, suggesting that these polymorphisms could also influence the response to cyclosporine treatment in psoriatic patients [27, 28]. There was only one pharmacogenetic study performed on psoriasis patients treated with cyclosporine, and it focused only on *ABCB1* polymorphisms (**Table 2**). In this study, rs1045642 (3435C>T) was associated with response to cyclosporine (OR = 2.995; $p = 0.0075$). The frequency of the minor T allele was found to be higher in the non-responders group, which means that T allele carriers have lower chance of good response [29].

2.3. Acitretin

Acitretin is a vitamin A derivative that belongs to the second-generation retinoids [30]. It reduces proliferation of epidermal keratinocytes and promotes their differentiation. It is also used as an anti-inflammatory agent. It is administered orally in doses of 0.5–0.8 mg/kg daily. Usually, it is used in combination with topical treatment as well as phototherapy [9]. Studies pointing out positive associations between polymorphisms and response to acitretin in psoriasis are listed in **Table 3**. The most widely studied polymorphisms lie in the gene coding for vascular epidermal growth factor (*VEGF*). Angiogenesis, especially inappropriate vascular expansion, is indeed a common pathogenic component of psoriasis. Two polymorphisms within *VEGF*, rs2010963 and rs833061, have been implicated in diseases with strong angiogenic background [31]. Beside the influence on treatment response, they may also influence the time of onset of the disease [32, 33]. rs833061 was associated with response to treatment in patients with early onset chronic plaque psoriasis. The frequency of rs833061TT genotype was higher in patients who were non-responsive to acitretin compared to

Genes	Variants	*p*-value	Predicted effect	Reference
Efficacy				
ABCB1	rs1045642 c.3435C>T p.Ile1145=	0.0075	Minor T allele associated with poor response to cyclosporine	[29]

Table 2. Genetic polymorphism associated with response to cyclosporine treatment in patients with psoriasis.

good responders ($p = 0.04$). Patients with the TT genotype were almost twice as likely to not respond to therapy as to respond. On the other hand, rs833061 TC genotype frequency was increased in the group of patients that responded well to acitretin compared to non-responders ($p = 0.01$). Patients with TC genotype were almost twice as likely to respond to therapy as to fail [31]. However, no association was found between rs2010963 and therapeutic response [31].

Another study performed on a group of Italian patients found an association between the *HLA-G* genotype and response to acitretin. *HLA-G* 14 bp del allele ($p = 0.008$; OR = 7.74) and del/del genotype ($p = 0.05$) were more frequent in responders compared to non-responders [34]. Another pharmacogenetic study investigated polymorphisms in the gene coding for apolipoprotein E (*APOE*). No association with treatment response was found for polymorphisms *APOE* rs429358 and rs7412 [35].

2.4. Biologic drugs

Biologic drugs specifically bind to their target, usually inflammation mediators or their receptors, and inhibit their action, which results in anti-inflammatory effect. Biologics used in treatment of psoriasis mainly inhibit tumour necrosis factor alpha (TNFα) and several interleukins (IL)—IL17, IL12 and IL23. Among the biologics used for psoriasis treatment, infliximab, adalimumab, etanercept are TNFα inhibitors, while ustekinumab is an IL12/23 inhibitor and secukinumab is IL17 inhibitor [36, 37].

Biologic drugs are relatively safe and well tolerated. Adverse events occur only in approximately 15% of patients, but the symptoms are usually not severe and are not the reason for discontinuation [38]. The most common adverse events are injection-site reaction (pain, erythema, itching and haemorrhage) and different infections, mostly of upper respiratory tract [9]. However, according to a study performed by Levin et al., 48% of patients discontinue treatment due to reasons not related to toxicity [8].

Genes	Variants	*p*-value	Predicted effect	Reference
Efficacy				
VEGF	rs833061 c.-958C>T	0.04	TT genotype increased the risk of poor response to acitretin	[31]
		0.01	TC genotype increased the chance of favourable response to acitretin	
HLA-G	14 bp DEL	0.008	DEL allele associated with better response to acitretin	[34]
		0.05	DEL/DEL genotype is associated with better response to acitretin	

Table 3. Genetic polymorphisms associated with response to acitretin treatment in patients with psoriasis.

A study conducted in 2015 that included 4309 patients treated with different biologics for 12 months showed that patients experienced dose escalations and discontinuations, restarting the same biologic or switching to a different one. Approximately one-third of patients had their doses increased until month 6 and 39% until month 12 of treatment. On the other hand, half of these patients also discontinued the biologic drug or reduced the dose [6]. This indicates that many patients do not achieve sufficient response or lose an initially favourable response over time. Pharmacogenetic studies have investigated several polymorphisms in genes coding for the targets of biologic drugs and their signalling pathways regarding their contribution to interpatient and intrapatient variability in treatment response to biologics in patients with RA, PsA, Chron's disease and spondyloarthritis (SA). However, such studies have been rarely performed exclusively in psoriasis patients [39].

2.4.1. Pharmacogenetics of anti-TNFα treatment

The most widely used biologic drugs for systemic psoriasis treatment are TNFα blockers. It is therefore not surprising that the majority of pharmacogenetic studies focused on polymorphisms in the gene coding for TNFα (*TNF*). TNFα levels are increased in affected skin and serum of patients and correlate well with disease severity measured with PASI score. TNFα inhibition can reduce the symptoms of the disease [40]. Studies pointing out positive associations between polymorphisms and response to anti-TNFα therapy in psoriasis and PsA are listed in **Table 4**.

Genes	Variants	*p*-value	Predicted effect	Reference
Efficacy				
TNFα	rs1799724 c.-857C>T	0.002	C allele associated with better response to etanercept	[49]
		0.004	Patients with CT/TT genotypes showed greater improvements in PASI score	[47]
	rs361525 c.-238A>G	0.049	Patients with GG genotype achieved PASI75 more frequently after 6 months of anti-TNFα therapy	[47]
		0.03	G allele associated with better response to etanercept	[48]
	rs1799964 c.-1031T>C	0.041	Patients with TT genotype demonstrated superior improvements in PASI after 6 months of therapy	[47]
	rs80267959 c.186+123G>A	0.0136	G allele favours better response to etanercept in PsA patients	[63]
	rs1800629 c.-308G>A	0.001	GG genotype associated with better response to etanercept	[48]
TNFRSF1B	rs1061622 c.676T>G p.Met196Arg	0.001	T allele associated with better response to etanercept	[49]
		0.05	G allele associated with poor response	[52]

Genes	Variants	*p*-value	Predicted effect	Reference
TNFAIP3	rs610604 c.987-152G>T	0.05	G allele associated with better response to anti-TNFα therapy	[53]
		0.007	T allele associated with better response to etanercept	[54]
TRAILR1	rs20575 c.626G>C p.Arg209Thr	0.048	CC genotype associated with better response to infliximab in PsA	[66]
TNFR1A	rs767455 c.36A>G p.Pro12=	0.04	AA genotype associated with better response to infliximab in PsA	
IL23R	rs11209026 c.1142G>A p.Arg381Gln	0.006	Patients with GG genotype achieved more frequently PASI 90 at 6 months	[47]
IL6	rs1800795 c.-237C>G	<0.05	Carriers of t C allele respond better to therapy	[55]
IL-17F	rs763780 c.482T>C p.His161Arg	0.0044	TC genotype associated with no response to adalimumab at 6 months	[56]
		0.023	TC genotype associated with better response to infliximab at 3 months	
		0.020	TC genotype associated with better response to infliximab at 6 months	
IL17RA	rs4819554 c.-947G>A	0.03	AA genotype associated with better response at12 weeks	[67]
HLA-C	rs10484554 g.2609009C>T	0.007	C allele associated with better response to adalimumab	[54]
TRAF3IP2	rs13190932 c.220C>T p.Arg74Trp	0.041	G allele associated with better response to infliximab	
HLA-A	rs9260313 g.1428637T>C	0.05	TT genotype associated with better response to adalimumab	
FCGR2A	rs1801274 c.497A>G p.His131Arg	0.03	Patients homozygous for high-affinity allele had a higher chance of achieving PASI75 after 3 months of therapy	[57]
		0.034	PsA patients with high-affinity genotype respond better to anti-TNFα drugs (etanercept) after 6 months of therapy	[64]
FCGR3A	rs396991 c.841T>C p.Val158Phe	0.02	Patients homozygous for high-affinity allele had a higher chance of achieving PASI75 after 3 months of therapy	[57]
		0.018	T allele associated with better response to etanercept	[58]
PDE3A-SLCO1C1	rs3794271 c.50+1078G>A	0.0031	AA genotype associated with better response to etanercept	[59]
		0.00034	A gender-specific (males) association between G allele and poor response found in PsA patients	[65]
CD84	rs6427528 c.*1738A>G	0.025	GA genotype associated with better response to etanercept	[60]

Genes	Variants	*p*-value	Predicted effect	Reference
SPEN	rs6701290 c.84-10630G>A	<0.05	Associated with anti-TNFα drug response in a GWAS	[62]
JAG2	rs3784240 c.475+782C>T			
MACC1	rs2390256 c.*2687G>A			
GUCY1B3	rs2219538 c.77+2269G>A			
PDE6A	rs10515637 c.2507-1067T>C			
CDH23	rs10823825 c.2290-538T>C			
SHOC2	rs1927159 c.704-13438A>C			
LOC728724	rs7820834 g.129238197T>C			
ADRA2A	rs553668 c.450+33966C>T			
KCNIP1	rs4867965 c.88+96839A>C			
Toxicity				
IL23R	rs11209026 c.1142G>A p.Arg381Gln	0.005	AG genotype associated with development of paradoxical psoriasiform reactions	[61]
FBXL19	rs10782001 c.1361+720G>A	0.028	GG genotype associated with development of paradoxical psoriasiform reactions	
CTLA4	rs3087243 c.*1421G>A	0.012	AG/GG genotype associated with development of paradoxical psoriasiform reactions	
SLC12A8	rs651630 c.1706-272C>T	0.011	TT genotype associated with development of paradoxical psoriasiform reactions	
TAP1	rs1800453 c.1307A>G	0.018	AG genotype associated with development of paradoxical psoriasiform reactions	

Table 4. Genetic polymorphisms associated with response to anti-TNFα therapy in patients with psoriasis or psoriatic arthritis.

The most frequently investigated candidate gene is *TNF* and rs1800629 (c.-308G>A) within it. The polymorphism, which is located in the promoter region of *TNF* gene, gained attention because it was associated with TNFα secretion and circulating levels [21]. Many studies have reported the association of this polymorphism with different traits, such as increased susceptibility to psoriasis and PsA, earlier onset of the disease or poor prognosis of the disease [41]. Zhu et al. performed a meta-analysis of 26 studies, which included 2159 psoriasis patients, 2360 patients with PsA and more than 2000 controls. They evaluated three SNPs in promoter region of *TNFα*, rs1800629 (c.-308G>A), rs361525 (c.-238A>G) and rs1799724 (c.-857T>C). They confirmed a protective influence of the polymorphic allele c.-308A. The polymorphic alleles of the other two frequently investigated polymorphisms also showed association with increased risk for psoriasis and PsA [42]. Another meta-analysis included nine studies with a total of 692 patients with RA. The main objective was to determine the influence of the *TNF* c.-308A allele on the response to TNFα inhibitors. The frequency of the *TNF* c.-308A allele was 22% in responders and 37% in patients not responding to treatment, irrespective of the choice of the TNFα inhibitor, which indicates that presence of c.-308A was associated with a poor response to the drug ($p = 0.000245$) [43]. This observation was in agreement with the findings of Mugnier et al. that showed better response to infliximab in RA patients with c.-308 GG genotype as compared to the patients with c.-308 AA/AG genotype [44]. Moreover, Guis et al. observed that RA patients homozygous for c.-308 G allele respond better to etanercept than heterozygous patients [45]. Seitz et al. evaluated response of RA, PsA and SA patients to infliximab, adalimumab and etanercept and came to the same conclusion as the above mentioned studies [46].

Other *TNF* promoter polymorphisms besides rs1800629 (c.-308G>A) were also investigated, among them were rs361525 (c.-238A>G), rs1799724 (c.-857T>C) and rs1799964 (c.-1031T>C). Better improvement in PASI score after 6 months of treatment with anti-TNFα drugs was achieved in psoriasis patients with *TNF* -238GG, -857CT/TT and -1031TT genotypes [47]. SNPs in *TNF* promoter were evaluated also by De Simone et al., and rs361525 (-238G allele; $p = 0.03$) and rs1800629 (-308GG genotype; $p = 0.001$) were found to be associated with good drug response [48].

Researchers expanded their interests also to polymorphisms in other genes in TNFα pathways. A study performed on 80 Greek patients with psoriasis investigated polymorphisms in *TNF* (c.-238G>A, c.-308G>A and c.-857C>T), tumour necrosis factor receptor superfamily 1A gene (*TNFRSF1A* rs7674559, c.36A>G) and tumour necrosis factor receptor superfamily 1B gene (*TNFRSF1B* rs1061622, c.676T>G). In total, 63 patients were responders and 17 non-responders. Carriers of *TNF -857C* ($p = 0.002$) and/or *TNFRSF1B 676T* ($p = 0.001$) alleles responded significantly better to etanercept treatment than non-carriers, while no SNPs were associated with response to infliximab or adalimumab [49]. Ongaro et al. reported poorer response to anti-TNFα therapy in RA patients with *TNFRSF1* 676TG genotype as compared to patients with 676TT genotype [50]. Recently, a meta-analysis investigated *TNFRSF1B* (rs1061622) and *TNFRSF1A* (rs7674559) polymorphisms in psoriasis patients. The investigated *TNFRSF1A* polymorphism showed no association with treatment response, but *TNFRSF1B* 676T allele was associated with better response [51]. Another recent study published in 2015 included 518 psoriasis patients and 480 healthy controls, but only 90 patients were treated with biologic drugs. In agreement with previous studies, they also observed higher frequency of *TNFRSF1B* 676G allele in non-responders, and rs1061622 polymorphism was shown to be associated with higher risk for the disease and poor response to anti-TNFα and anti-IL12/23 drugs [52].

Polymorphisms within gene coding for tumour necrosis factor alpha-induced protein 3 (*TNFAIP3*) were also associated with the response to biologics. A cohort of 433 patients with psoriasis and PsA was tested for two *TNFAIP3* SNPs, rs2230926 and rs610604. The results showed that rs610604G allele was associated with better response to etanercept, infliximab and adalimumab, when patients treated with all these drugs were analysed together ($p = 0.05$; OR = 1.50), but only to etanercept, when each drug treatment was analysed separately ($p = 0.016$; OR = 1.64). In addition, rs2230926 T allele and rs610604 G allele were also predictors of a better outcome. Unfortunately, researchers were unable to reproduce these results in a smaller cohort [53].

Furthermore, polymorphisms in genes encoding several interleukins and their receptors were investigated in psoriasis patients treated with anti-TNFα drugs. A study that included 109 psoriasis patients investigated polymorphisms in *IL12B* (rs6887695 and rs3212227) and *IL23R* (rs7530511 and rs11209026). Carriers of the rs11209026 GG genotype showed better response at 6 months of anti-TNFα treatment compared to non-carriers. This study also showed the association of *HLA-Cw6* haplotype with worse outcome [47]. Another association with HLA loci was observed by Masouri et al. who reported the association of *HLA-C* rs10484554 polymorphism with good response to adalimumab (CC or CT genotype, $p = 0.007$). In the same study, also *TRAF3IP2* rs13190932, *TNFAIP3* rs610604 and *HLA-A* rs9260313 were associated with good response to infliximab, etanercept and adalimumab, respectively [54]. In another small study of 60 psoriasis patients, a polymorphism in the *IL6* promoter (rs1800795) was investigated. Homozygotes and heterozygotes for *IL6* rs1800795 C allele responded better to therapy [55]. *IL-17F* rs763780 was also investigated for the association with treatment outcome. This SNP was associated with no response to adalimumab after 6 months (TC genotype, $p = 0.0044$) and with better response to infliximab after 3 and 6 months (TC genotype; $p = 0.023$ and $p = 0.020$, respectively) [56]. *IL17RA* rs4819554 polymorphism was associated with better response after 12 weeks in carriers of AA genotype compared to AG and GG carriers ($p = 0.03$).

Genes for Fc gamma receptors were also investigated for their association with response of psoriasis patients to anti-TNFα drugs. Patients homozygous for high-affinity alleles of two variants *FCGR2A-H131R* (rs1801274) and *FCGR3A-V158F* (rs396991) had a higher chance of achieving PASI75 after 3 months of therapy [57]. *FCGR3A* rs396991 was also evaluated by Mendrinou et al. who showed that T allele could be a marker of better response to etanercept [58]. Moreover, a positive association was found between *PDE3A-SLCO1C1* rs3794271AA genotype and PASI score in patients treated with etanercept [59]. Association between the *CD84* genotypes and response to biologics was also evaluated. *CD84* rs6427528 polymorphism with its heterozygous GA genotype ($p = 0.025$) was associated with better response to treatment with etanercept [60].

A study performed by Cabaleiro et al. revealed an association between certain polymorphisms and occurrence of paradoxical psoriasiform reactions after treatment with anti-TNFα therapy. Polymorphisms in five genes: *IL23R* rs11209026, *FBXL19* rs10782001, *CTLA4* rs3087243, *SLC12A8* rs651630 and *TAP1* rs1800453 were associated with the development of this adverse reaction to anti-TNFα treatment [61].

Another approach to identify novel loci and SNPs associated with response to anti-TNFα drugs included genome-wide association study (GWAS) approach. A small GWAS study was recently performed that included 65 psoriasis patients prospectively followed for 12 weeks. This study identified 10 SNPs in 10 different genes that could be associated with drug response: cadherin-related 23 (*CDH2*), soc-2 suppressor of clear homolog (*SHOC2*), adrenoceptor alpha

2A (*ADRA2A*), phosphodiesterase 6A (*PDE6A*), Kv channel interacting protein 1 (*KCNIP1*), spen family transcriptional repressor (*SPEN*), jagged 2 (*JAG2*), metastasis associated in colon cancer 1 (*MACC1*), guanylate cyclase 1, soluble, beta 3 (*GUCY1B3*) and long intergenic non-protein coding RNA 977 (*LOC728724*) gene [62]. However, all these SNPs still await to be replicated in independent patient cohorts.

Several studies have also investigated association of genetic polymorphisms with anti-TNFα treatment outcome in PsA cohorts. A study investigating the association of an intronic polymorphism at the position c.+489 of *TNF* gene (rs80267959) with response to treatment with etanercept reported better response in PsA patients carrying G allele compared to non-carriers ($p = 0.0136$) [63]. Furthermore, PsA patients with high-affinity FCGR2A His/His and His/Arg genotypes responded better to anti-TNFα drugs (etanercept) at 6 months of treatment compared to patients with low-affinity genotypes ($p = 0.034$) [64]. A gender-specific association between polymorphic rs3794271 G allele and poor response was reported at the *PDE3A-SLCO1C1* locus ($p = 0.00034$) [65]. Other candidate genes for prediction of treatment response were suggested, including genes coding for death receptors, such as tumour necrosis factor-related apoptosis inducing ligand receptor 1 (*TRAIL-R1*). *TRAIL-R1* (rs20575, 626G>C) and *TNFR1A* (rs767455, 36A>G) were investigated in a study of 55 PsA patients treated with TNFα blocker infliximab. This study concluded that *TRAILR1* 626CC ($p = 0.048$) and *TNFR1A* 36AA ($p = 0.04$) genotypes may be associated with better response after 3 months of infliximab treatment [66].

2.4.2. IL12/23 inhibitors

Ustekinumab is a human monoclonal antibody directed against interleukins IL12 and IL23. Studies of polymorphisms affecting patients' response to these inhibitors are scarce, but some of them, listed in **Table 5**, pointed out positive associations. A cohort of 51 patients with psoriasis treated with ustekinumab was tested for three polymorphisms, including the *HLA-Cw6* positivity, *TNFAIP3* rs610604 polymorphism and *LCE3B/3C* gene deletions. Better and faster response to ustekinumab was observed in *HLA-Cw6* positive patients, while no significant association with response was observed for the other two investigated genes [68]. Another larger study confirmed the role of *HLA-Cw6* as Chui et al. reported that *HLA-Cw6* positive patients were more likely to achieve PASI50, 75 and 90 after 28 weeks of treatment [69]. On the other hand, Galluzzo et al. suggested that a combination of genetic factors predicts response to ustekinumab better than a single factor. The presence of *IL12B* rs6887695 GG genotype in the absence of *IL12B* rs3212227 AA genotype in HLA Cw6 positive patients increased the chance of better treatment outcomes [70].

Another study found association between the *TNFRSF1B* rs1061622 G allele and poor response to anti-IL12/IL23 drugs ($p = 0.05$) [52]. Furthermore, study in a cohort of 70 psoriasis patients treated with ustekinumab reported an association between the *IL-17F* rs763780 TC genotype and no response to ustekinumab after 3 and 6 months of treatment ($p = 0.022$ and $p = 0.016$, respectively) [56]. *IL12B* rs3213094 polymorphism was also investigated for association with response to ustekinumab and CT genotype was recognized as a predictor of better response to the drug ($p = 0.017$) [60]. In the same study, *TNFAIP3* rs610604 GG genotype was associated with poor response to ustekinumab ($p = 0.031$) [60]. Association between two polymorphisms in *ERAP1*gene, rs151823 and rs26653, and good response to ustekinumab was also reported [54].

Genes	Variants	*p*-value	Predicted effect	Reference
Efficacy				
IL-17F	rs763780 c.482T>C p.His161Arg	0.022	TC genotype associated with no response at 3 months	[56]
		0.016	TC genotype associated with no response at 6 months	
IL12B	rs3213094 c.89-432G>A	0.017	CT genotype associated with favourable response	[60]
TNFAIP3	rs610604 c.987-152G>T	0.031	GG genotype associated with poor response	
HLA-C	Cw6POS/NEG	0.008	Cw6POS patients respond better and faster	[68]
		0.035	Cw6POS patients respond better	[69]
TNFRSF1B	rs1061622 c.676T>G p.Met196Arg	0.05	G allele associated with poor response	[52]
ERAP1	rs151823 c.-454-1169A>C	0.026	CC genotype associated with better response	[54]
	rs26653 c.380G>C p.Arg127Pro	0.016	GG genotype associated with better response	

Table 5. Genetic polymorphisms associated with response to ustekinumab in patients with psoriasis.

3. Future perspectives

Large heterogeneity in patients' response to therapy calls for new molecular predictors of treatment response. We have searched the current literature to compile a comprehensive review of today's knowledge on genetic variants that may influence the outcome of psoriasis systemic treatment. A rather small number of studies were performed so far, and, although some of the results are encouraging, even larger number of studies shows inconsistent or even conflicting results. The investigated patient cohorts were with a few exceptions rather small and the number of evaluated polymorphisms limited. The future studies should expand the range of polymorphisms investigated by either looking into other pathways besides the ones directly involved in drug mechanisms, such as metabolism and transport, though they certainly are important in treatment response. Great interindividual variability in treatment outcome among patients could also be associated with heterogeneous pathology. Not all of the patients have the same pathogenesis, although they present with similar symptoms. Genetic defects in various pathways could be causative of the disease or support disease occurrence, and these defects in so-called susceptibility genes should also be checked regarding their influence on treatment outcome. The heterogeneity in pathogenesis could also be the reason for inconsistency in pharmacogenetic studies conducted so far. The hypothesis-free approach of the GWAS studies could help to overcome these obstacles and help to elucidate genetic factors associated with both disease pathways and treatment responses; however, such studies should include large number of well-characterized patients. Furthermore, the identified predictors of the course of the disease and of the treatment response should be validated in independent patient samples.

Such validated pharmacogenetic biomarkers would enable us to characterize patients with psoriasis by their genetic characteristics and not just their phenotype and would allow for a more targeted approach to pharmacotherapy. The patients could be stratified according to their genetic defects affecting the molecular mechanisms of the disease in combination with genetic defects in pathways of drug metabolism and transport as well as in drug targets and effector pathways. Pharmacogenetic factors should also be combined with clinical data to find the most suitable way of stratifying patients into groups eligible for certain treatment strategies. If a physician would be able to predict patient's response based on pharmacogenetic polymorphisms, problems of inefficacy and toxicity could be overcome by choosing the right drug and dose for a particular patient. This would also help to lower the cost of the treatment and, what is more important, relieve some of the patient's psychological burden, which is often overlooked in psoriasis. Methods for genotyping are fast, reliable, relatively cheap and suitable for use in diagnostic laboratories. Despite the costs that would be spent on implementation of new genetic analysis methods into everyday clinical practice, pharmacogenetics-based personalized treatment approach would probably lower the expenses of psoriasis treatment due to more rational pharmacotherapy.

4. Conclusions

Personalized medicine is emerging as the innovative approach also in psoriasis treatment. A general belief that every drug can help every patient is getting obsolete. However, to be able to properly tailor the patient's treatment, consistent biomarkers of the treatment outcome must be identified and validated. In psoriasis treatment, the search for such biomarkers is still in its beginnings. In this chapter, we summarized the current knowledge on genetic predictors of response to MTX, cyclosporine, acitretin and biologic drugs. Several studies have already identified some of the genetic variants associated with response to a particular drug, but none of the genetic polymorphisms within these genes were recognized as specific enough to be used in clinical practice so far. However, some promising candidates for predictors of treatment response were identified that could be used in personalized treatment of psoriasis patients if validated in further studies.

Author details

Sara Redenšek and Vita Dolžan*

*Address all correspondence to: vita.dolzan@mf.uni-lj.si

Pharmacogenetics Laboratory, Institute of Biochemistry, Faculty of Medicine, University of Ljubljana, Slovenia

References

[1] Ryan C, Kirby B. Psoriasis is a systemic disease with multiple cardiovascular and metabolic comorbidities. Dermatol Clin. 2015;33(1):41–55. Epub 2014/11/22.

[2] Reich K. The concept of psoriasis as a systemic inflammation: implications for disease management. J Eur Acad Dermatol Venereol. 2012;2:3–11.

[3] Mease PJ, Armstrong AW. Managing patients with psoriatic disease: the diagnosis and pharmacologic treatment of psoriatic arthritis in patients with psoriasis. Drugs. 2014;74(4):423–41.

[4] Dauden E, Castaneda S, Suarez C, Garcia-Campayo J, Blasco AJ, Aguilar MD, et al. Clinical practice guideline for an integrated approach to comorbidity in patients with psoriasis. J Eur Acad Dermatol Venereol. 2013;27(11):1387–404.

[5] Voiculescu VM, Lupu M, Papagheorghe L, Giurcaneanu C, Micu E. Psoriasis and Metabolic Syndrome—scientific evidence and therapeutic implications. J Med Life. 2014;7(4):468–71. Epub 2015/02/26.

[6] Feldman SR, Zhao Y, Navaratnam P, Friedman HS, Lu J, Tran MH. Patterns of medication utilization and costs associated with the use of etanercept, adalimumab, and ustekinumab in the management of moderate-to-severe psoriasis. J Manag Care Spec Pharm. 2015;21(3):201–9.

[7] Nelson PA, Keyworth C, Chisholm A, Pearce CJ, Griffiths CE, Cordingley L, et al. 'In someone's clinic but not in mine'—clinicians' views of supporting lifestyle behaviour change in patients with psoriasis: a qualitative interview study. Br J Dermatol. 2014;171(5):1116–22. Epub 2014/07/02.

[8] Levin AA, Gottlieb AB, Au SC. A comparison of psoriasis drug failure rates and reasons for discontinuation in biologics vs conventional systemic therapies. J Drugs Dermatol. 2014;13(7):848–53.

[9] Pathirana D, Ormerod AD, Saiag P, Smith C, Spuls PI, Nast A, et al. European S3-Guidelines on the systemic treatment of psoriasis vulgaris. J Eur Acad Dermatology Venereol. 2010;24(1):117–8.

[10] Sutherland A, Power RJ, Rahman P, O'Rielly DD. Pharmacogenetics and pharmacogenomics in psoriasis treatment: current challenges and future prospects. Expert Opin Drug Metab Toxicol. 2016;12(8):923–35.

[11] Ray-Jones H, Eyre S, Barton A, Warren RB. One SNP at a time: moving beyond GWAS in Psoriasis. J Invest Dermatol. 2016;136(3):567–73.

[12] Dolžan V. Genetic polymorphisms and drug metabolism. Zdravniški vestnik. 2007; 76:II-5-II-12

[13] Venter JC, Adams MD, Myers EW, Li PW, Mural RJ, Sutton GG, et al. The sequence of the human genome. Science. 2001;291(5507):1304–51.

[14] Li A, Meyre D. Jumping on the train of personalized medicine: a primer for non-geneticist clinicians: Part 1. Fundamental concepts in molecular genetics. Curr Psychiatry Rev. 2014;10(2):91–100.

[15] Chandran V, Siannis F, Rahman P, Pellett FJ, Farewell VT, Gladman DD. Folate pathway enzyme gene polymorphisms and the efficacy and toxicity of methotrexate in psoriatic arthritis. J Rheumatol. 2010;37(7):1508–12.

[16] Foulkes AC, Warren RB. Pharmacogenomics and the resulting impact on psoriasis therapies. Dermatol Clin. 2015;33(1):149–60.

[17] Woolf RT, Smith CH. How genetic variation affects patient response and outcome to therapy for psoriasis. Expert Rev Clin Immunol. 2010;6(6):957–66.

[18] Cutolo M, Sulli A, Pizzorni C, Seriolo B, Straub RH. Anti-inflammatory mechanisms of methotrexate in rheumatoid arthritis. Ann Rheum Dis. 2001;60(8):729–35.

[19] Bohanec Grabar P, Logar D, Lestan B, Dolzan V. Genetic determinants of methotrexate toxicity in rheumatoid arthritis patients: a study of polymorphisms affecting methotrexate transport and folate metabolism. Eur J Clin Pharmacol. 2008;64(11):1057–68.

[20] Campalani E, Arenas M, Marinaki AM, Lewis CM, Barker JN, Smith CH. Polymorphisms in folate, pyrimidine, and purine metabolism are associated with efficacy and toxicity of methotrexate in psoriasis. J Invest Dermatol. 2007;127(8):1860–7.

[21] O'Rielly DD, Rahman P. Pharmacogenetics of psoriasis. Pharmacogenomics. 2011;12 (1):87–101.

[22] Warren RB, Smith RL, Campalani E, Eyre S, Smith CH, Barker JN, et al. Outcomes of methotrexate therapy for psoriasis and relationship to genetic polymorphisms. Br J Dermatol. 2009;160(2):438–41.

[23] Wessels JA, van der Kooij SM, le Cessie S, Kievit W, Barerra P, Allaart CF, et al. A clinical pharmacogenetic model to predict the efficacy of methotrexate monotherapy in recent-onset rheumatoid arthritis. Arthritis Rheum. 2007;56(6):1765–75.

[24] Grabar PB, Rojko S, Logar D, Dolzan V. Genetic determinants of methotrexate treatment in rheumatoid arthritis patients: a study of polymorphisms in the adenosine pathway: Ann Rheum Dis. 2010;69(5):931–2. doi: 10.1136/ard.2009.111567.

[25] Warren RB, Smith RL, Campalani E, Eyre S, Smith CH, Barker JN, et al. Genetic variation in efflux transporters influences outcome to methotrexate therapy in patients with psoriasis. J Invest Dermatol. 2008;128(8):1925–9.

[26] Haider AS, Lowes MA, Suarez-Farinas M, Zaba LC, Cardinale I, Khatcherian A, et al. Identification of cellular pathways of "type 1," Th17 T cells, and TNF- and inducible nitric oxide synthase-producing dendritic cells in autoimmune inflammation through pharmacogenomic study of cyclosporine A in psoriasis. J Immunol. 2008; 180(3):1913–20.

[27] Keown P, Landsberg D, Halloran P, Shoker A, Rush D, Jeffery J, et al. A randomized, prospective multicenter pharmacoepidemiologic study of cyclosporine microemulsion in stable renal graft recipients. Report of the Canadian Neoral Renal Transplantation Study Group. Transplantation. 1996;62(12):1744–52.

[28] Zhang Y, Benet LZ. The gut as a barrier to drug absorption: combined role of cytochrome P450 3A and P-glycoprotein. Clin Pharmacokinet. 2001;40(3):159–68.

[29] Vasilopoulos Y, Sarri C, Zafiriou E, Patsatsi A, Stamatis C, Ntoumou E, et al. A pharmacogenetic study of ABCB1 polymorphisms and cyclosporine treatment response in patients with psoriasis in the Greek population. Pharmacogenomics J. 2014;14(6):523–5.

[30] Prieto-Perez R, Cabaleiro T, Dauden E, Ochoa D, Roman M, Abad-Santos F. Pharmacogenetics of topical and systemic treatment of psoriasis. Pharmacogenomics. 2013;14 (13):1623–34.

[31] Young HS, Summers AM, Read IR, Fairhurst DA, Plant DJ, Campalani E, et al. Interaction between genetic control of vascular endothelial growth factor production and retinoid responsiveness in psoriasis. J Invest Dermatol. 2006;126(2):453–9.

[32] Barile S, Medda E, Nistico L, Bordignon V, Cordiali-Fei P, Carducci M, et al. Vascular endothelial growth factor gene polymorphisms increase the risk to develop psoriasis. Exp Dermatol. 2006;15(5):368–76.

[33] Young HS, Summers AM, Bhushan M, Brenchley PE, Griffiths CE. Single-nucleotide polymorphisms of vascular endothelial growth factor in psoriasis of early onset. J Invest Dermatol. 2004;122(1):209–15.

[34] Borghi A, Rizzo R, Corazza M, Bertoldi AM, Bortolotti D, Sturabotti G, et al. HLA-G 14-bp polymorphism: a possible marker of systemic treatment response in psoriasis vulgaris? Preliminary results of a retrospective study. Dermatol Ther. 2014;27(5):284–9.

[35] Campalani E, Allen MH, Fairhurst D, Young HS, Mendonca CO, Burden AD, et al. Apolipoprotein E gene polymorphisms are associated with psoriasis but do not determine disease response to acitretin. Br J Dermatol. 2006;154(2):345–52.

[36] Choy EH, Panayi GS. Cytokine pathways and joint inflammation in rheumatoid arthritis. N Engl J Med. 2001;344(12):907–16.

[37] Horiuchi T, Mitoma H, Harashima S, Tsukamoto H, Shimoda T. Transmembrane TNF-alpha: structure, function and interaction with anti-TNF agents. Rheumatology. 2010;49(7):1215–28.

[38] Day R. Adverse reactions to TNF-alpha inhibitors in rheumatoid arthritis. Lancet. 2002;359(9306):540–1.

[39] O'Rielly DD, Rahman P. Pharmacogenetics of rheumatoid arthritis: Potential targets from susceptibility genes and present therapies. Pharmgenomics Pers Med. 2010;3:15–31.

[40] Mizutani H, Ohmoto Y, Mizutani T, Murata M, Shimizu M. Role of increased production of monocytes TNF-alpha, IL-1beta and IL-6 in psoriasis: relation to focal infection, disease activity and responses to treatments. J Dermatol Sci. 1997;14(2):145–53.

[41] Balding J, Kane D, Livingstone W, Mynett-Johnson L, Bresnihan B, Smith O, et al. Cytokine gene polymorphisms: association with psoriatic arthritis susceptibility and severity. Arthritis Rheum. 2003;48(5):1408–13.

[42] Zhu J, Qu H, Chen X, Wang H, Li J. Single nucleotide polymorphisms in the tumor necrosis factor-alpha gene promoter region alter the risk of psoriasis vulgaris and psoriatic arthritis: a meta-analysis. Plos One. 2013;8(5):e64376.

[43] O'Rielly DD, Roslin NM, Beyene J, Pope A, Rahman P. TNF-alpha-308 G/A polymorphism and responsiveness to TNF-alpha blockade therapy in moderate to severe rheumatoid arthritis: a systematic review and meta-analysis. Pharmacogenomics J. 2009;9(3):161–7.

[44] Mugnier B, Balandraud N, Darque A, Roudier C, Roudier J, Reviron D. Polymorphism at position -308 of the tumor necrosis factor alpha gene influences outcome of infliximab therapy in rheumatoid arthritis. Arthritis Rheum. 2003;48(7):1849–52.

[45] Guis S, Balandraud N, Bouvenot J, Auger I, Toussirot E, Wendling D, et al. Influence of -308 A/G polymorphism in the tumor necrosis factor alpha gene on etanercept treatment in rheumatoid arthritis. Arthritis Rheum. 2007;57(8):1426–30.

[46] Seitz M, Wirthmuller U, Moller B, Villiger PM. The -308 tumour necrosis factor-alpha gene polymorphism predicts therapeutic response to TNFalpha-blockers in rheumatoid arthritis and spondyloarthritis patients. Rheumatology. 2007;46(1):93–6.

[47] Gallo E, Cabaleiro T, Roman M, Solano-Lopez G, Abad-Santos F, Garcia-Diez A, et al. The relationship between tumour necrosis factor (TNF)-alpha promoter and IL12B/IL-23R genes polymorphisms and the efficacy of anti-TNF-alpha therapy in psoriasis: a case-control study. Br J Dermatol. 2013;169(4):819–29.

[48] De Simone C, Farina M, Maiorino A, Fanali C, Perino F, Flamini A, et al. TNF-alpha gene polymorphisms can help to predict response to etanercept in psoriatic patients. J Eur Acad Dermatol Venereol. 2015;29(9):1786–90.

[49] Vasilopoulos Y, Manolika M, Zafiriou E, Sarafidou T, Bagiatis V, Kruger-Krasagaki S, et al. Pharmacogenetic analysis of TNF, TNFRSF1A, and TNFRSF1B gene polymorphisms and prediction of response to anti-TNF therapy in psoriasis patients in the Greek population. Mol Diagn Ther. 2012;16(1):29–34.

[50] Ongaro A, De Mattei M, Pellati A, Caruso A, Ferretti S, Masieri FF, et al. Can tumor necrosis factor receptor II gene 676T>G polymorphism predict the response grading to anti-TNFalpha therapy in rheumatoid arthritis? Rheumatol Int. 2008;28(9):901–8.

[51] Chen W, Xu H, Wang X, Gu J, Xiong H, Shi Y. The tumor necrosis factor receptor superfamily member 1B polymorphisms predict response to anti-TNF therapy in patients with autoimmune disease: a meta-analysis. Int Immunopharmacol. 2015;28(1):146–53.

[52] Gonzalez-Lara L, Batalla A, Coto E, Gomez J, Eiris N, Santos-Juanes J, et al. The TNFRSF1B rs1061622 polymorphism (p.M196R) is associated with biological drug outcome in Psoriasis patients. Arch Dermatol Res. 2015;307(5):405–12.

[53] Tejasvi T, Stuart PE, Chandran V, Voorhees JJ, Gladman DD, Rahman P, et al. TNFAIP3 gene polymorphisms are associated with response to TNF blockade in psoriasis. J Invest Dermatol. 2012;132(3 Pt 1):593–600.

[54] Masouri S, Stefanaki I, Ntritsos G, Kypreou KP, Drakaki E, Evangelou E, et al. A pharmacogenetic study of psoriasis risk variants in a greek population and prediction of responses to anti-TNF-alpha and anti-IL-12/23 agents. Mol Diagn Ther. 2016;20(3):221–5.

[55] Di Renzo L, Bianchi A, Saraceno R, Calabrese V, Cornelius C, Iacopino L, et al. -174G/C IL-6 gene promoter polymorphism predicts therapeutic response to TNF-alpha blockers. Pharmacogenet Genomics. 2012;22(2):134–42.

[56] Prieto-Perez R, Solano-Lopez G, Cabaleiro T, Roman M, Ochoa D, Talegon M, et al. The polymorphism rs763780 in the IL-17F gene is associated with response to biological drugs in patients with psoriasis. Pharmacogenomics. 2015;16(15):1723–31.

[57] Julia M, Guilabert A, Lozano F, Suarez-Casasus B, Moreno N, Carrascosa JM, et al. The role of Fcgamma receptor polymorphisms in the response to anti-tumor necrosis factor therapy in psoriasis A pharmacogenetic study. JAMA Dermatol. 2013;149(9):1033–9.

[58] Mendrinou E, Patsatsi A, Zafiriou E, Papadopoulou D, Aggelou L, Sarri C, et al. FCGR3A-V158F polymorphism is a disease-specific pharmacogenetic marker for the treatment of psoriasis with Fc-containing TNFalpha inhibitors. Pharmacogenomics J. 2016;5(10):16.

[59] Julia A, Ferrandiz C, Dauden E, Fonseca E, Fernandez-Lopez E, Sanchez-Carazo JL, et al. Association of the PDE3A-SLCO1C1 locus with the response to anti-TNF agents in psoriasis. Pharmacogenomics J. 2015;15(4):322–5.

[60] van den Reek JM, Coenen MJ, van de L'Isle Arias M, Zweegers J, Rodijk-Olthuis D, Schalkwijk J, et al. Polymorphisms in CD84, IL12B and TNFAIP3 are associated with response to biologics in patients with psoriasis. Br J Dermatol. 2016;26(10):15005.

[61] Cabaleiro T, Prieto-Perez R, Navarro R, Solano G, Roman M, Ochoa D, et al. Paradoxical psoriasiform reactions to anti-TNFalpha drugs are associated with genetic polymorphisms in patients with psoriasis. Pharmacogenomics J. 2016;16(4):336–40.

[62] Nishikawa R, Nagai H, Bito T, Ikeda T, Horikawa T, Adachi A, et al. Genetic prediction of the effectiveness of biologics for psoriasis treatment. J Dermatol. 2016;43(11):1273–7.

[63] Murdaca G, Gulli R, Spano F, Lantieri F, Burlando M, Parodi A, et al. TNF-alpha gene polymorphisms: association with disease susceptibility and response to anti-TNF-alpha treatment in psoriatic arthritis. J Invest Dermatol. 2014;134(10):2503–9.

[64] Ramirez J, Fernandez-Sueiro JL, Lopez-Mejias R, Montilla C, Arias M, Moll C, et al. FCGR2A/CD32A and FCGR3A/CD16A variants and EULAR response to tumor necrosis factor-alpha blockers in psoriatic arthritis: a longitudinal study with 6 months of followup. J Rheumatol. 2012;39(5):1035–41.

[65] Julia A, Rodriguez J, Fernandez-Sueiro JL, Gratacos J, Queiro R, Montilla C, et al. PDE3A-SLCO1C1 locus is associated with response to anti-tumor necrosis factor therapy in psoriatic arthritis. Pharmacogenomics. 2014;15(14):1763–9.

[66] Morales-Lara MJ, Canete JD, Torres-Moreno D, Hernandez MV, Pedrero F, Celis R, et al. Effects of polymorphisms in TRAILR1 and TNFR1A on the response to anti-TNF therapies in patients with rheumatoid and psoriatic arthritis. Joint Bone Spine. 2012;79(6):591–6.

[67] Batalla A, Coto E, Gomez J, Eiris N, Gonzalez-Fernandez D, Gomez-De Castro C, et al. IL17RA gene variants and anti-TNF response among psoriasis patients. Pharmacogenomics J. 2016;27(10):70.

[68] Talamonti M, Botti E, Galluzzo M, Teoli M, Spallone G, Bavetta M, et al. Pharmacogenetics of psoriasis: HLA-Cw6 but not LCE3B/3C deletion nor TNFAIP3 polymorphism predisposes to clinical response to interleukin 12/23 blocker ustekinumab. Br J Dermatol. 2013;169(2):458–63.

[69] Chiu HY, Wang TS, Chan CC, Cheng YP, Lin SJ, Tsai TF. Human leucocyte antigen-Cw6 as a predictor for clinical response to ustekinumab, an interleukin-12/23 blocker, in Chinese patients with psoriasis: a retrospective analysis. Br J Dermatol. 2014;171(5):1181–8.

[70] Galluzzo M, Boca AN, Botti E, Potenza C, Malara G, Malagoli P, et al. IL12B (p40) Gene Polymorphisms Contribute to Ustekinumab Response Prediction in Psoriasis. Dermatology. 2016;232(2):230–6.

Chapter 10

The Role of Methotrexate in Psoriatic Therapy in the Age of Biologic and Biosimilar Medication: Therapeutic Benefits versus Toxicology Emergencies

Carolina Negrei and Daniel Boda

Additional information is available at the end of the chapter

http://dx.doi.org/10.5772/67793

Abstract

Used in the psoriasis therapy for over 30 years, methotrexate belongs to the non-biological medication class. Its continued use must be studied in the context of the modern unprecedented powerful pharmacological and medical development, due to the particularly, even uniquely fast development of biologicals, which assume an extremely important role in cutting-edge medicine. This status has turned biosimilars and all related matters into an outstanding challenge not only for researchers worldwide but also for other medicinal product-associated fields such as development of regulatory standards and pharmacovigilance, to mention the most important. However, against a comparable high-risk background, compounded by the additional danger of serious cumulative toxicity, methotrexate therapy continues to be recommended mainly for patients suffering from severe psoriasis, seriously affecting their quality of life.

Keywords: methotrexate, biosimilars, psoriasis, benefit, toxicology

1. Introduction

Known since ancient times (judging by descriptions of typical lesions found in mummified bodies, as early as the Christian era), psoriasis is a frequent autoimmune disease mostly causing chronic inflammation of the skin, through other manifestations are not uncommon. Psoriasis is mediated by T-cells and as such is the more frequently encountered human disease of its class. Since the very beginning and as far as the late Middle Ages, because of its mistaken diagnosis as leprosy and subsequent isolation of patients, it was accompanied by significant social and economic burden. Further in history, at the beginning of the nineteenth century, scientists finally observed and mentioned its association with joint impairment (now known as arthropathic psoriasis) (1818, Jean-LouisAlibert) [1, 2]. The socio-economic impact of psoriasis has however been preserved [3], in the context of the generally severely impaired quality of life, as well as of forms refractory to treatment and frequent occurrence of comorbidities, accentuated by the fact that permanent cure for psoriasis is a goal yet to be accomplished.

Nowadays, some 2–3% of the population is affected, with too little dissimilarity between the two genders. From the perspective of race factors, studies conducted worldwide have shown 0.7% prevalence among individuals of African descent, relatively low frequency in native South-American populations as well as bimodal distribution as regards the age for its onset [4].

With regard to psoriasis-associated risks suggested by the results of epidemiological studies, the prevalence of various comorbidities and mortality seems rather high [5, 6]. Among the related comorbidities, mentioning due to psoriatic arthritis, chronic inflammatory intestinal disease and psychiatric and psychosocial disorders, as the most common; however, cardiovascular comorbidities (obesity, diabetes, dyslipidemia, hypertension as well as coronary disease) [7–10] have also more recently been shown to arise from psoriasis-induced metabolic changes. In this respect, research has found increased myocardial infarction risk for younger patients suffering from severe forms of psoriasis [11].

The clinical profile in psoriasis consists of erythematous and scaling lesions, distributed in various patterns and regions of the body. At the same time, a range of individual clinical phenotypes may be noted such as vulgar, pustular, inverted, erythrodermic and guttate. In 5–20% of the cases, psoriasis involves the joints and the nails [12]. A comparative look at premature onset or type I and type II or delayed onset psoriasis (arising between the ages of 50 and 60 or later), one should notice the former's more frequent family background of DR7 and HLA-Cw6 and the disease, as well as type I tendency to more significant dissemination and more frequent relapses [4, 12].

Psoriasis is known to be triggered and/or aggravated by such factors as trauma, drugs, infections, alcoholism and smoking [13, 14]. Given that psoriasis may not be yet cured, progress has mainly focused on suppression of the systemic inflammatory response and general disease signs, which are considered sufficient to allow symptom-free conditions for longer periods of time, as well as on development of therapies for accompanying diseases.

Not all has been fully clarified in relation to psoriasis pathogenesis mainly due to the involvement of complex factors of immunologic, environmental and genetic nature. Immune contribution to pathogenesis may be derived from the finding that former bone marrow transplant recipients from a donor with psoriasis also developed the disease; this has been further corroborated with the improvement of the disease observed subsequent to ablation followed by bone marrow transplant from psoriasis-free patients as well as by successful therapy using methotrexate, TNF-α inhibitors and cyclosporine [15–17].

Keratinocyte dysfunction is a result from tissue damage triggered by anomalous immunological response. This dysfunction can be observed in the more than 50 times increase of the mitotic activity of basal keratinocytes in the psoriatic skin, resulting in reduced migration time (3–5 days as compared to the regular 28–30 days) from the basal to the corneal stratum [15, 18]. Histopathological examinations typically reveal parakeratosis, acanthosis, hyperkeratosis, accompanied by loss of the granular layer, elongation of epidermal ridges, vascular dilation, dermal-epidermal infiltrate and angiogenesis. In addition, which is a key for histopathological diagnosis, Munro's micro-abscesses are present, consisting of a sub-corneal aggregation of neutrophils [16, 19].

2. An overview of psoriasis therapy

Depending on the type and degree of severity as well as on the area of skin involved, age of the patient, costs, therapeutic management of psoriasis mainly consists of phototherapy, involving UV exposure of the skin, topical approaches and systemic medication but selection of the most effective treatment from the numerous therapeutic approaches is challenging.

Mainly consisting of application of ointments and creams to the skin, topical therapy is generally resorted to in cases of mild disease and formerly relied on use of keratolytic agents or emollients intended to help shed off or hydrate the skin. In keeping with further research developments, this type of treatment has increasingly targeted underlying proliferation of T-cell, therefore including vitamin D, coal tar, retinoids and topical calcineurin inhibitors.

For more severe forms, light-therapy and systemic treatments have been developed. Medication with systemic action administered orally or by injection includes the use of conventional drugs such as cyclosporine, acitretin, methotrexate and hydroxyurea, however associates with more prominent risk of serious adverse reactions, particularly for long-term treatment. One approach that has proved successful in improved and prompter effectiveness has consisted in combining all such therapies, achieving suppression of the disease and mitigation of adverse reactions. More recently, this has further been boosted by development of new, more targeted drug carrier systems. Development and increase of biological drugs and gene therapy have currently further supplemented therapeutic approaches with essentially ground-breaking new modalities, though none of them curative.

3. Medicinal products for systemic medications

3.1. Non-biological medication

3.1.1. Methotrexate – Overview

Methotrexate (MTX), a folic acid antagonist, has been used as non-biological medication in psoriasis therapy for longer than 30 years. Its use has proved successful in both treatment of psoriasis as such and of psoriatic arthritis and nail disease.

Though first used before introduction of routine conduct of randomized clinical trials and therefore still wanting in efficacy and safety data MTX is widely used in both mono- and combination dermatologic therapy predominantly for psoriatic arthritis and psoriasis, but also for dermatomyositis, sarcoidosis and pyoderma gangrenosum [17, 20, 21].

First authorised for psoriatic therapy in 1972, methotrexate was accordingly indicated, with no specification of the minimum body surface, for severe, refractory to topical therapy and phototherapy, and debilitating forms, therefore used in patients with functional disability arising from unresponsive scalp disease, palmoplantar disease or other severe, limited psoriasis forms.

Used in line with the standards established in guidelines published as early as 1972 and continually updated up to 1998 [22], MTX has proved successful in the treatment of pustular, plaque, guttate and erythrodermic psoriasis.

Furthermore, in 1988, MTX further received approval for the treatment of rheumatoid arthritis, the dedicated standards developed by the American College of Rheumatology (ACR), not requesting prior liver biopsy, which in fact were later eliminated from the guidelines for dermatologic use as well. However, the latter do not mention mandatory patient monitoring for possible liver toxicity resulting from methotrexate use [23]. At the same time, the issue of possible MTX liver toxicity is counteracted by such means as appropriate individual evaluation of patients' medical status, disease severity, quality of life, and psychological standing for proper selection and monitoring.

At the same time, MTX is used for cancer treatment, although in much larger dose than for dermatologic purposes:

Common approaches for MTX administration are as follows [24]:

- *Conventional low-dose therapy*, as follows:

- dose: 15–50 mg/m^2 body surface area;

- frequency: weekly, as one/several doses;

- administration route: intramuscularly/intravenously.

Head and neck cancer:

- dose: 40–60 mg/m^2 body surface area;

- frequency: weekly, once;

- administration route: intravenous bolus injection.

- *Intermediate-dose therapy*, as follows:

- dose: 100–1000 mg/m^2 body surface area;

- frequency: single dose.

Cancer of the bladder, advanced squamous epithelial: intermediate dose, 100–200 mg/m^2.

http://dx.doi.org/10.5772/67793

- *High-dose therapy*, as follows:

- mostly in malignant diseases, e.g. acute lymphatic leukaemia, malignant lymphoma, metastatic choriocarcinoma, osteogenic sarcoma;

- dose: 1000 mg or more/m^2 body surface area;

- frequency: over a 24-hour period.

Folinic acid should be started at 10–15 mg (6–12 mg/m^2), 12–24 hours after MTX therapy initiation.

Since 1998, a therapeutic approach of psoriasis has undergone remarkable changes, brought about by unprecedented expansion of basic and clinical research, leading to development of biologic agents such as alefacept, efalizumab, etanercept, infliximab, adalimumab and ustekinumab, which have all been approved for the treatment of psoriasis.

In comparison to biological drugs, even considering the costs of pre-treatment liver biopsy and blood monitoring, MTX is significantly less expensive, which explains why proof of intolerance or lack of responsiveness to methotrexate is a prerequisite for certain insurance companies.

However, considering the long-term aspect of psoriasis management and the associated issue of possible haematologic or hepatic toxicity with methotrexate, and not withstanding reduced costs, targeted therapies allowed by biologic drugs are more viable alternative treatment options to methotrexate.

3.1.2. Efficacy of methotrexate in the treatment of psoriasis

MTX has been used effectively on patients suffering from widespread forms of psoriasis, unresponsive to phototherapy or topical therapy or disabling psoriasis [22].

The pharmacological action of MTX interferes with DNA consists and suppresses the immune system, resulting in notable slowing down the accumulation of dead skin cells.

Regarding actual administration, MTX is taken orally, in one weekly dose, either as a single dose or as three doses separated by 12 hours. Folic acid (a B vitamin) may also be administered as a concomitant supplement.

Generally, to reduce MTX toxicity, 5–10 mg folic acid weekly is recommended by most relevant reviews and guidelines; however, there is general agreement among them that 'the evidence base is insufficient to determine the optimum dose' and that there may be 'potential need for higher dosages, with the currently higher dosed methotrexate' [25].

Effects on the disease can be observed within several weeks from treatment initiation, as the condition of the skin starts to improve, full improvement to set in regularly in 2–3 months' time. To completely clear the disease, possible remaining plaques may be treated by topical application of other specific medication or UVB/PUVA phototherapy may be applied. This is also recommended when the MTX dose has to be reduced for toxicity reasons, combination with additional medication, e.g. a retinoid, is also an option.

Patients on MTX require close monitoring consisting of chest X-rays, regular blood tests or liver biopsy for more conclusive outcomes, as a result of possible damage to the liver and kidney functions or decrease of the body's capacity to produce white and red blood cells and platelets. Also, it should be borne in mind that MTX and specific metabolites intracellular accumulation leads to depletion of the folate store [26, 27].

The risk of adverse reactions may be dose dependent or vary with the route of administration (lower in parenteral administration) [28]. However, care should be exercised since doses under 15 mg/week may prove ineffective considering the therapeutic goal for disease control.

3.1.3. MTX contraindications and adverse reactions

Generally, MTX use is restricted by the risk of organ toxicity. Therefore, use of MTX for psoriasis is an absolute contraindication in:

(a) Pregnancy or by women planning to become pregnant and their partners, because of MTX teratogenic effect. In fact, conception is to be avoided both during methotrexate therapy and for at least 3 months afterwards for males or for one ovulatory cycle for females;

(b) Nursing;

(c) Significant leukopenia, anaemia or thrombocytopenia.

In a number of cases, MTX may not be reasonably used for psoriasis treatment. Thus, MTX should be avoided for patients with [29]:

(a) Active or recurrent hepatitis, cirrhosis or markedly deteriorated liver function, in the context of known liver toxicity potential of MTX; therefore, function tests are standard, as well as close monitoring in the case elevations are observed.

    In the same respect, excessive alcohol consumption is also an issue—despite the scarcity of data to substantiate any definite limits for alcohol, which allows recommendations to vary from total prohibition of alcohol to permitted consumption of no more than drinks/day, liver damage associated with a history of alcoholism is undeniably problematic.

    Also, in relation to MTX potential for liver toxicity, the drug is contraindicated in the case of other hepatotoxic drugs are used at the same time, which usually requires even closer liver function monitoring;

(b) Abnormal kidney functioning; a significantly lower dose may be required, taking into account that the kidneys are the main excretion route for MTX (ca. 85%);

(c) Active forms of infectious diseases, particularly chronic infections such as advanced HIV infection or active untreated tuberculosis, prone to exacerbation resulting from MTX immunosuppressive effects; therefore, in the case of patients on MTX developing an infection, the drug may be withheld temporarily.

http://dx.doi.org/10.5772/67793

The same may apply for immunosuppressed patients, but not to those using biologic therapies, for instance.

(d) Obesity, with >30 body mass index;

(e) Diabetes mellitus;

(f) Recent vaccination, particularly for live vaccines;

(g) Unreliable patient, which once more highlights the importance of psychological evaluation for patient selection for MTX therapy.

In the context of the above relative contraindications, cases may however arise when the benefits of MTX outweigh its inherent risks. Therefore, therapy decisions should be made for each individual patient, based on their specific status and background. For an obese patient with diabetes, for instance, who would benefit from short-term MTX therapy, the relative contraindication may be waived due to the short-term character of the therapy.

In MTX, there are three primary concerns for the physician, i.e. myelosuppression, hepatotoxicity and pulmonary fibrosis, as shown in a study conducted by the United Kingdom Committee on the Safety of Medicines on 164 possibly methotrexate-associated deaths reported during 1969–2004. Among these, 41% were attributable to myelosuppression, 18% to pulmonary fibrosis and only 0.5% to liver toxicity [30]. Though the risk of MTX-associated pulmonary fibrosis in the treatment of psoriasis is much lower than for rheumatoid arthritis (explaining why chest X-rays are not mandatory for routine baseline studies), development of pulmonary symptoms should be duly taken into account and pulmonary fibrosis should be considered [31, 32].

Hepato- and haematologic MTX effects may commonly manifest such as anorexia, nausea, stomatitis, malaise and fatigue, mainly right on administration. As shown by clinical experience, such manifestations may be avoided or alleviated by changing the administration route to subcutaneous or intramuscular injection or the time of administration to bedtime, supplementation of folates or dose-splitting.

Other adverse reactions have lately been identified and researched due to the more thorough study of the disease triggered by the introduction of biologic therapy and more sustained conduct of post-marketing surveillance studies, formerly obscured by the lack of closer scrutiny of MTX. Thus, such reactions as reactivation of hepatitis and tuberculosis and development of lymphoma (especially associated with the Epstein-Barr virus) have also been added to the list of potential toxicities [33–36].

In addition, as reported from a recent study conducted in the general population, a 50% increased risk of malignancy could also be observed, more precisely, the respective rise related to a fivefold increase in non-Hodgkin lymphoma, a threefold increase in melanoma and an almost threefold increase in lung cancer [37], which requires mandatory increased physician care for the unexpected in patients on immunosuppressive therapy in general.

Unexpected benefits are also possible in MTX side effects, such as its demonstrated protective effect as anti-inflammatory medication against cardiovascular disease in certain patients [38, 39], which is important for the overall benefit/risk balance of MTX.

3.1.4. MTX haematologic toxicity

In respect of haematologic toxicity, the main recognised risk factors of MTX therapy are renal impairment, advanced age, absence of folate supplementation, drug interactions as well as medication errors. Given that most part of the data on myelosuppression has been derived from patients with rheumatoid arthritis, the relative risk of myelosuppression in MTX treatment for psoriasis may only be inferred. Current literature suggests that, in properly monitored psoriasis patients and in the absence of risk factors for haematologic toxicity, cases of clinically significant myelosuppression only rarely occur. Even with low-dose weekly MTX, however, rare, pancytopenia and significant cytopenia are a permanent possibility in the presence haematologic risk factors, impaired renal function or even medication errors [40, 41]. This once again speaks for the importance of regular monitoring of haematologic toxicity by complete blood cell counts. For patients without risk factors, the monitoring routine should consist of a first repeat laboratory check within a 2-week period. Taking into account the possibility of pancytopenia in 4–6 weeks after increase of the MTX dose, as reported in some cases, monitoring should become more frequent in dose changes; in fact, according to some experts' opinion, complete blood cell counts should be best undertaken at least every 4 weeks [29]. Overtime and in patients with consistently stable conditions, the frequency of laboratory monitoring may decrease to 1–3-month intervals.

Given the higher significant renal impairment risk even at single weekly MTX doses, the glomerular filtration rate should be calculated even for patients with normal blood creatinine and urea nitrogen levels but at renal insufficiency risk because of age or decreased muscle mass considerations. In patients with known or at risk of impaired kidney function, careful monitoring should be a permanent concern and second doses or any dose increases should only be given after prior laboratory checks.

As medication interactions are an important source of adverse effects as well, in order to avoid error, patients should routinely be instructed to the proper use of MTX therapy.

3.1.5. MTX hepatotoxicity

In respect of MTX hepatotoxicity, the issue of liver biopsy has remained a subject of debate among physicians involved in MTX therapies for both rheumatoid arthritis and psoriasis. The opinion prevails among rheumatologists that, particularly in healthy patients, liver biopsy is not necessary [42]. To that stricter dermatology guidelines argue that hepatic toxicity is greater in psoriasis patients, partly relying on the confirmed higher incidence of rheumatoid arthritis among women, less in the habit of alcohol consumption and therefore at liver damage risk than men. On the other hand, as confirmed by recently published updates, higher liver damage incidence for psoriasis patients results from common risk factors such as obesity, diabetes, alcoholism as well as previous exposure to hepatitis and liver toxins [42–45].

This is corroborated with histopathologic features of MTX-induced liver toxicity, which are roughly similar to the liver histology pattern common in hyperlipidemic, obese or diabetic patients or to non-alcoholic steatohepatitis (NASH). Clinical practice has in fact shown that, compared to no-risk psoriasis patients, NASH risk factors likely aggravate pre-existing NASH and eventually contribute to development of liver fibrosis even at lower MTX cumulative doses for psoriasis therapy. Such risk factors may represent inherent psoriatic patient phenotypes increasing hepatotoxicity risk. Provided controls of such confounding variables were introduced in studies conducted, MTX-associated liver injury rate in psoriatic patients would probably be roughly similar to that encountered in rheumatoid arthritis patients [43, 46, 47]. All the above come to highlight that the necessity of the liver biopsy is a matter of individual patient condition and medical background and should be judged on a case-by-case ground.

As current guideline standards recommend for practice, based on their risk factors for liver injury, patients intended for MTX therapy should be divided into two groups, i.e. no-risk versus risk patients. In the former group, the risk of fibrosis is lower and similar to rheumatoid arthritis, which makes them eligible for application of ACR criteria for MTX monitoring (i.e. liver function evaluation every 1–3 months and liver biopsy in the case of elevation of 5–9 serum AST levels over a 12-month period or of serum albumin decline below the normal range against normal nutritional status and well-controlled disease), a practice-validated routine schedule allowing for safe reduction of biopsies performed [48].

According to other recent data, the first liver biopsy in patients without pre-existing hepatotoxicity risk factors should be performed on use of a 3.5–4.0 g in place of the 1.0–1.5 g cumulative MTX, routinely recommended for pre-existing risk factors [43, 49, 50]. In low-risk patients on MTX, for normal values found in history of liver conditions, physical examination and liver laboratory tests, the decision whether or not to perform liver biopsies should be individual and rely on relative risk evaluation. Further monitoring options for patients on 3.5–4.0 g cumulative dose consist of application of ACR guidelines and continued monitoring with no biopsy, conduct of a first biopsy at the 3.5–4.0-g level, or stopping MTX altogether or, if feasible, switching the therapy to some alternative treatment, if possible. In the case of normal results in the first biopsy, further liver biopsies in low-risk patients are conducted in line with the ACR guidelines-recommended timeframes.

It is generally agreed that management of patients with one or several hepatic fibrosis risk factors should be conducted in line stricter guidelines. Therefore, the presence of significant risk factors should first of all trigger consideration of the feasibility of therapy consisting of a different systemic agent. Next, a risk/benefit evaluation should be undertaken for each individual risk patient, to weigh the benefits against the risks of MTX therapy.

In the case of likely MTX benefits exceeding possible risks, liver biopsy is advisable on inception of the therapy. Biopsy results permitting, MTX may be started although, in a small number of patients, it would likely stop in 2–6 months after initiation mostly because of adverse effects or lack of clinical efficacy. In light of this possibility, the pre-treatment liver biopsy may be postponed until after this 'trial' period, as there are no data indicative of clinically significant liver disease triggered by short or several-month MTX treatment. In the case of anticipated long-term therapy or for patients with persistent significant abnormalities in laboratory liver values, the initial biopsy is recommendable. In patients with acknowledged risk factors for liver disease, the liver biopsy should be repeated at a 1.0–1.5 g cumulative dose. Higher risk patients also require repeated biopsy with every MTX additional 1.0–1.5 g. However, as liver biopsy is not without risks, the procedure may not be appropriate or may be referred to another time in case, for the individual in question, risks of the biopsy *per se* outweigh the benefits; anyway, the risk of advanced fibrosis and that of liver biopsy complications should be carefully balanced.

However, although an important matter in itself, there is no screening tool for liver fibrosis available, allowing for relatively safe and effective decision on whether or not to use liver biopsy in the management of patients on MTX or at least decrease its need. Various other means have been tested in that respect, such as ultrasonographic tests and radiographic imaging techniques, but these have been mostly unsuccessful. More recently, measurement of a potential marker has been also tried, i.e. the amino-terminal peptide of procollagen III (PIIINP), and comparative results have shown a sevenfold decrease in the number of biopsies in the group managed with application of the Manchester PIIINP guidelines as compared to the group for which the 1998 American Academy of Dermatology guidelines were applied [51]. Such results were later supported by an additional study showing the possibility of complete biopsy exclusion provided the PIIINP values remained stable [52]. Accordingly, this test is used as a monitoring tool for hepatic fibrosis by most practicing dermatologists in the UK and formal testing is currently put on hold in the US. One other additional aspect highlighted by the British study on PIIINP is the difference in characteristics among commercially available PIIINP kits [53, 54].

Lately, the potential MTX-associated hepatic fibrosis and cirrhosis have been shown to be considerably less aggressive than initially estimated [55, 56]. At the same time, there is an observable tendency for adverse events to mostly occur in patients with internal abnormalities associated with other diseases. More specifically, risks such as gallbladder perforation, hemoperitoneum subcapsular haemorrhage and pneumothorax are lower in psoriatic patients than in those with other diseases [57].

3.2. Therapies involving biological and biosimilars

In the same way as for rheumatoid arthritis, development of biologicals has been a groundbreaking event for the treatment of psoriasis, leading to unprecedented success in therapeutic approach of moderate-to-severe forms of psoriasis and psoriatic arthritis. In that respect, even if not considered first-line treatments, biologic agents such as etanercept, adalimumab, infliximab and ustekinumab have been approved as second-line therapies for psoriasis, whereas golimumab has been approved for psoriatic arthritis therapy.

Clinical practice with biologicals has revealed their higher efficacy and tolerability in comparison to traditional systemic therapies [58], even in cases of refractory disease and expressly indicated for use in the so-called high-need patients, unresponsive or intolerant to all other available and approved systemic agents, MTX and cyclosporine included, or who cannot possible use such conventional systemic agents for reason of pre-existing disease [59].

In addition, biologicals do not generally carry the same toxicity burden of toxic chemical or pharmacological adverse effects. Most related side effects are due to the specific biological properties of a given preparation, and result from neutralization of the biological activity of their target molecules, such as TNF-α or IL-12/IL-23.

Psoriasis treatment can now rely on agents such as the TNF-α antagonist etanercept, adalimumab and infliximab, and on ustekinumab, a p40-antagonist. An additional issue brought about by immunological properties of the novel biological therapies is the occasional need to switch between therapies because of immunological side effects such as severe local reactions or secondary loss of activity [60].

In fact, developments have been both rapid and uneven: on the one hand, biologicals mentioned above are currently standard for a certain group of psoriatic patients, and specific guidelines have been developed [60, 61] whereas, on the other hand, in spite of their undeniable usefulness, biological drugs are yet not in wide use for psoriasis treatment [61], partly because of practitioner's lack of awareness about their use for psoriasis and more importantly because of their comparative high costs.

This issue of cost effectiveness (the same benefit obtained with lower treatment costs) has prompted development of biosimilar alternatives following expiry of patents for biologicals; thus, in the context of a cost minimisation process, the appropriate products would be determined by price only [59]. Such so-called biosimilars as erythropoietin preparations and growth hormones have been developed in recent years for use in certain indications [62, 63]. In fact, an increasing range of pharmaceutical companies, mostly Asian, have already developed biosimilar drugs relying on evidence derived from controlled clinical trials [64].

In biosimilars, the therapeutic protein is obtained by recombinant technology, and its structure is similar to that of the original biological product ('the reference drug'); this accounts for their very name—'biosimilars'. In addition, the pharmacological effects of the biosimilar as well as its mechanism of action are presumed identical to those of the reference [65].

If compared to drugs developed by chemical synthesis, the molecular weight of biosimilarsis is higher and their molecular structure is very complex. Although identical to amino acid sequence, their tertiary and quaternary structures may be heterogeneous, impacting their respective efficacy and safety profiles. Although similar in concept, biosimilars as copies of biologicals and generics as copies of chemically synthesized drugs must be treated in the same way, a fact clearly recognised by regulatory measures for assessment of preclinical data of both the EMA and the FDA.

In the same way as for generics and original drugs, since their very proposal as alternatives, the issue has been raised with regard to the extent that a structurally similar imitation of a drug could actually present identical efficacy and safety as the original [66]. It has been argued that variations in manufacturing processes may result in alterations of clinically relevant properties, likely to affect the finished product and subsequently monoclonal antibodies. But even if successful in part only, biosimilars would lead to significant reduction in drug costs as well as to a re-structuring of the pharmaceutical market.

The limitations of biosimilars would thus consist of possibly diminished reduced efficacy and higher risk potential from new side effects arising from such manufacturing variations [67]. Critical assessment of functional differences between biosimilars and their reference biological drug is essential for successful therapy and treatment safety.

Biosimilars display several biological characteristics, giving rise to specific consequences for clinical use. In biologicals and accordingly in biosimilars as well, proteins are formed by protein folding, resulting in a complex three-dimensional structure [65]. The biotechnological manufacturing process may induce batch-to-batch variations in the tertiary and quaternary structure even within a single production line [53, 65]. In addition, change in conditions at the manufacturing site or even switch from one site to another have often negatively impacted the quality and stability of biological drugs (according to [68]). The case has become known of the transfer to a company's new facility of the manufacture of efalizumab, a biological drug specifically designed for psoriasis treatment, which induced differences of such a scale in biological characteristics that prompted an FDA request for new phase III study meant to assess and reconfirm bioequivalence [69].

Such clinically relevant variations in manufacture of a biosimilar have also been reported for erythropoietin, for instance, with the alteration of protein characteristics, resulting from different properties of ionic bonding [70].

Respective risk of the modified therapeutic effect is even greater in the case of biosimilars introduced as a *de novo* production line.

However, the reverse is also true, and biosimilars may have improved properties in comparison to the original, and this is the case of the so-called biobetters, provided improvements are subjected to systematic research and implementation.

With regard to the ability of biological drugs to elicit an intended or unintended immunological response (immunogenicity), this is of special importance for this type of medicines, due to their marked immunogenic capacity resulting from their molecular structure (protein, polypeptide) [71]. Typically, the immunogenicity and biological functions of proteins are a result of both covalent bonds and their native tertiary structure [72]. From the perspective of biosimilars, though not yet fully demonstrated, it cannot reasonably be assumed that alterations to the tertiary structure, however structurally minimal but significant as regards function, are unable to determine changes in immune responses, giving rise to autoimmune or allergic complications [70, 72–74]. On the other hand, the possibility also exists for the biological drug to prove excessively effective or become inactivated form of an immune reaction.

In the context of the high specificity of processes for the manufacturing of biologicals, they cannot possibly be fully replicated for manufacture of their biosimilars. The differences may arise from various sources, such as selection of production site as well as of cell lines, the manner of cell nutrition, fermentation conditions, the production temperature and environment, etc. [66] and they can each alter the recombinant drug's effectiveness, stability and tolerability [75, 76]. Even when subjected to close monitoring and careful compliance with strict quality in the production process, variability in product quality (i.e. the integrity of the finished product) cannot be routinely excluded [77].

In addition, variability of biological activity may also derive from its marked sensitivity to such environmental physical conditions as phases, temperature or shearing forces, to changes in the manufacturing process resulting in variable enzyme activity as well as to formulation changes [78]. Under the circumstances, it may reasonably be assumed that the drug's safety may also undergo some degree of influence and safety studies are therefore needed to test their behaviour in everyday use [79, 80].

In order to specifically determine the implications for clinical practice with biosimilars in psoriasis treatment, longitudinal studies are necessary, which has prompted both dermatologists and rheumatologists to require study of biosimilars in long-term registries as per their indications for use [68, 81]. An initiative in the respect is the PsoBest, conducted in Germany [82] as well as worldwide, with comparable registries [83, 84].

To counteract the possibility of diminished reduced efficacy and higher risk potential from new side effects in biosimilars, as early as 2004, the European Medicines Agency (EMA), followed by the U.S. Food and Drug Administration (FDA) developed legal and regulatory requirements (the consolidated Directive 2001/83/EC) and guidelines applicable to their development, evaluation and marketing, based on submission of preclinical data and clinical characteristics. As the time for patent expiry for biological drugs approved for psoriasis treatment draws nearer (e.g. the U.S. patents for etanercept was issued in 2012, for adalimumab in 2016 and infliximab in 2014), the market will be open for biosimilars, which requires urgent clarification of actual meaning and implications for healthcare regulation in general and for dermatology in particular. Therefore, a description is useful related to future introduction of biosimilars in the treatment of psoriasis and psoriatic arthritis, making use of current regulatory requirements and published data.

The same as for conventional medication, EU regulations require authorisation of biologicals and biosimilars. Centrally, scientific assessment is conducted by the European Agency's Committee for Medicinal Products for Human Use (CHMP) [85]; assessment may result in a recommendation on whether the medicine should be marketed, adopted by the EMA and transmitted to the European Commission which grants a marketing authorisation, applicable to all EU member states.

However, when it comes the evaluation of clinical bioequivalence, the EMA and the FDA have different perspectives: the EMA only requires evidence of pharmacodynamic and pharmacokinetic equivalence, with additional evidence of clinical bioequivalence from randomized clinical studies being necessary in uncertain cases only [68], whereas the FDA insists on bioequivalence being supported by clear factual information, resulting from clinical studies.

The EMA and FDA approaches for post-marketing surveillance are similar in that both require conduct of non-interventional safety trials after marketing.

EMA guidelines have been developed in relation to the quality of biologicals, stating preclinical and clinical requirements, as well as product specifications [76–88]. According to EMA guidelines, biosimilars should be deemed specifically different from generics and use of approval procedures for generics is prohibited in relation to biosimilars. Further provisions regard the manufacturer's obligation to conduct clinical studies [89] seeking to demonstrated similarity of quality, safety and efficacy between the biosimilar and its biological reference drug. The same similarity must apply to the formulation, concentration and mode of administration of the therapeutic substance. Such data are derived for assessment purposes from preclinical experiments, both *in vitro* and *in vivo*, as well as from clinical studies conducted on patients or healthy volunteers; however, the amount of data required for biosimilars is less extensive than for the original biological.

At the same time, the biosimilar manufacturer is required to submit a risk management plan, focusing on safety specifications as well as a pharmacovigilance plan and a risk minimisation plan.

A further regulatory request for biosimilars is that they should allow for clear identification, for instance by use of distinct brand names or non-proprietary names, which allow for clear documentation, particularly in what concerns reports of potential adverse reactions and side effects.

The EMA's appointed (co)-rapporteurs undertake a scientific assessment of the documentation submitted in support of the application for biosimilar authorisation, on a case-by-case basis. Positive assessment opinion results in grant of a marketing authorisation by the European Commission.

Provided certain conditions are met, the EMA allows for extrapolation of initially approved clinical indications for which they can provide evidence. This is of particular importance for psoriasis, which, because of the widely varying characteristics of the disease, patient features and similarities of risk profiles between psoriasis and rheumatoid arthritis, for instance, requires critical evaluation of claims of analogies between indications [81, 90, 91].

Exchangeability and substitution are also of importance with regard to the biological reference drug-biosimilar relation; exchangeability is the term used to refer to the possibility of replacement based on medicinal and pharmaceutical characteristics between a drug developed for a specific indication and a different substance with identical effects. This is only feasible when the substitute drug has same quality, safety and efficacy features as the substituted one. In pharmaceutical practice in Germany, for instance, drugs may be substituted if the substitute has been approved in relation to reference product, and no difference could be established with regard to original substance or their manufacturing process. In that context, taking into account the differences in manufacturing processes of biosimilars and their resulting immunological and pharmacological characteristics, identity with the reference in terms of active ingredients may be ruled out [92].

Currently, the clinical consequences of repeated substitutions with biosimilars, either between themselves or for a biological, are only reviewed in few clinical studies [92]. This has prompted the EMA recommendation that the decision as to which of the two, the original biological drug or its biosimilar, should be given should be the sole choice of the treating physician. This has been preceded by measures of national authorities such as the Drug Commission of the German Medical Association, which has issued a warning against substitution of biotechnological drugs for one another in the absence of medical reviews. Substitution of an original biological product with its biosimilars is only possible on explicit request by the patient's physician.

Also pertaining to substitution and exchangeability, one very important aspect is that, particularly where patients with chronic disease and clear immunological origins such as psoriasis are involved, uncontrolled product switching and the so-called 'product hopping' should be avoided.

With regard to the pharmacovigilance aspects of biologicals and biosimilars, their total range of immunogenicity and associated reactions remains yet to be researched and described: data from clinical studies and trials need to be complemented with information from actual healthcare practice [93]. The capacity of biosimilars to induce immune responses needs to be studies after their actual placement on the market and the same pharmacovigilance provisions should apply to biosimilars as to their reference. This obligation requires conduct of post-marketing studies, mainly designed as controlled patient registries. In that respect, the EMA has also developed a comprehensive post-marketing pharmacovigilance program applicable to biosimilars, consisting of performance of a post-marketing safety study and implementation of a risk management plan, including:

- Spontaneous reporting of potential side effects associated with use of a biosimilar after their reporting by patients themselves or healthcare professionals;
- Preparation of Periodic Safety Update Reports (PSURs);
- Preparation of post-authorisation safety studies (PASS) (also known as phase IV studies) [94].

Pricing issues are also relevant for biosimilars, which, although considered less costly in comparison to their biopharmaceutical reference, because of the considerable research and development financial investments (currently, 80–120 million Euros), to which costs of biotechnological production sites must be added, do not in fact bring about a very great difference as price is concerned (not exceeding 20–25% less than the biopharmaceutical reference).

All the aspects considered, introduction of biosimilars into therapy, psoriasis treatment included, will undergo constant increase after patent expiry for original. The process will however increase the need for information from healthcare professionals, carers and patients alike.

4. MTX therapeutic benefits versus toxicology emergencies

In psoriasis therapy, low MTX doses are rarely associated with toxicity, and in most cases this only occurs because of non-compliance with the recommended guidelines [95].

However, the risk of MTX toxicity increases when additional MTX is administered sooner than provided for by the routine planned weekly dose [96], as, for instance, in the case of out of self-administration outside therapeutic protocol of a higher, consecutive dose, acting as precipitating factor.

MTX toxicity may be observed by its effects on the skin (ulcerations), the gastrointestinal mucosa, as well as at liver, kidney and bone marrow levels. Limitation of toxicity-related skin ulcerations to psoriatic plaques is likely the result of higher MTX uptake by the hyperproliferative psoriatic plaques as compared to the normal skin. The influence of toxicity may be assessed by both evaluation of change of membrane fluidity at the cellular level [97, 98], as well as *in vivo*, by confocal microscopy [99].

MTX-induced pancytopenia may occur in renally impaired patients as well as in cases of folic acid deficiency, infection and hypoalbuminemia but also as a result of concomitant drug use (e.g. trimethoprim) and advanced age [100].

Additional features of MTX toxicity are mucositis and myelosuppression, the likely cause of the latter being advanced age [101], concomitant NSAID use and careless use of the prescribed MTX dose; in other cases, this may be a result of renal dysfunction not identified prior to treatment initiation. However, inadvertent MTX dosage is the major contributory factor for MTX toxicity found in clinical practice, which strongly speaks for mandatory avoidance of MTX self-administration and appropriate patient instruction in that respect as well against combination of MTX with other drug without prior medical counselling.

MTX toxicity potential may be enhanced by use of generally renotoxic drugs which either decrease MTX renal elimination (e.g. cyclosporine, aminoglycosides, nonsteroidal anti-inflammatory agents, probenecid, sulfonamides, salicylates, colchicines, penicillins and cisplatin) or induce MTX displacement from protein binding sites in the plasma (as is the case of salicylates, sulfonamides, probenecid, phenytoin, barbiturates, sulfonylureas, retinoids and tetracyclines). Use of NSAID for joint pain can contribute to MTX toxicity.

Methods for MTX quantification also exist, as both a parent compound and mostly as MTX polyglutamate forms, responsible for its effect [102, 103].

To avoid toxicity, over-the-counter availability of MTX should be prohibited.

5. Discussion

Development of biological medicines has brought about new therapeutic options for psoriasis and other inflammatory diseases, which have proved successful in the therapy of moderate-to-severe and severe forms of plaque psoriasis alike.

Although giving rise as novel therapeutic agents to concerns related to their efficacy and safety, innovative pharmacobiologicals such as etanercept, adalimumab, infliximab, ixekizumab, ustekinumab and secukinumab, to mention a few, clinical practice has proved their short- and long-term efficacy and remarkable tolerability.

The process is currently replicated with regard to emerging biosimilars, developed for treatment of the same conditions as their original reference. Suspicions as to their safety and efficacy should be lifted by the undeniable outcomes derived from in-depth clinical trials already conducted and clinicians should more resolutely make use of their demonstrated capacities.

In an overall context of unmatched medical and pharmacological development, mainly characterised by the uniquely fast pace of research and findings in the area of biologicals and biosimilars, these currently play a remarkable role in advanced medicine. However, this has also raised a challenge for both international researchers, developers, manufacturers and for other drug-related regulatory fields such as the development of standards and pharmacovigilance, as the most important. This is further enforced by the expectation that, at least in Europe, biosimilars would lead to 15–30% cost reduction in use of biological therapeutic agents.

With regard to the therapeutic benefits-toxicological emergencies ratio particularly in psoriatic patients, there is a common concern related to possible association of MTX therapy with toxicity in various forms, of which some are serious and, in rare cases, may even include patient death.

Because of their implication for clinical practice, two aspects should be particularly outlined in relation to MTX toxicity: firstly, there is their potential to manifest at any time during the treatment, which calls for constant monitoring; secondly, the importance of the MTX dose or the dosing frequency for determining the risk for both toxicity and its severity.

MTX-induced toxic effects of special concern are severe skin reactions, hepatotoxicity (with both acute and chronic forms, with liver fibrosis and cirrhosis), acute haematological toxicity, lymphoproliferative disorders and severe opportunistic infections, lung disease and serious gastrointestinal toxicity.

Given this relatively high-risk context, further complicated by the additional threat posed by the potential for serious cumulative toxicity, MTX therapy is generally to be used mainly for patients with severe psoriasis, whose quality of life is seriously affected by their disease as well as for cases where proper disease control cannot be accomplished by use of topical therapies. As a further minimisation measure, MTX dose reductions and off-treatment periods should be applied whenever possible.

Undeniably, a therapeutic advantage due to relatively low costs of therapy complemented by ease of oral administration, in the presence of potential to achieve reasonable safety and tolerance, use of MTX has to be considered against its serious toxicity potential, which may be kept under control by careful patient selection and individual assessment of the benefit-risk balance for each psoriasis patient, accompanied by routine monitoring and strict compliance with monitoring guidelines.

Acknowledgements

This paper is financed by the Romanian Government under grant number PNII-PT-PCCA-2013-4-1386 (Project 185/2014).

Author details

Carolina Negrei[1]* and Daniel Boda[2]

*Address all correspondence to: carolina.negrei@outlook.com

1 Department of Toxicology, "Carol Davila" University of Medicine and Pharmacy, Bucharest, Romania

2 Centre of Excellence in Dermato-Oncology, "Carol Davila" University of Medicine and Pharmacy, Bucharest, Romania

References

[1] Henseler T, Christophers E. Disease concomitance in psoriasis. J Am Acad Dermatol. 1995;32:982–6.

[2] Davidson A, Diamond B. Autoimmune diseases. N Engl J Med. 2001;345:340–50.

[3] Arruda LHF, Campbell GAM, Takahashi MDF. Psoríase. An Bras Dermatol. 2001; 76: 141–167.

[4] Christophers E. Psoriasis—epidemiology and clinical spectrum. Clin Exp Dermatol. 2001;26:314–20.

[5] Ortonne JP. Psoriasis, metabolic syndrome and its components. Ann Dermatol Venereol. 2008;135 (Suppl 4):S235–42.

[6] Späh F. Inflammation in atherosclerosis and psoriasis: common pathogenic mechanisms and the potential for an integrated treatment approach. Br J Dermatol. 2008;159 (Suppl 2):10–7.

[7] Gisondi P, Girolomoni G, Sampogna F, Tabolli S, Abeni D. Prevalence of psoriatic arthritis and joint complaints in a large population of Italian patients hospitalised for psoriasis. Eur J Dermatol. 2005;15:279–83.

[8] Persson PG, Leijonmarck CE, Bernell O, Hellers G, Ahlbom A. Risk indicators for inflammatory bowel disease. Int J Epidemiol. 1993;22:268–72.

[9] Gupta MA, Gupta AK. Psychiatric and psychological co-morbidity in patients with dermatologic disorders: epidemiology and management. Am J Clin Dermatol. 2003;4:833–42.

[10] Neimann AL, Shin DB, Wang X, Margolis DJ, Troxel AB, Gelfand JM. Prevalence of cardiovascular risk factors in patients with psoriasis. J Am Acad Dermatol. 2006;55:829–35.

[11] Gelfand JM, Weinstein R, Porter SB, Neimann AL, Berlin JA, Margolis DJ. Prevalence and treatment of psoriasis in the United Kingdom: a population-based study. Arch Dermatol. 2005;141:1537–41.

[12] Kormeili T, Lowe NJ, Yamauchi PS. Psoriasis: immunopathogenesis and evolving immunomodulators and systemic therapies; U.S. Experiences. Br J Dermatol. 2004;151:3–15.

[13] Kremers HM, McEvoy MT, Dann FJ, Gabriel SE. Heart disease in psoriasis. J Am Acad Dermatol. 2007;57:347–54.

[14] Lapeyre H, Hellot MF, Joly P. Motifs d'hospitalisation des malades atteints de psoriasis. Ann Dermatol Venereol. 2007;134:433–6.

[15] Sabat R, Philipp S, Höflich C, Kreutzer S, Wallace E, Asadullah K, et al. Immunopathogenesis of psoriasis. Exp Dermatol. 2007;16:779–98.

[16] Nickoloff BJ, Nestle FO. Recent insights into the immunopathogenesis of psoriasis provide new therapeutic opportunities. J Clin Invest. 2004;113:1664–75.

[17] Veien NK, Brodthagen H. Cutaneous sarcoidosis treated with methotrexate. Br J Der matol. 1977;97:213–6.

[18] Schön MP, Henning WB. Psoriasis. N Engl J Med. 2005;352:1899–912.

[19] Lowes MA, Bowcock AM, Krueger JG. Pathogenesis and therapy of psoriasis. Nature. 2007;445:866–73.

[20] Malaviya AN, Many A, Schwartz RS. Treatment of dermatomyositis with methotrexate. Lancet. 1968;2:485–8.

[21] Teitel AD. Treatment of pyoderma gangrenosum with methotrexate. Cutis. 1996;57:326–8.

[22] Roenigk HH Jr, Auerbach R, Maibach H, Weinstein G, Lebwohl M. Methotrexate in psoriasis: consensus conference. J Am Acad Dermatol. 1998;38:478–85.

[23] American College of Rheumatology Subcommittee on Rheumatoid Arthritis Guidelines. Guidelines for the management of rheumatoid arthritis: 2002 update. Arthritis Rheum. 2002; 46:328–46.

[24] The electronic Medicines Compendium: eMC. https://www.medicines.org.uk/emc/medicine/ 26959

[25] Menting SP, Dekker PM, Limpens J, Hooft L, Spuls PI. Methotrexate dosing regimen for plaque-type psoriasis: a systematic review of the use of test-dose, start-dose, dosing scheme, dose adjustments, maximum dose and folic acid supplementation. Acta Derm Venereol. 2016;96(1):23–8.

[26] Kamen BA, Nylen PA, Camitta BM, et al. Methotrexate accumulation and folate depletion in cells as a possible mechanism of chronic toxicity to the drug. Br J Haematol. 1981;49:355–360.

[27] Hendel J, Nyfors A. Impact of methotrexate therapy on the folate status of psoriatic patients. Clin Exp Dermatol. 1895;10:30–35.

[28] Roenigk HH, Bergfed FW, Curtis GH. Methotrexate for psoriasis in weekly oral doses. Arch Dermatol. 1969;99:86–93.

[29] Kalb RE, Strober B, Weinstein G, Lebwohl M. Methotrexate and psoriasis: national psoriasis foundation consensus conference. J Am Acad Dermatol. 2009;60(5):824–37.

[30] MacDonald A, Burden AD. Noninvasive monitoring for methotrexate hepatotoxicity. Br J Dermatol. 2005;152:405–8.

[31] Belzunegui J, Intxausti JJ, De Dios JR, López-Domínguez L, Queiro R, González C, et al. Absence of pulmonary fibrosis in patients with psoriatic arthritis treated with low dose weekly methotrexate. Clin Exp Rheumatol. 2001;19:727–30.

[32] Kremer JM. Toward a better understanding of methotrexate. Arthritis Rheum. 2004; 50:1370–82.

[33] Maruani A, Wierzbicka E, Machet MC, Abdallah-Lotf M, de Muret A, Machet L. Reversal of multifocal cutaneous lymphoproliferative disease associated with Epstein-Barr virus after withdrawal of methotrexate therapy for rheumatoid arthritis. J Am Acad Dermatol. 2007;57 (Suppl):S69–71.

[34] Clarke LE, Junkins-Hopkins J, Seykora JT, Adler DJ, Elenitsas R. Methotrexate-associated lymphoproliferative disorder in a patient with rheumatoid arthritis presenting in the skin. J Am Acad Dermatol. 2006;56:686–90.

[35] Binymin K, Cooper RG. Late reactivation of spinal tuberculosis by low-dose methotrexate therapy in a patient with rheumatoid arthritis. Rheumatology. 2001;40:341–2.

[36] Gwak GY, Koh KC, Kim HY. Fatal hepatic failure associated with hepatitis B virus reactivation in a hepatitis B surface antigen-negative patient with rheumatoid arthritis receiving low dose methotrexate. Clin Exp Rheumatol 2007;25:888–9.

[37] Buchbinder R, Barber M, Heuzenroeder L, Wluka AE, Giles G, Hall S, et al. Incidence of melanoma and other malignancies among rheumatoid arthritis patients treated with methotrexate. Arthritis Rheum. 2008;59:794–9.

[38] Prodanovich S, Ma F, Taylor JR, Pezon C, Fasihi T, Kirsner RS. Methotrexate reduces incidence of vascular diseases in veterans with psoriasis or rheumatoid arthritis. J Am Acad Dermatol. 2005;52:262–7.

[39] van Halm VP, Nurmohamed MT, Twisk JW, Dijkmans BA, Voskuyl AE. Disease-modifying antirheumatic drugs are associated with a reduced risk for cardiovascular disease in patients with rheumatoid arthritis: a case control study. Arthritis Res Ther. 2006;8(5):R151.

[40] Yang C-P, Kuo M-C, Guh J-Y, Chen H-C. Pancytopenia after low dose methotrexate therapy in a hemodialysis patient: case report and review of literature. Renal Failure. 2006;28:95–7.

[41] Jih DM, Werth VP. Thrombocytopenia after a single test dose of methotrexate. J Am Acad Dermatol. 1998;39:349–51.

[42] Herron MD, Hinckley M, Hoffman MS, Papenfuss J, Hansen CB, Callis KP, et al. Impact of obesity and smoking on psoriasis presentation and management. Arch Dermatol. 2005;141:1527–34.

[43] Langman G, Dela M, Hall P, Todd G. Role of nonalcoholic steatohepatitis in methotrexate induced liver injury. J Gastroenterol Hepatol. 2001;16:1395–401.

[44] Rosenberg P, Urwitz H, Johannesson A, Ros AM, Lindholm J, Kinnman N, et al. Psoriasis patients with diabetes type 2 are at high risk of developing liver fibrosis during methotrexate treatment. J Hepatol. 2007;46:1111–8.

[45] Kent P, Luthra HS, Michet CJ Jr. Risk factors for methotrexate-induced abnormal laboratory monitoring results in patients with rheumatoid arthritis. J Rheumatol. 2004; 31:1727–31.

[46] Zachariae H. Have methotrexate-induced liver fibrosis and cirrhosis become rare? Dermatology. 2005;211:307–8.

[47] Henning JS, Gruson LM, Strober BE. Reconsidering liver biopsies during methotrexate therapy. J Am Acad Dermatol. 2007;56:893–4.

[48] Erickson A, Reddy V, Vogelgesang S, West SG. Usefulness of the American College of Rheumatology recommendations for liver biopsy in methotrexate treated rheumatoid arthritis patients. Arthritis Rheum. 1995;38:1115–9.

[49] Aithal GP, Haugk B, Das S, Card T, Burt AD, Record CO. Monitoring methotrexate-induced hepatic fibrosis in patients with psoriasis: are serial liver biopsies justified? Aliment Pharmacol Ther. 2004;19:391–9.

[50] Thomas JA, Aithal GP. Monitoring liver function during methotrexate therapy for psoriasis: are routine biopsies really necessary? Am J Clin Dermatol. 2005;6:357–63.

[51] Chalmers RJ, Kirby B, Smith A, Burrows P, Little R, Horan M, et al. Replacement of routine liver biopsy by procollagen III aminopeptide for monitoring patients with psoriasis receiving long-term methotrexate: a multicentre audit and health economic analysis. Br J Dermatol. 2005;152:444–50.

[52] Maurice PD, Maddox AJ, Green CA, Tatnall F, Schofield JK, Stott DJ. Monitoring patients on methotrexate: hepatic fibrosis not seen in patients with normal serum assays of aminoterminal peptide of type III procollagen. Br J Dermatol. 2005;152:451–8.

[53] Collin B, Srinathan SK, Finch TM. Methotrexate: prescribing and monitoring practices among the consultant membership of the British Association of Dermatologists. Br J Dermatol. 2008;158:793–800.

[54] Khan S, Subedi D, Chowdhury MM. Use of amino terminal type III procollagen peptide (P3NP) assay in methotrexate therapy for psoriasis. Postgrad Med J. 2006;82:353–4.

[55] Berends MA, Snoek J, de Jong EM, van de Kerkhof PC, van Oijen MG, van Krieken JH, et al. Liver injury in long-term methotrexate treatment in psoriasis is relatively infrequent. Aliment Pharmacol Ther. 2006;24:805–11.

[56] Zachariae H. Liver biopsies and methotrexate: a time for reconsideration? J Am Acad Dermatol. 2000;42:531–4.

[57] Al Knawy B, Shiffman M. Percutaneous liver biopsy in clinical practice. Liver Int. 2007; 27:1166–73.

[58] Radtke MA, Schäfer I, Blome C, et al. Patient Benefit Index (PBI) in the treatment of psoriasis—results of the National Care Study "PsoHealth". Eur J Dermatol. 2013;23:212–7.

[59] Nast A, Boehncke WH, Mrowietz U, et al. Deutsche Dermatologische Gesellschaft (DDG); Berufsverband Deutscher Dermatologen (BVDD). S3-Guidelines on the treatment of psoriasis vulgaris (English version). Update. J Dtsch Dermatol Ges. 2012; 10: S1–95.

[60] Sterry W, vande Kerkhof P. Is "class effect" relevant when assessing the benefit/risk profile of a biologic agent? J Eur Acad Derm. 2012;26 (Suppl 5):9–16.

[61] Augustin M, Glaeske G, Schäfer I, et al. Processes of psoriasis health care in Germany—long-term analysis of data from the statutory health insurances. J Dtsch Dermatol Ges. 2012;10(9):648–55.

[62] Tsiftsoglou AS, Ruiz S, Schneider CK. Development and regulation of biosimilars: current status and future challenges. BioDrugs 2013;27(3):203–11.

[63] Schellekens H. How similar do "biosimilars" need to be? Nat Biotechnol. 2004;22:1357–9.

[64] Declerck PJ. Biosimilar monoclonal antibodies: a science-based regulatory challenge. Expert Opin Biol Ther. 2013;13:153–6.

[65] Schellekens H. Biosimilar therapeutics—what do we need to consider? NDT Plus. 2009;2:27–36.

[66] Subramanyam M. Clinical development of biosimilars: an evolving landscape. Bioanalysis. 2013;5(5):575–86.

[67] Ebbers HC, Pieters T, Leufkens HG, et al. Effective pharmaceutical regulations needs alignment with doctors. Drug Discov Today. 2012;17:100–3.

[68] Dörner T, Strand V, Castañeda-Hernández G, et al. The role of biosimilars in the treatment of rheumatic diseases. Ann Rheum Dis. 2013;72(3):322–8.

[69] Adis Insight. Efalizumab: anti-CD11a monoclonal antibody-Genentech/Xoma, HU 1124, hu1124, xanelim. Drugs R&D 2002; 3(1): 40–3; http://adisinsight.springer.com/drugs/800007491

[70] Gershon SK, Luksenburg H, Coté TR, et al. Pure red-cell aplasia and recombinant erythropoietin. N Engl J Med. 2004;351:1403–8.

[71] Strand V, Kimberley R, Isaacs JD. Biologic therapies in rheumatology: lessons learned, future directions. Nat Rev Drug Discov. 2007;6:75–92.

[72] Schellekens H. Biosimilar therapeutic agents: issues with bioequivalence and immunogenicity. Eur J Clin Invest. 2004;34:797–9.

[73] Atzeni F, Talotta R, Benucci M, et al. Immunogenicity and autoimmunity during anti-TNF therapy. Autoimmun Rev. 2013;12:703–8.

[74] Ramos-Casals M, Brito-Zerón P, Munoz S, et al. Autoimmune diseases induced by TNF-targeted therapies: analysis of 233 cases. Medicine. 2007;86:242–51.

[75] Schellekens H. Bioequivalence and the immunogenicity of biopharmaceuticals. Nat Rev Drug Discov. 2002;1:457–62.

[76] Mellstedt H, Niederwieser D, Ludwig H. The challenge of biosimilars. Ann Oncol. 2008;19:411–9.

[77] Chrino AJ, Mire-Sluis A. Characterizing biological products and assessing comparability following manufacturing changes. Nat Biotechnol. 2004;22:1383–91.

[78] Jefferis R. Glycosylation as a strategy to improve amtibody-based therapeutics. Nat Rev Drug Discov. 2009;8:226–34.

[79] Jahn EM, Schneider CK. How to systemically evaluate immunogenicity of therapeutic proteins-regulatory considerations. N Biotechnol. 2009;25:280–6.

[80] Brockmeyer C, Seidl A. Binocrit: assessment of quality, safety and efficacy of biopharmaceuticals. EJHP Practice. 2009;15:38–44.

[81] Strober BE, Armour K, Romiti R, et al. Biopharmaceuticals and biosimilars in psoriasis: what the dermatologist needs to know. J Am Acad Dermatol. 2012;66:317–22.

[82] Augustin M, Spehr C, Radtke MA, et al. Deutsches Psoriasis-Register PsoBest: Zielsetzung, Methodik und Basisdaten. J Dtsch Dermatol Ges. 2014;12(1):48–58.

[83] Papp KA, Strober B, Augustin M, et al. PSOLAR investigators and Steering Committee. PSOLAR: design, utility, and preliminary results of a prospective, international, disease-based registry of patients with psoriasis who are receiving, or are candidates for, conventional systemic treatments or biologic agents. J Drugs Dermatol. 2012;11(10):1210–7.

[84] Ormerod AD, Augustin M, Baker C, et al. Challenges for synthesising data in a network of registries for systemic psoriasis therapies. Dermatology. 2012;224(3):236–43.

[85] European Medicines Agency. Guideline on similar biological medicinal products containing biotechnology-derived proteins as active substance: quality issues. 2006.

[86] European Medicines Agency, Committee for Medicinal Products for Human Use (CHMP): Draft: Guideline on immunogenicity assessment of biotechnology-derived therapeutic proteins. EMA/CHMP/BMWP/14327/2006. London, 24 January 2007.

[87] European Medicines Agency, Committee for Medicinal Products for Human Use (CHMP): Guideline on comparability of biotechnology-derived medicinal products after a change in the manufacturing process. Non-clinical and clinical issues. EMA/CHMP/BMWP/101695/2006. London, 19 July 2007.

[88] European Medicines Agency, Committee for Medicinal Products for human Use (CHMP): Guideline on similar biological medicinal products containing biotechnology-derived proteins as active substance: Non-clinical and clinical issues. EMA/CHMP/BMWP/42832/2005. London, 22 February 2006.

[89] European Medicines Agency. Questions and answers on biosimilar medicines (similar biological medicinal products). 27–9–2012, 18–11–2012.

[90] Lee H, Yim DS, Zhou H, et al. Evidence of effectiveness: how much can we extrapolate from existing studies? AAPS J. 2005;7:E467–74.

[91] Ratiu MP, Purcarea I, Popa F, Purcarea VL, Purcarea TV, Lupuliasa D, Boda D. Escaping the economic turn down through performing employees, creative leaders and growth driver capabilities in the Romanian pharmaceutical industry. Farmacia. 2011;59(1):119–130.

[92] Romer T, Zabransky M, Walczak M. Effect of switching recombinant human growth hormone: comparative analysis of phase 3 clinical data. Biol Ther. 2011;1:5.

[93] Joshi SR. Biosimilar peptides: need for pharmacovigilance. J Assoc Physicians India. 2011;59:44–7.

[94] Casadevall N, Edwards IR, Felix T, et al. Pharmacovigilance and biosimilars: comsiderations, needs and challenges. Expert Opin Biol Ther. 2013;13(7):1039–47.

[95] Roenigk Jr. HH, Maibach HI, Weinstein GD. Use of methotrexate in psoriasis. Arch Dermatol. 1972;105(3):363–365.

[96] Bleyer WA., Methotrexate: clinical pharmacology, current status and therapeutic guidelines. Cancer Treat Rev. 1977;4(2):87–101.

[97] Negrei C, Arsene AL, Toderescu CD, Boda D, Ilie M. Acitretin treatment may influence the cell membrane fluidity. Farmacia. 2012;60(6):767–72.

[98] Boda D, Negrei C, Nicolescu F, Balalau C. Assessment of some oxidative stress parameters in methotrexate treated psoriasis patients. Farmacia. 2014;62(4):704–10.

[99] Căruntu C, Boda D, Căruntu A, Rotaru M, Baderca F, Zurac S. *In vivo* imaging techniques for psoriatic lesions. Rom J Morphol Embryol. 2014;55 (Suppl 3):1191–6.

[100] Kaplan DL, Olsen EA. Erosion of psoriatic plaques after chronic methotrexate administration. Int J Dermatol. 1988;27(1):59–62.

[101] Căruntu C, Grigore C, Căruntu A, Diaconeasa A, Boda D. The role of stress in skin diseases. Intern Med. 2011;8:73–84.

[102] Negrei C, Căruntu C, Ginghină O, Burcea Dragomiroiu GTA, Toderescu CD, Boda D. Qualitative and quantitative determination of methotrexate polyglutamates in erythrocytes by high performance liquid chromatography. Rev Chim. 2015;66(5):607–10.

[103] Negrei C, Ginghină O, Căruntu C, Burcea Dragomiroiu GTA, Jinescu G, Boda D. Investigation relevance of methotrexate polyglutamates in biological systems by high performance liquid chromatography. Revista de Chimie. 2015;66(6):766–8.